Accident and Emergency Nursing

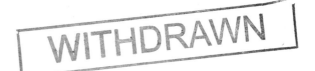

Dedication

This book is dedicated to the memory of my father, Bernard Francis Walsh, who died the day this edition was completed. Whatever abilities I may have as a writer are largely due to him and his gift with words.

Accident and Emergency Nursing

Fourth edition

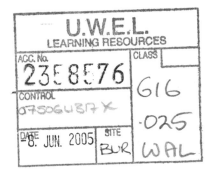

Mike Walsh PhD BA (Hons) RGN PGCE DipN (London) A&E Cert (Oxford)
Reader in Nursing
St Martin's College, Carlisle, UK
and
Andrew Kent MA RGN ENB199 ENB998 MIMGT
Clinical Nurse Manager
Accident & Emergency Department, Carlisle Hospitals, UK

U.W.E.L.
LEARNING RESOURCES

ACC. No.
23 8576

CLASS
616
.025

CONTROL
0750643177 X

DATE
8. JUN. 2005

SITE
BUR

WAL

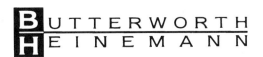

BUTTERWORTH
HEINEMANN

EDINBURGH LONDON NEW YORK OXFORD PHILADELPHIA ST LOUIS SYDNEY TORONTO 2001

Butterworth-Heinemann,
an imprint of Elsevier Science Limited,
Robert Stevenson House, 1-3 Baxter's Place,
Leith Walk, Edinburgh EH1 3AF

First published 2001
Reprinted 2002, 2003

British Library Cataloguing in Publication Data
Walsh, Mike, 1949–
    Accident and emergency nursing. – 4th ed.
    1   Emergency nursing
    I   Title   II   Kent, Andrew
    610.7'3'61

ISBN 0 7506 4317 X

Library of Congress Cataloging in Publication Data
A catalog record for this book is available from the Library of Congress

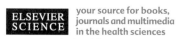

your source for books,
journals and multimedia
in the health sciences
www.elsevierhealth.com

Typeset by E & M Graphics, Midsomer Norton, Bath

Printed in China
B/03

CONTENTS

ACKNOWLEDGMENTS

A big thank you is due to the library staff of the Education Centre, Cumberland Infirmary, for all their assistance in researching this updated 4th edition. We would also like to say thank you to the various A & E staff we have worked with along the way in our careers, and especially the staff of the Cumberland Infirmary A & E Department, Carlisle, for their contribution, however unwitting that may have been!

The environment

Chapter 1

SOCIAL FACTORS AND A & E ATTENDANCE

In the most recent year for which statistics are available, 1996, 15.055 million people attended A & E departments in England and Wales (Annual Abstract of Statistics, 1999). This represents a 5% increase on 1993 and there is no reason to suspect that similar increases have not been registered in Scotland and Northern Ireland. A & E nurses deal annually with a population equal to that of a major country such as Australia. This implies that, in their work, A & E nurses will meet the full range of human society in terms of class, age, religion, ethnicity and culture. It is important, therefore, to place A & E nursing in its sociological perspective, as it is from this extensive and varied tapestry of the human condition that our patients originate and to which we will return them.

In every tapestry, certain colours dominate and characteristic shapes and patterns are discernible as individual fibres are woven into the final complex picture. So it is with the sociological make-up of a typical day's patients in an A & E department. There will be certain accident patterns that dominate (e.g. alcohol-related accidents, motorbike accidents, assaults) and the patterns will shift and change with the time of day. Furthermore, a large number of patients will have factors in common, such as occupation, age and class. These factors will give the A & E picture a characteristic social colouring. Looked at this way, therefore, A & E patients constitute a group from which striking sociological patterns emerge. These patterns demand the attention of the nurse if care is to be carried out in the patient's best interest.

For example, a discerning nose in A & E after 10 p.m. will detect the smell of alcohol on the breath of most patients. There is clearly a link between alcohol use and trauma, especially late at night. A glance through the register of any A & E department will show that certain districts or streets crop up with remarkable frequency. This suggests there is a link between where people live (and therefore social class) and their probability of attending A & E (Walsh, 1990a,b).

The woman with a bruised and battered face, the baby with a broken arm, the overdosed teenager vomiting in a cubicle, the drug-dependent youth and the depressed middle-aged alcoholic person are all familiar figures in A & E. They may seem to have very different problems, but could the root cause be the same? The breakdown and disintegration of normal family and interpersonal relationships lies behind many such presentations.

The alert A & E nurse will quickly perceive these sorts of patterns. They represent only a few strands, however, of the sociological mix that goes to make up the A & E caseload. The rest of this chapter will attempt to flag up some of the key themes which the nurse may choose to pursue further.

Accidents, emergencies and social class

It is thought that there are two main causes of accidents – the environment and the behaviour of the individual. Both these causes are closely linked to social class. This link was initially explored in a pioneering study into health and society carried out under the chairmanship of Sir Douglas Black. This study, known as the Black Report, concluded that where you are in the social scale plays a major part in determining your health: 'Gender and class exert highly significant influences on the quality and duration of life in modern society' (Townsend and Davidson, 1982). Despite the passage of some 20 years since the Black Report was published, these gender- and class-related differences in health still persist and may be seen every day in A & E.

Table 1.1 Life expectancy by social class 1987/91

Class	Life expectancy at birth	
	Male	Female
I (Professional) and II (Managerial/minor profs)	74.9	80.2
IIIN (Skilled non-manual)	73.5	79.4
IIIM (Skilled manual)	72.4	77.6
IV (Semi-skilled) and V (Unskilled)	69.7	76.8

Source: Drever and Whitehead (1995)

Simply being male makes you more likely to die sooner than any comparable female. Life expectancy at birth has increased from 69.2 years to 72.3 between 1972 and 1991 for men. However, for women the figures are 75.1 and 77.9 respectively (Drever and Whitehead, 1995). These simple figures conceal marked variations related to social class. This is defined according to the Registrar General's system based upon occupation and the effects are shown in Table 1.1.

A similar trend is found when childhood mortality rates are considered. For children aged 1 to 15 in England and Wales, the mortality rate in social class V is 42 deaths per 100 000 compared to 18 for children in class I. For all classes the mortality rates are higher in boys than girls. Of particular importance to the A & E nurse is the fact that accidents are the biggest cause of death in children. The class gradient has actually become steeper with the passage of time, especially in the case of deaths involving fires. Here the rates have fallen between 1981 and 1991 for children in classes I and II but increased in classes IV and V, mainly due to residential fires. It is hard to disagree with Black's original verdict on these figures 'While the death of a single child may appear as a random misfortune, this overall distribution indicates the social nature of the phenomenon' (Townsend and Davidson, 1982). Several factors can explain this difference: the lack of safe play areas in the poorer parts of towns and cities; the more dangerous types of household heating and furnishing which tend to be found in poorer homes; the lack of health knowledge among poorer groups; and the lack of parental supervision. This is often due to situations where a single parent cannot take or is not granted time off from work to look after children who are on school holiday or absent from school ill.

When these mortality statistics are analysed by cause, striking class-related patterns emerge, especially among cases of death from trauma or the serious diseases which frequently present at A & E (Table 1.2).

Put simply, these figures are saying that a man in class V is some three to four times more likely to die from these causes than a man in class I. Class variation becomes even more pronounced when age is considered. For accidental death, the mortality rates in class V are five times higher than class I for the age range 25–34 and seven times higher for ages

Table 1.2 Standardized mortality ratios; men aged 20–64 England and Wales 1991–3

Social class	Stroke	IHD	Accidents	Suicide
I	70	63	54	55
II	67	73	57	63
IIIN	96	107	74	87
IIIM	118	125	107	96
IV	125	121	106	107
V	219	182	226	215
All	100	100	100	100
Total deaths	8350	52 219	10 275	9725

Table 1.3 Standardized mortality ratios for accidental death by social class, men aged 20–64, England and Wales 1991–3

Class	Accidents	Suicide	Homicide	Road accidents	Falls	Fire	Poisoning
I	54	55	25	66	61	25	28
II	57	63	43	65	56	41	36
IIIN	74	87	72	86	60	66	46
IIIM	107	96	80	113	109	91	90
IV	106	107	116	101	117	90	117
V	226	215	300	185	273	384	329
All	100	100	100	100	100	100	100
Total deaths	10 275	9725	482	5155	1196	369	1301

NB: Suicide statistics include those deaths where cause was undetermined
Source: Drever and Whitehead (1995)

40–44. Younger adults in class V are some seven to eight times more likely to commit suicide than those in class I. Table 1.3 gives some of the detail.

Nurses are, by definition, class II and are therefore likely to be from a different social class than many of their patients in A & E. But, as individualized patient care can only be achieved by considering the social background of the patient, the nurse must be able and willing to bridge that social gap. The A & E nurse must display empathy and be able to see the problem through the eyes of a single parent mother living on social security or a casual labourer who has lengthy spells on the dole in between jobs. Environment and class must be considered in nursing care as they affect the resources and health knowledge available to the patient on discharge from A & E. Patients are people and people are products of their environment. It is that environment which is a major determining factor as to who attends A & E and why.

Age, gender and accidents

There is a strong relationship between age, gender, social class and the probability of attending A & E after an accident. This is summarized in Table 1.4.

The high risk factors are clearly being male, belonging to a younger age group and being of lower social class. Where you are in society, therefore, is an important determinant of the probability that you will attend A & E following trauma.

Although the attendance rate decreases with age, it increases again among the age group 75 and over. The dramatic increase in the elderly population has serious implications for all aspects of health care, including A & E units.

Table 1.4 Accident rates per 1000 requiring medical treatment (England 1995–6)

Age	Male			Female		
	Manual	Non-manual	All	Manual	Non-manual	All
16–24	52	38	42	24	22	22
25–34	38	22	31	15	14	14
35–44	24	16	20	13	13	13
45–54	19	15	17	14	12	13
55–64	10	14	12	13	14	13
65–74	8	9	9	15	15	14
75+	13	12	12	16	22	20

Source: Office for National Statistics (1999)

In 1961, 2.11 million people were aged 75 or over in the UK. By 1997 this figure had risen to 4.13 million and is projected to rise to 4.87 million by 2011 (Office for National Statistics, 1999). The elderly are prone to accidents by virtue of failing faculties, degenerative changes in the musculoskeletal system and the increasingly poor conditions that many elderly people are forced to live in. This compounds the other health problems associated with ageing, leading to the elderly being a very important group of patients in A & E who have special needs (Chapter 12).

Road traffic accidents are a significant factor in accounting for the high number of young people seen in A & E and the marked bias towards males in the A & E population (Table 1.5).

There has been a steady decline in deaths from road traffic accidents (RTA) from just over 6000 in 1981 to 3700 in 1997, despite a substantial increase in traffic. Improved vehicle design, seat-belt wearing and the impact of drink–driving legislation have all contributed to this welcome decrease. However, failed breath tests are three times more likely in male drivers than female and twice as likely in men under 35 as those aged 35 or more (Office for National Statistics, 1999). Motorbikes remain the most dangerous form of transport as they are involved in more than eight times as many accidents as motor cars and 30 times as many deaths per kilometre travelled (Office for National Statistics, 1999). It is interesting to note that walking is the second most dangerous form of transport with a mortality rate of 54.3 deaths per billion km compared to 3.1 for cars! Motorways accounted for less than 5% of deaths from RTA, whereas open roads in rural areas are the most common site of fatal accidents. The greatest number of serious but non-fatal accidents tend to happen on roads in built-up areas.

The much higher male attendance rate at A & E in the under 64 age group can be partly explained by the more hazardous nature of male work and sport. However, the tendency to aggression and assertiveness undoubtedly underlies much male trauma leading, as it does, to more dangerous behaviour on the roads, increased alcohol consumption and violence. As male children are socialized into this aggressive/assertive role from childhood, nurses may speculate on how many accidents would be, in fact, preventable if we had different child-rearing practices, and it should be remembered that the victims of male aggression are frequently female.

Families, women and A & E

Marxists see traditional families as a tool of capitalist oppression as they create a large pool of cheap female labour. Feminists, on the other hand, see families as trapping women and denying them equal rights. The traditional role of women in the family is changing dramatically and the rapid increase in the divorce rate since the 1960s is one of the many factors driving such change. It is, for example, estimated that 25% of children born in 1979 had been affected by divorce by the time they were 16. Despite the growth in lone parent families from 2% of all UK households in 1961 to 7% in 1998, it has to be remembered that 80% of children still live in households with two parents who, in 90% of cases, are married (Office for National Statistics, 1999).

In the many families where the woman is the head there are special problems when either the woman or her children become A & E patients. It is very difficult for a lone mother to supervise her children if she is ill. This will mean that she may have to make special arrangements for someone to look after her children, or the A & E unit will have to step into the breach on a temporary basis. Alternatively, if one of the children is ill, the only way that the mother can accompany the child to A & E may be to bring the rest of the children along as well. This requires that the A & E unit be able to look after well children in addition to injured or ill children. One further

Table 1.5 Car user casualties by age and gender 1997 UK

Age	Drivers per 1000 population	
	Male	Female
17–21	7.6	5.3
22–39	4.4	4.1
40–59	2.5	2.1
60 and over	1.6	0.6

Source: Office for National Statistics (1999)

problem faced by women in the context of the family is that of violent partners. It is important for A & E nursing staff to realize that a woman's injuries may be due to violence from her partner, even though she may not admit this at first. A reluctance to leave the A & E unit after treatment for minor injuries suffered as a result of a 'fall' may be understood better in this light and A & E nurses should be alert for tell-tale signs of anxiety and inappropriate injuries when compared to the story of how they occurred. The existence of women's refuges should be known to the nurse together with the knowledge of how to contact one if needed. A battered woman may be more prepared to talk about her problems to a female nurse than to a male doctor. She is most unlikely to involve the law.

Another traditional role of the woman in the family is to look after aged relatives. However, increased family mobility, increased numbers of women in work, and the decline of the extended family have led to a decline in the numbers of women able to play this role. A & E units then face a dual problem – an increasing number of elderly people living alone and who are therefore more accident prone, and fewer situations where an elderly patient can be discharged home with someone to look after them. The A & E nurse should be non-judgemental at all times, and never more so than when dealing with the relatives of an elderly patient who refuse to take the patient home because they cannot look after him or her. The need is to see the problem from the family's perspective.

Increasing numbers of elderly people are now cared for in nursing homes. The A & E department will benefit from a good working relationship with such homes as when an elderly person is brought to A & E after a fall or collapse for example, it is essential to find out the patient's medical history, what medication they are taking and what their normal behaviour is like. Good liaison with the home is also essential if a smooth discharge back to the home is to be arranged, rather than admission to hospital.

Culture, ethnicity and A & E

The UK is fortunate in that it is a multiracial society and, as a result, has a rich and diverse cultural heritage and ambiance. If the A & E nurse is to give individualized patient care, then the ethnic and cultural background of the patient must be a major consideration. This in turn requires A & E nurses to familiarize themselves with cultural factors. It is a mistake for the nurse to judge the patient's beliefs against his or her own which usually will be Caucasian Christian. Such an ethnocentric approach will lead to a failure in individualized care.

It is strange to talk of individualized care when many nurses do not know the patient's correct name, a situation that often arises with the Asian community. In the case of Sikhs, Singh merely indicates male and Kaur female; either title will be preceded by a personal name and followed by the name of the subcaste which is borne by the whole family (equivalent to a surname): for example, Mohinder Singh Sandhu or Gurmit Kaur Sondh would be correctly addressed as Mr Sandhu or Mrs Sondh. Sometimes the last name is dropped, and only then is it correct to talk of Mr Singh or Mrs Kaur. Hindus use one or more personal names followed by the subcaste name (equivalent to a surname) but do *not* use the titles Singh or Kaur.

The Muslim naming system is more complex as there are many titles that are not names, for example, Abdul, Mohammed, Shah, Syed; other titles such as Ahmad, Ahmed and Rahman can become names when combined with other titles, for example, Abdul Rahman. Khan and Choudhery are common names in Pakistan but these too are titles rather than names, while Bibi, Begum and Khatoon all signify that the bearer is female and do not act as true names. It is quite usual for members of the same family to have different names, with no common family name.

Human behaviour is as much learnt as it is innate, therefore, the response to pain and illness will depend heavily upon upbringing. In other words, it will be a product of cultural background. This should lead the A & E nurse to realize that in dealing with patients from a different cultural background to the nurse, there will be significant differences in how the patient responds to illness and pain. Such differences are not to be interpreted as signs of weakness but rather as a normal learnt behaviour pattern. The whole concept of what is illness itself varies from one ethnic group to

Table 1.6 Standardized mortality rates (SMRs) for men aged 20–64 due to trauma by ethnic background (England and Wales 1991–3)

	Country of birth				
	All countries	Caribbean	Indian subcontinent	Scotland	Ireland
Non-manual (I,II,IIIN)	60	79	66	71	88
Manual (IIIM, IV, V)	119	131	95	268	228

Source: Drever and Whitehead (1995)

another, and from class to class within any group (Helman, 1990). That which is defined as illness by one group may be considered normal by another, thus illness becomes socially constructed; its perception and how you respond to it are relative to where you are in society.

This chapter has so far shown that various social factors are at work in determining the probability of any one person attending A & E. It is not surprising to note that ethnic background also has a significant influence over mortality rates from trauma as shown in Table 1.6.

Of particular concern in Table 1.6 are the high SMRs recorded by Scottish and Irish manual workers living in England and Wales. The combined effects of living away from home and family, heavy alcohol use and the hazardous nature of manual labour may all account for these figures. This is a particular group in need of urgent attention.

Alcohol-related accidents and emergencies

Alcohol-related problems will be considered in depth later in the book. However, at this stage, the A & E nurse should recognize the role of alcohol as one of the major causative factors leading to the front door of A & E. The effect of alcohol on drivers is well known, but it is also a major factor in pedestrian trauma. There is an overwhelming volume of statistics that shows the effects of alcohol on drivers, but McCoy *et al.* (1989) showed that 33% of fatally injured pedestrians had significant alcohol levels in their bloodstream. More recently, it has been shown that, in 1991, 22% of drivers killed in RTAs had blood alcohol levels over the legal limit (Social Trends, 1993).

Alcohol is frequently associated with acts of self-harm such as overdose and self-inflicted injury, while the depression of inhibition effect of alcohol leads to many acts of violence and other behaviour which results in trauma. The depression of inhibition may also result in behaviour which makes it impossible to treat a patient, and alcohol consumption will also delay the giving of an anaesthetic.

Individualized nursing care and social factors

The first step in nursing care is assessment. Social factors such as class, age, gender, housing, and cultural and ethnic backgrounds will all affect the A & E nurse's assessment of the patient. Furthermore, without these factors being considered in all stages of nursing there can be no individualized nursing care. This task is made more difficult by the fact that often the patient will be from a very different sociological grouping than the nurse. Therefore, it is necessary for the nurse to try to see things from the patient's point of view and level of understanding. Only if the nurse and patient are looking at the same problem in the same way is there hope for understanding and cooperation. The patient's perspective on a problem, because of class, gender, age, family, culture, religion and ethnicity, may be very different from the nurse's.

During assessment, an open-minded, non-judgemental attitude will help to bridge what may be a very wide gap between nurse and patient.

In planning care, nurses have to plan for what is possible and for what the patient sees as the problem. What is possible will be partly determined by the factors discussed so far; what the patient sees as the problem will be the result of an interaction between his or her previous life experience and beliefs, and what the nurse can explain and teach.

Our patient may have a beautifully applied plaster or burns dressing in the A & E department, but what are we sending him or her home to? Can a single mother look after two young children with a burns dressing on her hand? Does she understand what will happen if she removes the dressing and the hand becomes infected? Can an elderly lady look after herself (and her even more dependent elderly husband) with her leg in a below knee walking plaster? Is it reasonable to expect a family living 60 miles away with three young children to take on the care of a confused, incontinent elderly father who has not lived with his daughter for 20 years and who has a fractured humerus? Should we be surprised if an Asian lady will not allow intimate procedures to be performed by a male doctor?

The point is that in planning and carrying out care we have to plan for what is *socially* possible and be prepared to include a large amount of education and teaching in our care package, and make sure that the patient understands fully the importance of what is being done. After all, it is not what is taught that is important, it is what is learnt.

When we evaluate the success of our care, we must consider whether the goals set were socially attainable and realistic, and we must be prepared to alter our goals in accordance with experience and home environment.

In conclusion, the A & E nurse needs to realize how important environmental factors are in both the causation and care of the victims of trauma and sudden emergencies. In short, he or she must pay due care and attention to the home and social circumstances of the patient. For these reasons, A & E nursing belongs equally in the primary health care field as much as it does in the hospital.

References

Annual Abstract of Statistics (1999) London: National Office for Statistics.

CSO (1993) *Social Trends* 25, London: HMSO.

Drever F, Whitehead M (1995) Health Inequalities Decennial Supplement. London: Office for National Statistics.

Helman CG (1990) *Culture, Health and Illness*. Oxford: Butterworth-Heinemann.

Office for National Statistics (1999) *Social Trends* 29, London: HMSO.

Townsend P, Davidson N (1982) *Inequalities in Health*. Harmondsworth: Penguin.

Walsh M (1990a) Social factors and A & E attendance. *Nursing Standard*, 5:9, 29–32.

Walsh M (1990b) Geographical factors and A & E attendance. *Nursing Standard*, 5:8, 28–31.

Chapter 2

PATIENTS, PEOPLE AND NURSES – PSYCHOLOGY IN A & E

An understanding of psychology is essential for good nursing practice, for how can we truly individualize care unless we consider the mental processes of our patients? This chapter aims, therefore, to familiarize the reader with some of the areas of psychology that are most relevant to A & E and to show how psychological insights can make a real and beneficial impact on patient care.

Emotion

In A & E, nurses work in an emotion-charged atmosphere. They come into contact with depression and sadness, happiness and joy, and guilt and anger – in fact, with the full range of human emotion. The suddenness with which many patients are taken ill and the media image of the A & E department – as a place full of wailing sirens, flashing blue lights and life-saving heroics – combine to make sudden illness in the A & E department a highly emotional and anxiety-provoking experience for the general public.

Nurses sometimes overlook the emotional content of a patient or a relative in A & E, because they do not know what they are looking for. However, there is a useful body of research on the psychology of emotion that can be applied to the A & E department to improve nursing care and to prevent problems arising out of emotional behaviour.

In reviewing various classic experiments and theories of emotion, Atkinson *et al.* (1991) consider that emotion is triggered by an arousing event which leads to autonomic arousal. The emotional experience that follows is determined by a process known as cognitive appraisal. This term means the way we interpret the event, and this is heavily influenced by previous experiences and cues from the surrounding environment.

The sudden onset of illness or trauma followed by the rapid movement to A & E will certainly act as an emotionally arousing event leading to autonomic stimulation. Similarly, when a family is told that their relative has been 'rushed to hospital', their emotions will be aroused.

When the patient and the family arrive in the A & E, together or apart, the nurse will be one of the most potent sources of emotional cues. Much of the patient's emotional behaviour will therefore depend on the nurse's behaviour. If the nurse is anxious and hostile, the patient may well be anxious and hostile. Conversely, if the nurse is calm and confident, this manner will help bring a distressed patient to a clearer and calmer state of mind. The same applies to the nurse's interaction with the family.

In addition, nurses should remember the effect of previous experience on emotion and consider that a patient's apparently unreasonable emotions may have their origins in some previous unhappy experience. Furthermore, the experience undergone by patients today will have an important effect on their reaction to future hospitalization; this is especially true of young children and their fears of hospital.

A potent source of such cues will be A & E staff who are therefore in a good position, by their own emotional behaviour, to reduce anxiety, fear and anger among patients and relatives.

Grief and bereavement

Today some two-thirds of all deaths occur in institutions, with a high proportion of sudden deaths occurring in A & E departments. It is the suddenness of death in A & E and the age range involved that makes coping with death and the bereaved family and friends one of the most difficult aspects of A & E work.

Most nurses will have witnessed death

before coming to A & E, but these deaths will usually have been the result of a lengthy illness so that the act of dying is expected. In contrast, the dead person in the A & E department is often the cheerful child last seen by his mother setting off to school, the baby found in its cot, the husband and father collapsing at work or the teenager who never came home from a party. It is the stunning suddenness of this most final act of all that lends such a devastating dimension to the problem of caring for the bereaved in A & E.

The grief reaction consists of a cultural and an individual component. Nurses in A & E should remember that the cultural background of the bereaved may be very different from their own and, therefore, not be surprised if the relatives' behaviour is different from that which nurses expect as a result of their own cultural upbringing.

Descriptions of grief include shock, denial, anxiety, depression, guilt, anger and a wide range of somatic signs linked to anxiety. However, these manifestations should not be thought of as a strict succession of stages. Regression is also common.

It is a long walk from the resuscitation room to the relatives' waiting room when a patient has died. The response of relatives will vary with culture and individual factors, therefore their response may lie anywhere in a wide range of behaviours from stunned unbelieving silence through to collapse and a flood of emotion and on to stoical acceptance. The nurse should not be fooled by the stoical response, the grief is there and it has to be worked through in the long term. Stoicism certainly does not convey a lack of care for the dead person or an easy acceptance of the death.

The nurse must be prepared for many questions. 'Why me?' 'Why her?' 'Couldn't anything be done?' 'It's all my fault, isn't it?' These questions do not have answers in this context. A denial response may be observed with the relative simply refusing to believe the person is dead. This denial has to be overcome as an essential part of the grief work, if acceptance is to be reached. The relative should be shown the body and allowed to touch and feel the deceased in order to help with the grief work. This is especially true of mothers of children and infants who have died (particularly cot death infants). The mother should be encouraged to hold the dead baby in her arms to help her overcome the denial mechanism so that she may more readily come to terms with the death of her baby.

There has been considerable debate recently about allowing relatives into the resuscitation room during a resuscitation attempt. It is argued that whatever happens is probably not going to be as bad as they imagine and ultimately as the next of kin, they have the right to be there. Barratt and Wallis (1998) have carried out a survey which sheds interesting light on this argument. They contacted the next of kin of 35 patients who had died during cardiopulmonary resuscitation in A & E and 24 stated that they would have liked to have been asked whether they wished to be present (only four actually were). Of these 24 relatives, 15 stated unequivocally that if they had been offered the chance to witness the resuscitation, they would have taken it. When asked what they thought happens in the resuscitation room, the responses indicated that most relatives actually had little idea. Barratt and Willis observe that if relatives were present it would show them that everything possible had been done and help them with subsequent grief work, it might also help with the decision about when to discontinue resuscitation.

A single bereaved person should never be left alone in the department or left to go home alone. Somebody must sit with them until a relative or friend can be found. Providing human company at this most difficult hour of a person's life is a nursing responsibility. In providing that company, nurses provide the person with an opportunity to verbalize their grief and they protect the person from possible harm. If in the process of doing this, nurses themselves feel moved to tears, there is nothing wrong in that. It is an expression of human empathy, not inadequacy. The nursing care provided in the immediate aftermath of bereavement, however difficult it may be for the nurse, can greatly help the patient's grief work (Davies, 1997).

One important practical point concerns the identification of the deceased. Friends can mistakenly identify a person they have known for years under the stress of an A & E resuscitation room and in the aftermath of a resuscitation attempt on a badly injured patient. The result may be that the wrong relatives are informed.

If nurses find that they are upset by a death in A & E, they should know that this is a normal reaction to a very stressful event that is rather different from death in other hospital areas. Saines (1997) observes that nurses should be allowed to talk about their emotions after encountering sudden death and urges the establishment of a 'culture of caring' within A & E, rather than the traditional 'you'll get used to it approach'. Saines notes that this is one of the most difficult of all parts of A & E work for most nurses. We should, however, remember the successes we have in the resuscitation room to help balance the picture.

How we perceive others

How do patients perceive nurses and how do nurses perceive patients? Research into person perception suggests that the answer may be that they perceive each other very differently and that neither's perceptions may be very accurate. Nurses need to look carefully at how misperception occurs, for misperception may radically alter their assessment of the patient and accurate assessment is central to the process of nursing.

One view of perception sees it as depending heavily upon previous experiences, with judgements being inferred from the information available. In addition, however, we have systems of rules by which we understand what we perceive. These association rules are based on experience and culture. Some may in addition be unique to the individual. These rules create mental sets that act as pigeon-holes into which perceived information can be conveniently filed and rapidly understood.

We expect people to behave in certain ways because they conform to stereotypes. These are defined by Leyens and Codol (1988) as theories of personality that a group of people share about their own group or another group. Common to all stereotypes is that they deny the person's individuality.

The nurse who treats all elderly patients as deaf, confused and incontinent is not nursing people but stereotypes. That nurse is failing to deliver individualized nursing care. Quality nursing depends upon accurate assessment and that means we must look beyond the clothes a person wears, or the number of wrinkles in a person's skin, and treat each as an individual, avoiding the short cut of pigeon-holing them as 'a typical…'.

One final aspect of perception is the old cliché that 'first impressions count'. Luchins (1957) carried out the original research that showed there is a great deal of truth in this statement. In forming impressions of people, we do allow our first impression to control much of what follows, often leading to serious errors in perception. Atkinson *et al.* (1991) have summarized a mass of research data which confirms Luchin's original findings. If A & E nurses are aware of this trap, they will find it easier to put first impressions to one side and to spend time talking to patients, trying to get to know them a little better, before making an assessment. Their assessment will be more accurate for the time spent.

It should also be remembered that the same mechanisms that cause misperception are also at work in the patient who will be working with a stereotype of you as a nurse. Impressions of you will be formed based on the first minute of your interaction.

Accurate patient observation and assessment, therefore, depends upon the nurse being aware of factors that influence perception. In making observations of people and their behaviour, the nurse is inevitably led into seeking to explain that behaviour. The nurse therefore makes attributions or inferences about causality and in doing so, as psychologists have demonstrated, makes all sorts of mistakes or attribution errors (Atkinson *et al.*, 1991).

Humans tend to attribute behaviour to either factors within the individual (internal attribution) or situational, environmental factors outside the individual (external attribution). The fundamental attribution error that people make seems to be to overemphasize the importance of internal attribution. Consequently, in explaining behaviour, we tend systematically to ignore a range of possible environmental explanations and locate the reasons for behaviour within the individual. Internal attributions are linked to the notion of intent; in making such an attribution we also tend to assume that the person knew the likely consequences of their actions. A further key element of attribution theory is the suggestion that the more socially undesirable the consequences of an action the more we tend to attribute to the individual a disposition to behave in that way – an internal attribution is therefore made (Hewstone and Antaki, 1988).

In assessing A & E patients, attribution theory suggests nurses should be wary of how they interpret and explain observed behaviour. It seems as though we may consistently ignore the importance of the strange A & E environment and other situational factors in our assessment, attributing patient behaviour to a pathological cause or to their personality and hence making erroneous judgements about the type of person they are. We are also prone to assume that the patient knew the consequences of his or her actions. This is particularly true of the patient whose behaviour may be seen as antisocial such as a homeless person, a drug user, or a person who has committed an act of self-harm such as self-poisoning. Attribution theory underlines the importance of not making judgements about patients and therefore displaying attitudes lacking in the essential caring qualities that help define nursing as a profession. We should tread carefully and approach patients with an open mind in attempting to understand their behaviour.

How we perceive our environment – sensory deprivation in A & E

When a person is deprived of meaningful sensory input, they are said to be experiencing sensory deprivation. After a period of only a few hours, sensory deprivation can produce hallucinations, anxiety, fear and other mental disturbances.

Let us think of a typical A & E cubicle where a patient can remain for several hours. What sensory input does a patient have in that situation? There is no clock to tell the time. Often the patient cannot even tell if it is day or night. The walls are blank. Loose curtains block off the view beyond the end of the trolley. Overhead there is the ubiquitous neon strip lamp in an equally bare ceiling. If the patient has no friends or relatives present, and no nurse has the time to chat with her, how will she be able to assess the passage of time? We have put our patient into a state of sensory deprivation. It is possible that much apparent 'confusion' in elderly patients has its origins in sensory deprivation. Sensory deprivation will be even more profound if the patient is deaf or

wears spectacles and the hearing aid or spectacles have been left at home.

The patient will probably also be suffering from perceptual deprivation as we may be exposing her to stimuli that are meaningless: the X-ray machines, the ECG monitors, the strange sounds and the mysterious jargon of modern hospitals mean very little to most people. All this adds up to the patient being deprived of meaningful perceptions.

Many sudden mood changes and cases of apparent confusion, therefore, may be the result of the A & E environment depriving the patient of meaningful sensations and perceptions. If a patient is likely to be in A & E for any length of time, reality orientation must be a vital part of the care. Leave the curtain at the end of the cubicle pulled back a little so patients can see what is going on. Make sure spectacles and hearing aids are worn and working. Explain the sounds and sights of the A & E department so that patients have meaningful perceptions of it (the nurse as the interpreter of the hospital experience). These simple measures can greatly assist the patient. It is unfortunate, however, to find that according to Byrne and Heyman (1997) they are often not carried out as nurses feel they are too busy or they can provide sufficient psychological support by just 'keeping an eye on patients' rather than actually talking to them. This study was a small-scale qualitative piece of research and therefore not generalizable, however, these findings are worrying.

Learning and behaviour

Why do we behave the way that we do? This is a vast field that lies in the province of psychology, however, a few simple ideas are presented here as they are of relevance to the work of A & E nurses.

Behaviourism proposes that human behaviour is a product of learning experiences and of the environment and that it is not due to pre-programmed activity or instinct. This implies, therefore, that behaviour can be learned and can be changed. As nurses, we often need to do just that, change behaviour. Hence the importance of behaviourism to learning and to nursing care.

Learning can occur through operant conditioning. If an act is followed by desirable experiences, it is more likely to be repeated; the desirable consequences act as positive re-inforcement. If an act is followed by punish-ment, the effect is to suppress the behaviour, but not to eliminate it, for when the punish-ment is removed, the behaviour will reappear. A more effective way of eliminating behaviour is by *extinction*. In this case, positive reinforce-ment is withheld. This leads to a long-term removal of the behaviour.

These three ideas can be illustrated with a familiar example in A & E. A disturbed young woman with a disordered personality is a regular attender at A & E. She comes in regularly with self-inflicted minor lacerations on the arms, accompanied by attention-seeking and disruptive behaviour. The atten-tion that follows such actions acts as a positive reinforcement leading to repetition of this behaviour. If, however, the attention that the woman receives on each visit is denied .by simply ignoring her disruptive behaviour, then the extinction effect will be expected to lead to the patient reducing her self-harming and attention-seeking behaviour. On the other hand, an angry reaction from staff and a major scene will lead to further disruption and more positive reinforcement so the behaviour continues.

A further form of learning that comes under the heading of operant conditioning is negative reinforcement. In this case, behaviour leads to the removal of unpleasant or adverse situa-tions. Alcohol abuse is a good example of negative reinforcement; the patient drinks to avoid the difficult realities of everyday life. The difficult behaviour of some patients can also be explained in terms of avoiding problems of living by getting other people to perform various tasks for them.

Positive reinforcement is potentially a powerful tool for the nurse who seeks patient cooperation and for the nurse who wants to teach and motivate junior staff. In teaching a patient how to use crutches or how to do the essential finger exercises for an arm in plaster, we must reward correct actions with praise (positive reinforcement) if we want those actions to be repeated. Similarly, if a junior member of staff is being taught a skill or a junior nurse performs an intelligent or thoughtful piece of nursing care, then we should praise the nurse and say 'well done!'. Such positive reinforcement will help moti-vation and morale. Ignoring good work will produce extinction of that good work, while merely telling the nurse off for poor work (punitive reinforcement) will not bring about good care.

Having discussed operant conditioning, it now remains to look at classical conditioning, the origins of which lie in the famous work of Pavlov and his dogs (Fig. 2.1). Pavlov pre-sented food to a dog (unconditioned stimulus) and obtained a response of salivation (uncon-ditioned response) which was a reflex action. If he rang a bell at the same time (conditioned stimulus), he found that after a while the dog associated the bell with the food and salivated to the sound of the bell only. Salivation had become a conditioned response.

This form of learning has been demon-

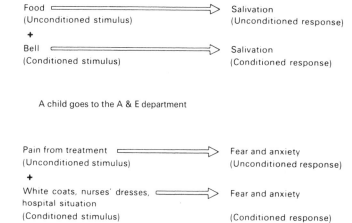

Food ➡ Salivation
(Unconditioned stimulus)   (Unconditioned response)
+
Bell ➡ Salivation
(Conditioned stimulus)   (Conditioned response)

A child goes to the A & E department

Pain from treatment ➡ Fear and anxiety
(Unconditioned stimulus)   (Unconditioned response)
+
White coats, nurses' dresses, ➡ Fear and anxiety
hospital situation
(Conditioned stimulus)   (Conditioned response)

Fig. 2.1 Pavlov's classic experiment and an A & E example: the unconditioned and conditioned stimulus become paired together to produce a conditional response.

strated in humans. Consider the example of the small child taken to A & E after an accident. The combined efforts of the nurses and a casualty officer may do a very good job of stitching his scalp back together, but this can be a very frightening experience for the child. The strange environment and those funny strangers in white coats and dresses will become associated with the pain and discomfort involved in having a wound stitched. The result will be that the next time the child has to attend hospital, white coats and nurses' dresses will act as a conditioned stimulus to produce the conditioned response of fear and anxiety. It is thought that the origins of many irrational fears and phobias lie in this mechanism, where the response to one stimulus is transferred onto another stimulus by classical conditioning. Examples range from fear of injections through to phobias about spiders and on to sexual fetishes.

If we want to prevent children developing fears about hospitals, the unconditioned stimulus must be reduced by reducing pain and discomfort to a minimum and the child's experience of A & E made as pleasant as possible. We can also remove the conditioning stimulus of white coats, nurses' uniforms and all the other hospital paraphernalia which, fortunately, has been done in many departments. Ideally there should be a special children's section in the A & E department with toys and a play area, where staff should be in ordinary clothes and where the hospital environment should, as far as possible, be minimized.

One other method of learning behaviour that needs discussion is learning by imitation (Bandura, 1986). The power of modelling as a means of learning behaviour is so potent that it is not surprising that the student copies what he or she has seen in the clinical setting. We are all teaching junior colleagues every day without realizing it, simply by the example we set.

Memory

How do we remember information? What can we do to improve recall? These two questions deserve our attention if we are to ensure optimum results from teaching patients prior to discharge about their dressings, exercises, plasters and other aspects of care. A patient who has had a Colles fracture reduced and plastered has enough problems to contend with. However, if s/he forgets the importance of exercising the fingers, maintaining the arm in a sling, looking out for signs of discoloration, excessive swelling or symptoms such as a tingling sensation, then all manner of neurovascular complications may arise.

Similar comments apply to a whole range of treatments, drugs and instructions with which we discharge patients every day from A & E. Nurses, therefore, need to know something of the work that has been done in the field of memory, for not only will it benefit patients but, incorporated into teaching, it will improve the way that student nurses learn.

Memory is thought of as consisting of two components, long-term memory (LTM) and short-term memory (STM). The short-term part of memory can only retain about seven items which are then either lost from STM by displacement by new items to remember or are passed on into LTM after appropriate rehearsal. We tend to remember better things that are said to us first and last while forgetting the material in between (Fig. 2.2). Our success in remembering the early parts of information we are given reflects the working of LTM and is called the primacy effect. Remembering the last thing we are told is due to the STM. However, LTM will diminish due to emotional upset and interference, where similar items get in the way of what we are trying to recall, hence the much poorer recall of the mid part of a piece of information. Improvements in LTM can be brought about by repetition of what is to be remembered and by the provision of cues to enable us to access information more readily in LTM.

A patient will tend to recall best what is said first and last. Therefore, we must put the most important information first and last. To help patients to remember what is said in the middle of a message, we can use repetition of key points coupled with cues to help memory. At the same time, we should try to avoid introducing spurious information that will only interfere with what has to be remembered, especially if it is similar in content. Emotional upset will interfere with memory also, so there is not much point expecting someone who is very anxious or distressed to remember detailed instructions, their emotional state has to be stabilized first. Finally, given the falli-

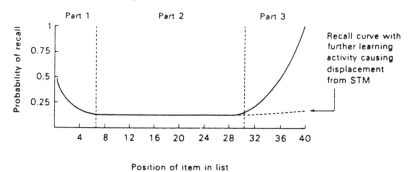

Fig. 2.2 Free recall curve (Murdock, 1962)

bility of human memory, simple pre-printed instruction cards should be given to patients on discharge for such things as care of plaster of Paris, wounds, anti-tetanus follow up and so on.

Pain

Pain is a subjective, psychological experience known only to the patient and which may bear little relationship to the tissue damage involved. Factors that are associated with pain include anxiety and fear, a sense of loss of control, isolation, learning of cultural and familial responses to pain and the individual's prior experiences (Rawal, 1998). Many of these factors are present in any A & E patient. Walsh (1993) has demonstrated the widespread prevalence of pain and anxiety among ambulatory A & E patients. He asked a sample of 200 adults who walked into a typical busy urban A & E unit to assess their pain and anxiety levels using a simple scale of 0–5, where 0 indicated the absence of pain or anxiety and 5 indicated the most severe pain or anxiety the person could imagine. Only 10% of patients stated they were pain free, while 52% rated their pain as 3, 4 or 5. Half the patients stated their anxiety levels as 3, 4 or 5. Statistically significant differences emerged indicating that the higher the pain level reported, the higher the degree of anxiety that the person was experiencing. This association between pain and anxiety is well documented in the literature (Thomas, 1997). Nurses in A & E can make a major contribution to relieving the patient's pain therefore by working to reduce fear and anxiety.

Pain and anxiety are therefore common problems in A & E patients. Evidence shows that nurses are not very good at assessing pain as they ignore its personal nature. This means it cannot be assessed reliably from physical signs such as the extent of trauma, raised blood pressure, pulse rate or even facial expression (Thomas, 1997).

Different cultures express pain in different ways and within any one culture there are different rules for male and female. The familiar phrase 'Now be a brave boy and don't cry' that is heard in A & E tells us a lot about our culture's views; it is permitted for females to cry but not males.

The nurse cannot know what the patient is feeling. It is a unique experience to that individual and the most reliable guide to a patient's pain is what the patient says it is. This must be a fundamental principle in A & E nursing. After our ABCD of resuscitation, pain should be the next thing to be assessed and it should be reassessed at regular intervals during the patient's stay in A & E. It is sad that some nurses still see patients' requests for pain relief as attention seeking, undesirable behaviour or use stereotypes to decide on pain relief, i.e. 'If it's a Colles fracture, the patient should have ...' rather than look at the individual person.

The provision of psychological care in A & E

This chapter has briefly introduced some well-known themes from psychology and demonstrated their relevance to A & E nursing. Many A & E departments, particularly in large cities during the winter, are under extreme pressure and therefore psychological care may be viewed as being of secondary importance under such conditions by some nurses. This is highly regrettable and actually, under these circumstances, psychological care assumes even greater importance.

Walsh and Dolan (1999) have provided evidence that caring is one of the casualties of the A & E pressure cooker environment. Their research involved using a well-validated tool which asked nurses to rate the importance of 25 statements about caring (the Caring Dimensions Inventory, CDI) and involved a sample of 156 A & E nurses attending a major national conference. These nurses rated being neatly dressed on duty (20th) as of almost equal priority as getting to know the patient as a person (19th) and more important exploring a patient's lifestyle (22nd). The fact that such important aspects of care were ranked 19th and 22nd out of a list of 25 items does raise questions about psychological care given in A & E, although it is reassuring that providing privacy for patients was ranked 2nd and listening to patients was ranked 4th. The short period of interaction with A & E patients may explain these findings. The performance of A & E nurses on the CDI tool was comparable with another large sample of ward nurses indicating that A & E nurses are no less caring than general ward nurses, however.

The heavy workload and stresses of A & E work do take their toll on A & E nurses. The evidence for this has also been provided by Walsh and Dolan (1998) who found significant levels of burnout in a large sample of A & E nurses (n = 134). Of particular concern were the high levels of depersonalization present which could adversely affect nurse–patient interaction.

Psychological care in A & E is not therefore an add-on optional extra, but a core element of A & E nursing. It is essential if we are to provide individualized, humane and effective care to help patients deal with the fear, pain and distress of serious illness, trauma or bereavement.

References

Atkinson R, Atkinson R, Smith E (1991) *Introduction to Psychology,* 19th edn. New York: Harcourt Brace Jovanovitch.

Bandura A (1986) *Social Foundations of Thought and Action.* Englewood Cliffs NJ: Prentice-Hall.

Barratt F, Wallis D (1998) Relatives in the resuscitation room: their point of view. *Journal of Accident and Emergency Medicine,* 15:109–11.

Byrne G, Heyman R (1997) Understanding nurses communication with patients in A&E departments using a symbolic interactionist perspective. *Journal of Advanced Nursing,* 26:93–100.

Davies J (1997) Grieving after a sudden death; the impact of the initial intervention. *Accident and Emergency Nursing,* 5:181–4.

Hewstone M, Antaki C (1988) Attribution theory and social explanations. In Hewstone M, Stroebe W, Codol J, Stephenson G (eds) *Introduction to Psychology.* Oxford: Blackwell.

Leyens JP, Codol J (1988) Social cognition in introduction to social psychology. In Hewstone M, Stroebe W, Codol JP, Stephenson G (eds) *Introduction to Psychology.* Oxford: Blackwell.

Luchins A (1957) Primacy-recency in impression formation. In Houland CI (ed.) *The Order of Presentation in Persuasion.* New Haven: Yale University Press.

Rawal N (1998) *Management of Acute and Chronic Pain.* London: BMJ Books.

Saines JC (1997) Phenomenon of sudden death (2). *Accident and Emergency Nursing,* 5, 205–9.

Thomas V (1997) *Pain; Its Nature and Management.* London: Bailliere Tindall.

Walsh M (1993) Pain and anxiety in A & E attenders. *Nursing Standard,* 7:26, 40–42.

Walsh M, Dolan B (1998) Burnout and stress amongst A&E nurses. *Emergency Nurse,* 6:2, 23–30.

Walsh M, Dolan B (1999) Emergency nurses and their perceptions of caring. *Emergency Nurse,* 7:4, 24–31.

Chapter 3

THE ROLE OF THE A & E NURSE

The role of the A & E nurse is one of the most varied in the profession. During a single shift you can nurse patients across the whole age range, from infants to the very elderly, and your work can vary between dealing with relatives who have lost a loved one through to applying a supportive stockinette to a sprained ankle.

The shifts may be hard. Dealing with the public at the cutting edge demands tact, mental agility and the ability to be flexible as what may happen in the next hour is totally unpredictable. A & E nursing is the front line fire-fighting service of the NHS. Much time and energy is spent keeping waiting times down to ensure a through flow of patients while, in winter, you have to offer a high standard of care to patients who may be waiting six to eight hours for a bed.

This tremendous variability means that the job is never boring. The quiet times can be used for teaching juniors, developing yourself or sharing experiences with colleagues. Whatever you are doing, a sense of humour helps. Career progression to senior nurse can be quicker than on general wards if you are prepared to move to gain differing experiences and pursue your continuing education

Patient focused care

A & E nurses have to remember to look at care from the patient's perspective as often care is far from focused on what the patient desires. Often the patient will see many members of staff and be frequently moved around the department before being moved on elsewhere (X-ray, Plaster Room etc.) for further treatment.

A move towards more patient focused care is to be welcomed. The traditional model of working within A & E needs to be revisited and the focus moved towards what works best for the patient. Staff should work around the injured or ill rather than organizing the department for the benefit of themselves. This is particularly true in planning care for those with minor injuries.

The generic A & E nurse

The A & E nurse is known for the specialist skills needed to deal with a wide range of injury and illness. It is important therefore for the nurse new to this field to gain experience within all areas of A & E. Caring for the critically ill may be the most exciting and dramatic part of A & E, but many experienced nurses get more enjoyment from working with patients who have had minor injuries. Another group of patients who need expert nursing care and where nursing really does make a difference are older people who are often waiting hours for a bed. They commonly have not only an acute problem, such as a fractured neck or femur or chest infection, but also have multiple other problems. Working with this group of patients teaches you the skills of assessment and communication, but it is also demanding and tiring. Their dependency on you as a nurse is high, yet their priority within A & E may be low. The instigation of critical care pathways has allowed these patients to be seen by nurses and transferred to the ward, by-passing the usual medical model of care.

Triage nurse

Triage is the most fundamental but demanding skill that the inexperienced A & E nurse has to learn. An experienced A & E nurse, however, makes it seem simple. The basic purpose of triage is to sort patients into categories in order that those who most need urgent care receive it first. An experienced A & E nurse rapidly assesses the patient's problems, decides a triage category and establishes the beginning of a treatment process including immediate analgesia for pain relief. Expanding roles now mean that many triage nurses can send the patient for an appropriate X-ray. In many departments the nurse also receives patients from the paramedic service and also then decides on the assessment category of the patient with more major complications. For a new nurse this responsibility may appear a daunting prospect.

However, around 40% of hospitals now use the 'Manchester Triage' system which allows even junior staff to deliver an acceptable level of assessment to the general public (Manchester Triage Group, 1997). The system is based on flow charts (algorithms) to facilitate decision making. The system follows a medical model despite triage being fundamentally a nursing activity in practice. The triage groups are colour coded and shown in Table 3.1, with the recommended waiting time for treatment.

This has led to much criticism from more senior nurses who feel that the Manchester Triage System is too closely tied into physiological findings with little consideration of psychosocial factors. If the system is used as a basis for assessment then it does, however, provide a safety net for junior staff. We believe therefore that the system is beneficial as it provides a minimum standard for assessment and brings all staff to a common level of competency. The more experienced nurse should be able to diverge from the pathway, to provide a more individual assessment. Divergence from algorithms and guidelines is acceptable providing that RNs remember they are accountable practitioners and therefore should

be able to justify their actions at all times (Walsh, 2000).

Other triage models do exist and, whatever model is used, the key thing is that it is used consistently and ensures that those patients who most need care receive it first. One of the most important issues around triage is that whatever scheme is used, it must be audited on a regular basis. If clinical managers are to argue for more resources, they must have good data on patient numbers and dependency.

The nurse in the resuscitation room

As the nurse begins his/her career within A & E, the most exciting area is the resuscitation room. The skill level, as everywhere else within A & E, is high. Anything can appear in this room with very little warning, and you have to be able to react promptly and effectively. A team approach to resuscitation has proved highly effective in reducing mortality rates (Vincent and Driscoll, 1992). This team approach to resuscitation is described in more detail in the resuscitation chapter.

Nurse-led X-ray

One of the most recent developments in A & E is that of the nurse practitioner (NP). The role has been extensively discussed by Walsh *et al.* (1999) who stress that the NP sees patients with undifferentiated presentations as the first point of contact and manages their condition with a high degree of autonomy. This has allowed experienced nurses to assess, treat and discharge patients without the traditional,

Table 3.1 Manchester Triage Scale

Number	Name	Colour	Target time (minutes)
1	Immediate	Red	0
2	Very urgent	Orange	10
3	Urgent	Yellow	60
4	Standard	Green	120
5	Non-urgent	Blue	240

Manchester Triage Group, 1997

lengthy delay caused by waiting for busy medical staff. In A & E, the ability to order and interpret X-rays is therefore fundamental to the NP role.

More than half the patients attending A & E will require an X-ray yet, research (Vincent, 1988) has shown that senior house officers were missing 39% of important clinical abnormalities. It is important therefore that, if nurse-led X-ray is to be implemented, then appropriate training must be given if we are to improve upon such figures. At the point of triage, nurses can assess specific injuries that may require an X-ray. A good clinical examination technique is therefore needed to avoid unnecessary X-rays. The Ottawa ankle tool is an example of a simple protocol which has allowed nurses to become accurate in their examination of the ankle and has led to more appropriate decisions on whether to order X-rays (Stiell, 1993).

Nurse-led X-ray though has had its difficulties. Tye (1998) showed that 84% of NPs could order X-rays but only 36% were allowed to interpret the findings. This study only looked at NPs and not at general nurse-led X-ray. It is a golden rule of radiology that you should never look at a radiograph without seeing the patient and never see the patient without looking at the radiograph.' If the nurse is allowed to interpret the films s/he ordered, immediate decisions can be made about treatment, which might include referral to a doctor. Alternatively, if the nurse has an immediate diagnosis of the films available from the radiologist or appropriately trained radiographer, s/he can also instigate immediate treatment. The problem is that if after a nurse orders an X-ray and s/he is not allowed to interpret it and/or proceed with treatment based upon that interpretation, the patient is left waiting to see a doctor in the traditional way. The doctor has to examine the patient (in line with 'Commandment 4') and review the X-ray and much of the time saved by the nurse ordering the X-ray is then lost. Instead of a lengthy wait to see a doctor *before* X-ray, the patient is left with a lengthy wait *after* X-ray. The queue of patients is effectively transferred to another area further into the department. Despite the fact that if nurses are not allowed to interpret X-rays or act upon interpretations carried out in the radiology department, much of the time saved can be lost, nurse-led X-ray

still does focus on the patients needs immediately on arrival. It has the benefit of ensuring that once the patient gets to see the doctor, all investigations are complete.

When considering nurse-led X-ray, the nurse must be appropriately trained in physical examination of the areas that they will be allowed to X-ray. Upon examination, the nurse must feel that an X-ray is appropriate. The question to ask is whether this investigation will affect the patient's management? If the answer is yes then an X-ray will be appropriate. If the answer is no, then the nurse should not send the patient for X-ray. The view that the doctor may send them for one anyway is avoiding a decision and equating your clinical practice with that of a junior doctor. The result is likely to be that if your department has an audit of nurse-led X-ray, you will come out with a high score for inappropriate X-rays. Some injuries require treatment in accordance with the findings of the clinical examination even though the X-ray may be negative, for example a suspected fracture of the scaphoid.

Pregnancy and X-ray

Protection of the fetus from radiation is of great importance. The primary responsibility for identifying women at risk lies with the person requesting the X-ray. This includes situations where the woman may not be aware that she is pregnant herself.

The Royal College of Radiologists (1998) recommends that if a woman of reproductive age requires radiographic investigation in which the primary beam irradiates directly, or by scatter, the pelvic region:

- She should first be asked if she is pregnant.
- If she cannot exclude the possibility, then she should be asked if her period is overdue.
- If the woman is definitely, or probably pregnant the justification for the investigation should be discussed either with a senior medical colleague or the on-call radiologist.

The X-ray request form

It is vital that the X-ray request form is filled in appropriately, clearly and legibly. Errors made here will continue throughout the patient's visit, and further, if not rectified. For example, if the name or date of birth is wrong, then old films of another patient may be found in error by the filing clerks. The nurse must also ensure an adequate history is written on the form. This will allow the radiologist to identify exactly where the patient may have been tender or bruised. Remember that the radiologist reporting the film will not have the luxury of the patient sat in front of him/her so that s/he can compare the film with the clinical presentation themselves. For example 'tender left ankle' is inadequate clinical information, whereas 'tender over posterior tip of left lateral malleous', gives the exact location of the pain. Finally, remember to write down the correct limb. All too often the form does not state which limb or may even identify the wrong side with potentially disastrous implications.

The A & E nurse and the law

The police are one agency with whom the A & E nurse will have many dealings, and such is the nature of police interest in some patients, that there are going to be occasions when difficult dilemmas of confidentiality arise. On the one hand, it is essential to have a good working relationship with the police, but on the other hand, there is the question of patient confidentiality and police access to information.

If a patient feels that what s/he tells a nurse is genuinely in confidence, and will not be immediately repeated to the police, vital clinical information may be forthcoming that would otherwise be withheld. Examples are in drug use, where it may be essential to know what drugs have been taken, the route and timing of administration and, in wounding cases, where information about the real manner in which the injury was sustained may be withheld, leading to inappropriate treatment and nursing care.

Nursing and medical records have been traditionally held as confidential. This includes the A & E Register which, on occasion, the police may wish to access. This should not be allowed without the consent of the hospital management. Where records have been computerized the close controls of the Data Protection Act also apply. Enquiries about the names and addresses of patients who have attended A & E are best passed on to management, although details of patients involved in a road traffic accident (RTA) may be released directly to the police as this is required under law. The police must also be immediately notified of incidents involving firearms and suspected terrorism.

On occasions staff may suspect that a patient has sustained injuries in the act of carrying out a crime which the police are either unaware of or are inquiring about. This is a most difficult situation (unless it involves firearms, terrorism or an RTA as mentioned previously) as the demands of patients' confidentiality are such that theoretically nothing should be said to the police. McHale *et al.* (1998) point out that the police have no automatic right to demand access to a patient's records. However, the nurse is also a citizen and, as a citizen, has certain responsibilities before the law. There can be no hard and fast rules and each case must be treated on its merits. If there is a strong suspicion that an individual has been involved in criminal activity, then you should discuss the case with the doctor responsible for the patient, and a joint approach should be made to a senior manager or the consultant in charge. The Police and Criminal Evidence Act permits the police in serious cases to compel the hospital to produce personal information and even samples of human tissue (McHale *et al.*, 1998).

An example will illustrate the point. A rather scruffy young man comes to A & E with a cut leg. There is a large laceration through the back of his right calf and also through his jeans. The wound is obviously fresh and still bleeding. The friend who is accompanying the patient disappears for coffee while the patient explains his injury in vague terms of 'falling through a hedge'. At this stage the nurse's suspicions are aroused as the wound and story do not match. Enter a policeman and a rather distressed young woman with the story that the woman has just come home to find two men burgling her flat. They broke a window in making their escape, and one of them cut himself in the process. The flat is only a few hundred yards from A & E and the police have followed the blood trail to the front door. Meanwhile, a nurse is applying a dressing to the leg, the wound having been sutured. A decision is needed quickly. This real example was dealt with by checking that the woman felt able to identify the men in question, followed by the suggestion that if the police wanted to wait by the main entrance, discreetly out of view, the young woman may be able to identify the men in question in the next few minutes. This was acceptable to the police who easily arrested the two men.

This example shows that, by using initiative and common sense, an awkward situation may be resolved satisfactorily.

Collecting evidence is another area of police work that the A & E nurse will come into contact with. Patient clothing may contain vital evidence and every effort should be made to preserve it. In the resuscitation room, it is often cut off the patient but, if possible, this should be done in such a way as to leave undisturbed existing tears or holes as these may give clues as to the weapon used in an assault, for example. Clothing offers clues in 'hit and run' cases as it may contain traces of paint from the offending vehicle, while in shootings there will be gunpowder stains on clothes if the gun is fired from a range of less than 1 m (approximately 3 feet). Such evidence is vital to corroborate verbal testimony. Even shoes offer potential evidence, for there may be footprints found near the scene of the crime.

All possessions and clothing must, therefore, be safely labelled and stored for, if such evidence is to be admissible in court, it must be possible to establish continuity, otherwise there is the possibility of the evidence being 'planted'. A & E staff will be required to make statements in order to establish continuity of evidence, so the nurse should make mental notes of what is done with clothing and patient possessions during the course of a resuscitation attempt if there is suspicion of foul play.

One problem that commonly occurs involving police is when they want to breathalyse a car driver injured in an accident. As in other cases, they must have the consent of the casualty officer before they can proceed to administer a breathalyser test. If the patient has suffered significant facial trauma, the doctor may refuse consent for a breathalyser if, in their opinion, the patient's injuries will interfere with the ability to give a full and proper breath sample. If blood tests are required by the police, a police surgeon will be called to the department to take the necessary samples.

It is essential that there should be a good working relationship between police and A & E nurses, and this relationship may be assisted by trying to see things from the other side's point of view.

Turning away from matters involving the police to more general considerations of legal matters, readers should note that the legal aspects of treating patients against their will are covered in Chapter 17. However, this only refers to the Mental Health Act (1983) and does not cover the situation where the patient is a child or young person under 18.

Young people aged 16 or 17 may give valid consent for any treatment but not for participation in a research project unless it can genuinely be considered to be part of the treatment (Dimond, 1990). For those aged under 16 the situation is no longer as clear cut as it used to be when it was assumed that parental consent was always necessary for treatment unless in an emergency. In 1985, the famous Gillick case led to a ruling in the House of Lords that, in some cases, mature minors under 16 who are capable of understanding the situation, can give valid consent. The safest course of action for the A & E nurse appears to be always to act in the best interest of the child, while recognizing the need for parental consent to be obtained normally, unless in emergencies.

In the rare case where parents refuse to consent to treatment which is clearly in the child's interests, the hospital authorities may apply to the courts for an interim care order or to have the child made a ward of court in order for treatment to proceed. This covers objections to blood transfusion on religious grounds for example. The difficult area of suspected child abuse will be covered in Chapter 11; suffice it to say here that every A & E unit should have a clearly understood policy drawn up with the local social services department and the police to cover such cases.

The situation may also arise where an adult patient refuses treatment, even though their life may be endangered by so doing. An example seen in A & E is the patient who has deliberately taken an overdose of medication or other drugs and who refuses treatment or admission. Davis (1993) points out that, although patients are legally entitled to refuse treatment, this right is poorly protected in law as the issue of how rational the patient is in making such a decision allows medical and nursing staff the opportunity to override the patient's wishes. There are strong professional arguments that make nurses and doctors attempt to intervene to prevent suicide, although Davis (1993) considers that if the suicidal patient is competent, then legally s/he could be left to die. Treatment that involves touching the patient without his or her consent, according to Young (1994), entitles the patient to sue for battery. Young (1994) considers that the law tends to support the patient's refusal of consent but without considering the nurse in such a situation negligent if s/he respects the patient's wishes.

Davis (1993) rightly considers the A & E nurse to be caught in a moral and legal minefield when considering various ethical principles, the law and the UKCC Code of Professional Conduct. She recommends that the A & E nurse tries to ensure that the patient fully understands the consequences of refusing treatment and assesses the patient's level of insight into the situation. In this way refusal of consent could be said to be a rational and informed act. However, if in doubt, Davis advises the nurse to err on the side of life and rely on the defence of necessity. It might be added that membership of a professional trades union will greatly assist such a defence in the event of an attempt to sue the nurse subsequently.

It is understandable that nurses are often concerned about the risk of legal action being taken against them for neglect or malpractice, although in practice it is always the Trust that will be sued under the principle of vicarious liability. This simply means that an employer is always held responsible for the actions of employees providing they were acting within their normal fields of employment and were not acting for personal gain. On many counts A & E nurses feel particularly vulnerable to legal action being taken against them, and certainly many general letters of complaint, which contain a wide range of allegations, are written to hospitals about A & E staff. Although all the nursing trade unions will support their members, it is strongly recommended here that all A & E staff belong to the Royal College of Nursing in order to obtain the benefit of their professional indemnity insurance cover and also to ensure that if complaints are made at local level, they are well repre-

sented by an RCN steward and/or officer. Such representation is essential if staff are to have a fair hearing. The RCN also has a very active A & E Association, a section formed specially for A & E nursing staff.

With regard to the problems of negligence, the legal view is that, provided a nurse behaves in such a way as could be *reasonably* expected for a nurse of that position then, whatever the outcome, they are not guilty of negligence. The whole issue hinges on the principle of the nurse's actions being *reasonable*: it is reasonable to expect a qualified nurse to recognize a patient in cardiac arrest, but not reasonable to expect a qualified nurse with no training in the skill to intubate that patient.

A key question concerns what it is reasonable to expect of a nurse when acting in new and expanded roles that have traditionally been seen as the medical domain. The answer is that the nurse is expected to be as competent as the doctor who would have previously performed the task in question (Walsh, 2000). Simply saying 'but I am only a nurse' is no defence when a law suit for negligence is brought against the Trust.

An argument that is frequently aired is whether a nurse who witnesses an accident or other emergency situation should stop to render first aid. The debate is about the nurse's competence in first aid. Castledine (1993) has rightly argued that the nurse must help in any way possible as s/he has a moral duty to do so and the UKCC Code of Conduct requires him/her to do so. Castledine cites the case of a nurse who walked past an accident and was reported to the UKCC for not helping. The UKCC found her guilty of professional misconduct and disciplined her, although not striking her off the register. It is incomprehensible that an A & E nurse could ignore an accident and not stop to help for fear of legal repercussions if something went wrong. Such an attitude is inconsistent with the caring ethic that underpins nursing.

The situation can be summarized by saying that you should always:

- Act in what is perceived to be the best interests of the patient.
- Only attempt to do things that could be reasonably expected of you in the light of your experience and training.
- Adhere to Trust policy and guidelines.

Health education and the A & E nurse

The National Health Service has been criticized for being a National Ill Health Service, i.e. for emphasizing treatment and attempting to cure once a person is ill and for not paying enough attention to the *prevention* of illness.

At present in many parts of the western world, the demand for health care is growing faster than the resources available to meet that demand; the UK is no exception. It is therefore essential to pursue vigorously a policy of prevention in order to try to reduce health demands. It should be noted here, however, that the other side of the coin is campaigning for greater resources to be made available for health care, which means becoming involved in the political process. A dual approach is needed, and nursing as the major caring profession has a responsibility to be in the forefront of both aspects of the campaign for better health.

Chapter 1 identified certain key groups within society who are most at risk of death from accidents or violence (such as children and young male adults), while the relationship between social class and ill health was also explored. These groups can be targeted by A & E departments for health education work. You will come in to contact with many more members of the general public in a day's work than will most other nurses. Furthermore, the people that A & E nurses are dealing with will tend to be motivated by the fact that they have just had a firsthand experience of illness or trauma; they will, therefore, in most cases, be receptive to advice about health or accident prevention.

Simple first aid is one obvious area in which the A & E nurse can carry out health education. Patients still come to A & E with burns covered in butter or toothpaste, with fractured arms where there has been no attempt at splintage, with dressings that are effectively tourniquets that lead to blue hands, or even with tourniquets to control bleeding from simple lacerations. The sight of a patient vomiting the hot sweet tea and brandy that was poured down their throat by a well-intentioned person is still all too common. The nurse has a major responsibility in explaining to the patient about the need to complete a course of anti-tetanus vaccine commenced in A & E, while patients starting a course of antibiotics must have the consequences of not completing the course explained to them. In addition to advice about first aid and medication, there are many other areas where the A & E nurse has a real preventative role, such as in advice about smoking, alcohol and drug problems, contraception, obesity and how to make the best use of social services and GPs.

In the future, health care will become increasingly a matter of prevention and the A & E nurse, far from being merely a 'picker-up of pieces', should use the opportunities that present themselves daily to promote health.

Summary

The role of the nurse in A & E has undergone dramatic change in the last two decades and will continue to evolve and develop into the future. It is important, therefore, to remember the two basic principles of always considering what is in the patient's best interests as the priority and also ensuring you are adequately trained and prepared for any new roles you may be expected to take on. This chapter has introduced you to the world of A & E nursing and shown that a career can be made from working within this specialized field. The roles described above are the most common. Other roles are emerging, such as in mental health provision, trauma coordinators and the nurse consultant role. All of these are likely to play a major part in the development of the service in years to come.

The emergence of the RCN Faculty of Emergency Nursing aims to structure career development further (RCN, 1999) and allow nurses to progress along a defined pathway, while maintaining clinical competency. The fact that the Royal College of Nursing is choosing the Accident and Emergency service to be the first pilot for this concept, ensures that A & E nursing will stay at the forefront of the nursing profession.

References

Castledine G (1993) Ethical implications of first aid. *British Journal of Nursing*, 2:239–41.
Davis J (1993) Ethical and legal issues in suicide. *British Journal of Nursing*, **2**:777–80.

Dimond B (1990) *Legal Aspects of Nursing*. London: Prentice-Hall.

Manchester Triage Group (1997) *Emergency Triage*. London: BMJ.

McHale J, Tingle J, Peysner J (1998) *Law and Nursing*. Oxford: Butterworth-Heinemann.

Royal College of Radiologists (1998) *Making the Best Use of a Department of Radiology*. London: Royal College of Radiologists.

Stiell I (1993) Decision rules for the use of radiology in acute ankle injuries. Refinement and prospective validation. *JAMA*, **269**:1127–32.

Tye C (1998) Emergency nurse practitioner services in major accident and emergency units: a United Kingdom postal survey. *Journal of Accident and Emergency Medicine*, **15**:31–4.

Vincent CA (1988) Accurate detection of radiographic abnormalities by junior doctors. *Arch. Emerg Med.*, **5**:101–9.

Walsh M, Crumbie A, Reveley S (1999) *Nurse Practitioners: Clinical Skills and Professional Issues*. Oxford: Butterworth-Heinemann.

Walsh M (2000) *Nursing Frontiers: Accountability and the Boundaries of Care*. Oxford: Butterworth-Heinemann.

Young A (1994) *Law and Professional Conduct in Nursing*. London: Scutari.

Critical care

Chapter 4

NURSING CARE OF THE CRITICALLY INJURED PATIENT

Introduction

In 1988 the Royal College of Surgeons produced a report discussing trauma care within Accident and Emergency Departments in the UK (1988). It suggested the development of the Advanced Trauma Life Support (ATLS) course within the UK. This course and its nursing counterparts have changed how critically ill patients are treated within the British system.

The course fundamentally showed how one doctor and one nurse could use a systematic approach to resuscitation and be skilled in delivering techniques that would allow the patient to survive. The template of primary assessment, resuscitation and secondary survey is now common vocabulary among doctors, nurses and paramedics throughout the western world. This approach has allowed patients to have better survival rates than previously. The ATLS course for doctors and the nursing versions of TNCC and ATNC have become standard qualifications for people wishing to pursue a career with A & E nursing.

The Airway, Cervical spine, Breathing, Circulation and Disability, are the major components upon which resuscitation should be based. Followed in sequence, the patient's life-threatening injuries can not only be identified, but corrected. If followed out of sequence the patient may well come to more harm.

The team approach to resuscitation best described by Driscoll et al. (1992b) showed that if a systematic approach was used with each team member performing an individual task, this reduces mortality. This system is best compared to a 'Formula One Pitstop' approach where each team member has a specific task, such as assessment and maintenance of the airway. Once completed the team leader needs to be informed so that the team may progress further (Fig. 4.1). Many teams now use three nurses for specific roles such as airway nurse, circulation nurse and finally recorder nurse. The first part of this chapter will therefore be structured around the broad headings of airway, cervical spine, breathing and circulation, as the key principles outlined under these heading are the fundamentals of treatment for the seriously injured patient.

Airway

If the patient's airway is obstructed, all other considerations are of secondary importance and immediate intervention to clear the airway is required. If a complete airway obstruction exists then the patient will be brain dead within 4 minutes. More commonly a partial obstruction exists. This causes hypoxia and eventually brain death but is totally avoidable with good basic airway technique. The common causes of obstruction are the tongue falling back against the epiglottis, vomitus, blood, inhaled material such as food or dentures, and soft tissue trauma affecting the neck or respiratory tract. This trauma can be caused by the inhalation of flames or of hot or noxious gases leading to burns of the trachea, by insect stings in the upper respiratory tract, or by a blow to the neck. The unconscious patient will be far less able to protect his or her airway than the patient who is conscious.

Assessment

Airway assessment is the first step in examining the patient. Obvious respiratory distress, cyanosis, stridor or snoring sounds and level of consciousness are all signs in assessing airway patency, together with a history of the event. The sound of the patient's voice is also important. Hoarseness may indicate airway problems and, in these circumstances, laryngoscopy should not be performed as it may provoke

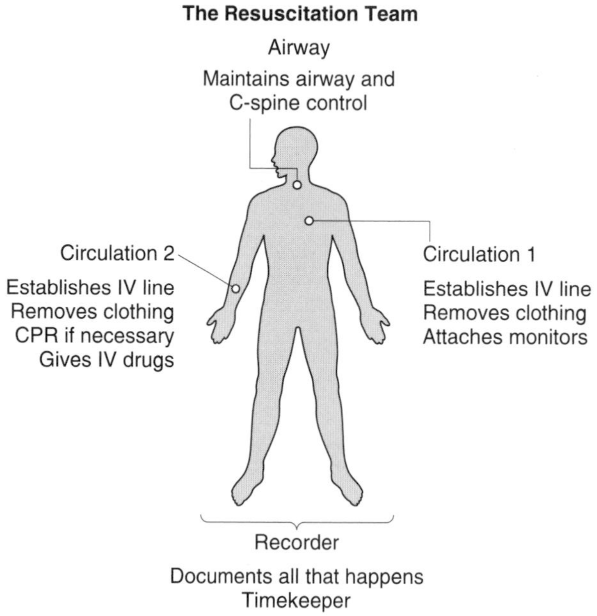

The Resuscitation Team

Airway

Maintains airway and
C-spine control

Circulation 2

Establishes IV line
Removes clothing
CPR if necessary
Gives IV drugs

Circulation 1

Establishes IV line
Removes clothing
Attaches monitors

Recorder

Documents all that happens
Timekeeper

Fig. 4.1 The resuscitation team

spasm of the epiglottis or vocal cords. Shining a pen torch into the open mouth is the most appropriate way to examine the upper respiratory tract. Frequency and depth of respirations are important parameters for the nurse to record. Remember that a completely obstructed airway is silent as no air can pass the vocal chords.

Intervention

The first intervention is to clear the airway for the patient. If the patient is able to respond verbally to the question, 'Are you all right?', the airway is fundamentally clear, you may then progress onto oxygen therapy. If you get no reply or a response such as stridor, gurgling or snoring, then the patient has a potential or real airway problem and you must react quickly. This can be done by first opening the airway. Three different methods are now acceptable. If no trauma to the neck is suspected, then head tilt, chin lift can be used. If trauma is suspected then chin lift or jaw thrust are the preferred methods. This action will pull the tongue away from the posterior pharynx. Currently, as this book goes to press, jaw thrust is the preferred method. After opening the airway you then must inspect the mouth. The airway should be inspected for foreign bodies, vomit or secretions. Suction

should be applied with the aid of a wide bore, rigid sucker (e.g. a Yankeur sucker). Dentures often cause obstruction if they have slipped out of place so, if they have, then remove them. If still secure then it is best leaving them, so that they help maintain the shape of the mouth and will help maintain a seal if you need to give assisted ventilation. Once you have cleared any obstruction, reassessment of the airway again is vital, this time it is to ensure that what you have done is correct. This is best done by looking for chest wall movement, listening for normal breath sounds, and feeling breath on your arm or face. If you have all these positive indicators you then have a clear airway and again you can progress to oxygen therapy. If you are still having problems, then you will need further medical assistance, while you try the airway adjuncts described below.

The two most common airway adjuncts are the oral pharyngeal airway and the nasal airway. Both are equally as good, although the latter is probably under used. Once *in situ* either may allow you to discontinue holding the airway open by a manoeuvre such as jaw thrust. In a seriously ill casualty you may have an adjunct in place and still need physically to maintain the airway. As a nurse you will certainly then need to be preparing for a rapid sequence induction with the anaesthetist. Oxygen will need to be administered to the patient throughout resuscitation, even though the airway has been secured. If the patient is spontaneously breathing then a non-re-breathing oxygen mask can be used. If the respiration rate is below 10 or above 29 then the bag/valve mask device is the best system, preferably with a two-person technique. This involves one nurse securing the airway and ensuring a good mask seal while the other squeezes the bag to ventilate the patient.

In serious cases of trauma to the neck region leading to an airway obstruction not amenable to clearance by manual or suction methods (e.g. soft tissue swelling), the medical staff may require assistance with a needle cricothyrotomy. Needle cricothyrotomy involves making a temporary (and possibly life-saving) entry into the trachea with a large bore (e.g. 14 G) IV cannula attached to a 10-ml syringe which applies a gentle negative pressure. The point of insertion is about 3 cm below the laryngeal prominence (the Adam's apple). After air is observed to fill the syringe, indicating entry into the trachea, the IV cannula can then be connected via an IVI giving set to an oxygen source. Baskett (1993) advocates using a second needle to facilitate exhalation. Such a procedure can 'buy' the time needed to set up for a tracheotomy. The A & E resuscitation room should have the equipment ready to perform both procedures, and the A & E nurse must know where the equipment is and what is required.

The most satisfactory way of maintaining the airway is intubation. In most hospitals, this is a medical task, although ambulance crews are now trained to intubate, and with the development of A & E clinical nurse specialists, it could easily become part of the nurse's role.

At present the A & E nurse must know how to assist with intubation (see Fig. 4.2 for equipment). The first requirement is a muscle relaxant drug, usually suxamethonium, which will be stored in a fridge. The endotracheal tube will often require cutting to length before insertion, so scissors should be kept ready. The laryngoscope blade is then passed on the right side of the midline with the neck extended. The blade is used to elevate the tongue and visualize the glottic opening by pulling forward the jaw at 45°, not by levering on the front teeth. The laryngoscope should be checked every morning to ensure it is working. The

tube is introduced into the glottic opening by the right hand. If the tube is too long, there is a danger that it will be introduced into the right bronchus, leaving the left lung unventilated. The cuff of the ET tube must be inflated using a 10-ml syringe, and a Spencer Wells clamp is used to ensure the air stays in the cuff. Once inflated, the cuff protects the airway from aspiration, deep bronchial suction is possible and efficient intermittent positive pressure ventilation (IPPV) may be performed. The muscle relaxant drugs given to permit intubation mean that the patient will now be unable to breathe. It is therefore essential to connect quickly the ET tube to a bag/mask device (e.g. Ambu bag) and an oxygen source via an adaptor and a catheter mount and commence hand ventilation. It is essential that the A & E nurse has the correct equipment to hand immediately, can connect it together promptly and, if need be, can take over ventilating the patient. The nurse should not forget the need for tape to tie and secure the ET tube in place.

Evaluation of the patency of the airway after intervention is crucial. The nurse should check whether the patient's colour improves, the respiratory rate and oxygen saturation level. In the case of an intubated patient check whether the chest expands with ventilation and whether there is air entry to both lungs.

Cervical spine

Pathology

The spinal cord is enclosed in a canal extending through the vertebral column with nerves branching off (motor) or entering (sensory) via openings in the vertebrae. The soft nature of the spinal cord makes it very vulnerable to injury with potentially disastrous consequences.

Injury occurs when either a vertebra is fractured and/or spinal ligaments (whose function is to hold the vertebrae in alignment) are ruptured which allows subluxation (partial dislocation) of the vertebrae. The result will be either compression of the cord or a partial or complete transection. All injuries should be assumed to be unstable until proven otherwise.

The forces causing the injury can be either flexion, extension or rotation, or any combination of these forces. For example, the injury

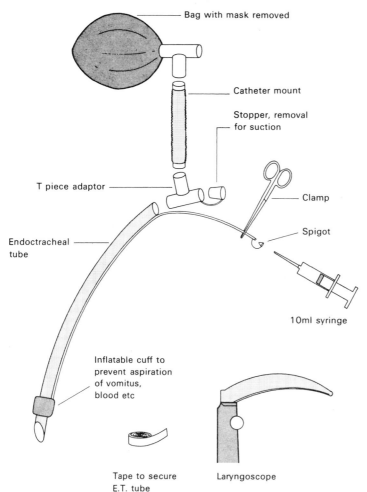

Bag with mask removed

Catheter mount

Stopper, removal for suction

T piece adaptor

Clamp

Spigot

Endoctracheal tube

10ml syringe

Inflatable cuff to prevent aspiration of vomitus, blood etc

Tape to secure E.T. tube

Laryngoscope

Fig. 4.2 Equipment for intubation and IPPV

known as a 'whiplash', which is seen in car occupants whose vehicle has been struck from behind, is an extension/flexion injury. Flexion/ rotation injuries are seen in accidents in sports such as rugby or gymnastics. These tend to be cervical injuries. The lumbar spine is typically injured in falls where the person lands feet first and a lumbar vertebra is either crushed or, if there is flexion as well, crushed into a wedge shape. Alternatively, the vertebra may shatter and produce a burst fracture. The thoracic spine is commonly injured by a direct blow such as a roof collapse in mining or when a person falls, landing on his or her back.

Complete transection of the cord is fortunately rare and, as Folman and Masri (1989) point out, it is very difficult to demonstrate clinically, citing studies of patients with apparent complete cord transection where some 10–20% made some degree of recovery. These authors have looked at a series of 70 patients with incomplete transection between the 4th cervical and 10th thoracic vertebrae and can find no better indicator of recovery than the amount of sensation and function present after the first few days. They urge A & E staff not to jump to conclusions about recovery based on a rapid assessment in A & E, particularly when the patient may be suffering the immediate effects of head injury and other trauma. A careful assessment carried out after a few days is the best indicator of recovery.

The difficulty of predicting outcomes is shown in a study of 410 patients with major blunt trauma carried out by Ross *et al.* (1992). The only significant predictors of unstable cervical injury were loss of consciousness, neurological deficit on assessment and neck tenderness. A total of 13 patients in this sample had an unstable injury, i.e. 6.1%.

Assessment

Complete transection of the cord produces a flaccid paralysis. It may also lead to spinal shock due to loss of vessel tone (an example of vasogenic shock). Sensation will also be lost. Male patients may display an erection in cord transection. If the injury is incomplete, there will be a mixed picture of sensory/motor loss. The nurse should, therefore, be looking for any weakness or any complaint by the patient of unusual sensations, tingling or numbness. The best way to assess weakness in the upper limbs is to ask the patient to squeeze both of your hands with their hands or to hold the arms out in front of the body for a period of time. If there is any motor weakness, the affected limb will be seen to fall away gradually after a few seconds. To assess lower limb weakness, the patient, lying flat, should be asked to push the nurse away while s/he presses against the soles of the patient's feet with the palms of the hands. Weakness may be perceived in one or both of the limbs. It is important in the case of neck injury to note how the patient is behaving, as there will be considerable muscle spasm involved in a serious injury. The patient will tend to hold their neck with both hands. Such behaviour in a patient should act as a warning sign of significant injury.

Immobilization of the spine

Much discussion occurred in the 1990s regarding the immobilization of the spine. Watson (1991) cites evidence to indicate there is a 5–10% chance of cervical injury in cases of blunt trauma to the head region. However, in the UK, severe spinal injury is relatively uncommon with approximately 17 new cases reported each week. It is safest to assume a cervical injury until proven otherwise and the head and neck should always be stabilized in a correct alignment.

In the early 1990s much immobilization occurred with the use of sandbags and tape. These proved unpopular with the fear of aspiration and gave way to the introduction of 'headblocks'. At the same time, the ambulance service introduced the 'spine board' to assist patient transfers. This is probably the worst name for the device as it does not immobilize the spine. In the USA and Europe they are known as rescue boards. It is important to note that these boards are hard and do cause pressure sores in the critically ill or elderly in a short space of time. Due to their flat surface area, they provide little or no spinal immobilization to the thoracic or lumbar spine. If the patient is left on a board with no strapping system, then a situation called the pendulum effect occurs. This is when the head is immobilized by the headblocks but the rest of the body is not. When the patient moves around then all the stress is placed on the neck point, causing further potential damage.

It is now recommended that the patient be removed from the rescue board as soon as possible. The nurse must also decide whether the headblocks should be left *in situ* or whether the patient should be left flat on the trolley with a collar in place. A study by Haughton *et al.* (1999) showed that collars at best give 30% immobilization and that leaving a patient with a set of headblocks on and no collar is equally as effective as the current trend of using both collar and headblocks. Remember that when dealing with a patient with a suspected spinal injury the manual hold is still the best method of immobilization within the A & E department, so long as you have the staff to do it.

Sexton (1999) discussed a set of guidelines that allow the removal of both the board and collar. This has added some sanity to the current trend of immobilizing all patients from even minor RTAs who may be suffering from whiplash injury. The protocol developed by Sexton states that the rescue board may be removed if there are no potential life-threatening injuries, no other interventions are required first, such as establishing an IV, and there are no neurological signs or symptoms. All three conditions must be satisfied. Cervical collars may be removed if *all* of the following criteria are satisfied:

- Patient alert, oriented and able to answer questions
- No neurological signs or symptoms present
- Patient has not taken alcohol or other drugs which alter mood

- There is no painful distracting injury elsewhere
- There is no midline tenderness of the neck on palpation.

Experience and audit has shown that these guidelines work very effectively and safely.

All head and multiply-injured patients must be assumed to have an unstable spinal injury until proven otherwise. This requires minimal movement of the patient, and then only in a carefully controlled way. In transferring them to the A & E trolley, the ambulance spinal or rescue board should be used if one is available. Otherwise a slide device can be used with extreme caution to maintain alignment of the spine. The head should be immobilized with headblocks where practicable, and a cervical collar applied. The soft foam type is less than 100% effective in immobilizing the neck and, therefore a semi-rigid collar should be used. Research by Ferguson *et al.* (1993) has measured a wide range of tissue interface pressures beneath different types of collars, some of which might be expected to cause jugular venous obstruction and hence raised intracranial pressure. Soft collars are again contraindicated by this research and staff are encouraged to think carefully of the dangers of applying collars too tightly.

The patient should be kept flat at all times, turning being accomplished using the log rolling technique. The principle of this is to move the patient in such a way that the spine remains in a straight line and no part of the spine moves relative to another. This will need four people to perform properly. The person in charge of the movement is the person who is bridging the injured part of the spine with their hands. As the patient is being cared for in a flat position, there should be a nurse with the patient at all times, and suction equipment must be immediately available in case of vomiting.

If the patient is conscious and aware of the possibility of spinal injury, the nurse must be prepared for anxious questions from the patient and also from the family. Such questions are very difficult to deal with, but they must be answered honestly and realistically. The patient will need a great deal of psychological support in this sort of situation.

In the A & E department the aim is to prevent any further worsening of the situation by not allowing displacement to occur in a potentially unstable injury. The immediate aim of the medical treatment after a detailed neurological exam and radiography will be to stabilize the spine. This may involve traction applied in the short term, while long-term options include operative fixation or the patient may be immobilized in halo traction. For the spine-injured patient, there will be many long-term problems involving bowel and bladder training, chest and urinary tract infections, pressure sores, rehabilitation, and social and psychological trauma.

There has been a major increase in less serious neck injuries over the last twelve years. The term acute neck sprain is more accurate than 'whiplash' as this latter term is only strictly applicable in a small number of RTA cases. Galasko (1993) has charted a rise in neck sprain injuries from 7.7% of RTA victims in 1981 through to 45.6% in 1991 and suggests this is related to driving standards and traffic flow patterns rather than seat-belt wearing. It should be remembered that many patients will have painful symptoms from neck sprain injury many years after the accident. Robinson and Cassar-Pullicino (1993) reported that 86% of patients in a sample of 21 followed up over 10 years later still had painful symptoms from acute neck sprain after an RTA.

Breathing

Pathology

Once the airway is cleared and the cervical spine is immobilized, the next question is – can the patient breathe normally? And if not, how can the patient be helped to achieve normal respiration? If the patient is making no respiratory effort, the procedure for respiratory arrest must be initiated at once with IPPV. However, the patient may be attempting to breathe but may be suffering from chest trauma which is interfering with normal respiration. If this trauma is serious, it may quickly prove fatal.

A common problem associated with serious chest trauma is pneumothorax in which air gains entry to the potential space of the pleura surrounding a lung. This will lead to the lung's collapse. A pneumothorax can arise spontaneously, without any trauma, due to the rupture of a weakness in the wall of the lung (Fig. 4.3a).

The most serious form of pneumothorax is a tension pneumothorax in which the hole into the pleura acts like a one-way flap valve, permitting air entry to the pleural space but prohibiting any escape of air (Fig. 4.3b). The result is a progressive build-up of pressure in the pleural space which will not only collapse the lung on the affected side, but will exert pressure on the uninjured side, leading to mediastinal shift, possible nipping of major blood vessels and collapse of the other lung.

If bleeding occurs into the pleural space, a haemothorax is said to be present. This, too, will prevent lung expansion, and often occurs in conjunction with a pneumothorax. The quantity of blood involved may be over one litre, so that in addition to serious respiratory impairment, there may also be hypovolaemic shock.

Rib fractures are an extremely painful condition – so painful that proper chest expansion and coughing will be severely restricted, greatly increasing the risk of chest infection. The very serious condition of a flail

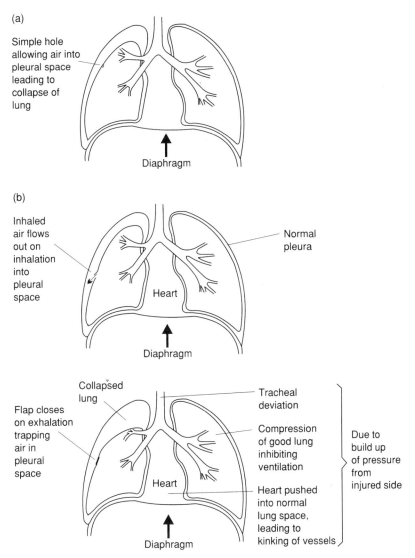

Fig. 4.3 (a) Spontaneous pneumothorax. (b) Tension pneumothorax

segment occurs if there are ribs with double fractures, as one segment of the chest wall will no longer be attached to the rest of the chest (Fig. 4.4). As a result, when there is a lowering of intrathoracic pressure (an essential step in respiration) brought about by expansion of the chest wall, the unattached flail segment collapses inwards under atmospheric pressure, as the atmospheric pressure will be greater than the pressure within the thorax. The inward collapse prevents lung expansion. Flail chest can be readily observed as it results in what are known as paradoxical respirations, i.e. a section of chest wall collapsing inwards when the rest of the chest is expanding outwards. A flail segment constitutes a potential life-threatening emergency, especially as it is often associated with a haemo- or pneumothorax.

Within the lung tissue itself, trauma can cause respiratory impairment in several ways. Major blood vessels may be damaged due to penetrating injury or severe deceleration stresses. Lung tissue may be contused, leading to the extravasation of blood into the parenchyma which, in turn, will cause anoxia of the tissue. If a high pressure blast wave passes through the lung, the Spalding effect will produce what amounts to implosion of the alveolar walls leading to massive damage and pulmonary oedema which can be rapidly fatal. This effect must be looked for in all victims of explosions. Finally, there is the possibility of the inhalation of material deep into the lung tissue. This material can range from water in drowning victims to noxious gases in burns cases.

Assessment

The chest must be fully visualized for examination. If necessary, clothing should be cut off. The respiratory rate must be recorded, together with the depth and pattern of respiration. The following should be watched for:

- Evidence of cyanosis.
- Notably shallow or deep respirations.
- The use of accessory muscles of respiration.
- Cheyne–Stokes breathing.
- Gulping, 'air hunger' type breathing (an indication of hypovolaemic shock).
- Stridor (an indication of airway obstruction).
- Pain (an indication of fractured ribs).

The chest wall should be examined for evidence of trauma, bruising and wounds. Crepitus, indicating rib fractures, may be inadvertently elicited while palpating for bony tenderness (the cardinal sign of a fracture). Surgical emphysema may be perceived as a crackling feeling. This is caused by air escaping into the tissues, typically into the upper part of

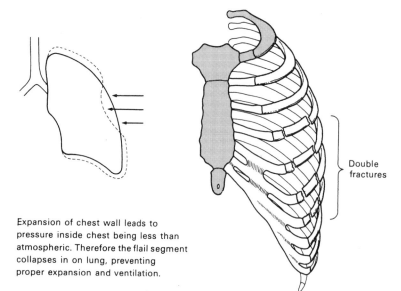

Expansion of chest wall leads to pressure inside chest being less than atmospheric. Therefore the flail segment collapses in on lung, preventing proper expansion and ventilation.

Double fractures

Fig. 4.4 Flail segment

the chest wall. Paradoxical respirations will usually be apparent if there is a flail segment.

Pulse oximetry is a widely used non-invasive monitoring procedure which measures arterial oxyhaemoglobin saturation (SaO_2) and therefore gives important information about the supply of oxygen to body tissues. It does not, however, provide the information about ventilatory status which might come from arterial blood gases, e.g. CO_2 tension or acid–base balance, and its accuracy is compromised by a range of factors such as patient motion, abnormal haemoglobin, dark skin pigmentation or nail polish (Durren, 1992). Adequate tissue oxygenation, according to Durren (1992), requires an SaO_2 of over 90% and adequate haemoglobin levels.

The medical staff's assessment will include the standard percussion and stethoscopic exam, chest X-rays (the area of lung collapse in pneumothorax is seen on an X-ray as a blank area without lung markings separating the lung margin from the chest wall) and arterial blood gases.

Intervention

If the patient is not breathing, IPPV must be commenced at once. Cardiac compression, however, should be withheld until an assessment has been made of cardiac output and the ECG. Using an oropharyngeal airway and a bag/mask connected to an oxygen supply, the A & E nurse should be able to ventilate the patient adequately. Watson (1991) suggests more effective ventilation occurs if a second person secures the mask on the face, as in this way a more airtight seal is achieved.

If the patient is exhibiting respiratory distress, 100% oxygen should be applied by mask at 6 l/mm. If possible, the sitting-upright position should be adopted to assist respiration. Chest injuries are very painful and adequate analgesia needs to be given as soon as possible. Subcutaneous analgesia or nerve blocks are becoming increasingly popular.

If the patient is conscious, it is likely that he or she will require a great deal of psychological support as difficulty in breathing is a very frightening experience. It is suggested that such a patient should not be left alone at any time for, in addition to the risk of deterioration going unnoticed, it may provoke great fear in the patient.

The need for pulse oximetry and continual monitoring of respiratory rate and effort cannot be overemphasized as this will give first warning of a deterioration in respiratory function. Cyanosis is a very late sign and, in a significant proportion of the population, i.e. the non-Caucasian population, it is an unlikely sign at all. In non-Caucasians, cyanosis can be seen in the mucous membranes. Drowsiness and confusion are associated with respiratory failure and are due to cerebral hypoxia. In multiple trauma victims, however, it may not be possible to differentiate between when these signs are caused by head injury and when they are due to respiratory failure.

The remaining area of nursing care for respiratory problems concerns supporting medical intervention. In the case of a pneumothorax or haemothorax, the requirement is for a rapidly introduced chest drain, together with an underwater seal, to drain off the air or blood that is compressing the lung (Fig. 4.5). Most of the equipment for this procedure should be ready in advance in the form of a CSSD pack in the resuscitation room. Great stress should be laid on asepsis during the procedure. Iodine in spirit is usually used as a skin preparation. Local anaesthetic will be administered around the area, followed by a small incision with a scalpel to facilitate the introduction of the chest drain. The nurse should have the bottle ready with a litre of sterile water and should ensure that the tubing is connected the correct way, i.e. the drain coming from the patient must be connected to the tube that ends underwater. Negative pressure is usually applied to the system by means of a specialized suction pump to facilitate drainage of blood. The chest drain will be sutured in place and the area around it should be dressed with a keyhole dressing secured with elastoplast. If it is correctly inserted, the nurse should observe air or blood draining into the bottle, and the fluid level in the drain will oscillate with the changes in intrathoracic pressure associated with the patient's breathing. The bottle should never be raised above the level of the patient because, if this is done, the contents of the bottle will syphon off through the drain into the chest with catastrophic results. The traditional practice of clamping the drainage tube before moving the patient is not necessary (Armstrong *et al.*, 1991).

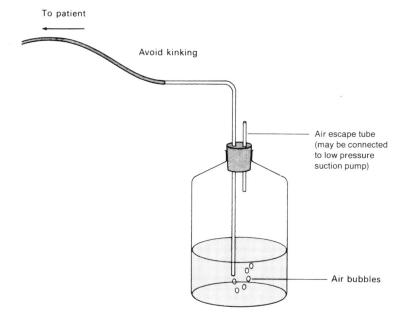

To patient

Avoid kinking

Air escape tube
(may be connected
to low pressure
suction pump)

Air bubbles

Fig. 4.5 Simplified diagram of chest drainage

A dramatic improvement in the patient's condition often follows chest drainage, the re-expanded lung being seen on a check X-ray immediately after the procedure. A nurse should accompany the patient during this X-ray, monitoring respiratory status and offering psychological support. If a haemothorax has been present, blood pressure and pulse need close observation because of the danger of hypovolaemic shock. The quantity of blood draining into the bottle needs to be recorded accurately.

In dealing with a large flail segment, it is likely that IPPV will be required, although the medical staff will not automatically resort to this measure; the patient's clinical condition is the key indication. The patient will require intubation for IPPV.

Evaluation

The effectiveness of interventions to improve breathing must be carefully evaluated. The most common successful way is by using the look, listen and feel approach. Simple mistakes can occur, such as having the oxygen mask connected to an oxygen point that is not turned on or to an empty cylinder. The chest drain can become kinked or blocked by clots and can therefore stop functioning. Patients may be placed in the correct position to help

their breathing, but that is no guarantee that they will stay there. They have a tendency to slip down the trolley!

Airway and breathing problems are very dramatic and desperate situations. It is very easy, therefore, for some simple error to occur with potentially fatal results. Continual evaluation must be the rule to be absolutely sure that things are going to plan and that the patient is benefiting from our interventions to ensure normal breathing.

Circulation

Pathology

The next priority in the nursing care of the critically injured person is circulation. Here the principal concern is the possibility of cardiac arrest or of insufficient circulation leading to shock. Therefore, while attention is being paid to the patient's airway and breathing, a nurse should also be assessing the patient's circulation.

The pathology of shock is very complex and there remains much still to be learnt of its nature. However, the main common denominator in all types of shock is reduced cellular perfusion, i.e. insufficient oxygen reaches the tissues of the body. If this condition is not

Table 4.1 Classification of shock by cause

Type of shock	Cause
1. Hypovolaemic	
Haemorrhagic	Blood loss due to soft tissue bleeding, fractures, wounds, etc.
Burns	Loss of plasma in burn exudate.
Dehydration	Major body fluid loss, e.g. due to prolonged vomiting, diarrhoea, or metabolic disorders such as diabetic ketoacidosis.
2. Cardiogenic	Failure of cardiac pump leading to inadequate cardiac output, although the blood volume is normal, e.g. after myocardial infarction.
3. Vasogenic	
Septic	Endotoxins from Gram-negative bacteria can cause massive vasodilatation in certain infective conditions.
Anaphylactic	Severe allergic reaction; histamine release increases capillary permeability and leads to dilatation of capillaries and arterioles.
Neurogenic	Loss of sympathetic control leading to dilatation of venules, capillaries and arterioles.

corrected, it will eventually set in train a series of complex physiological changes which will result in irreversible shock and death (Fig. 4.6). There are three main types of shock – hypovolaemic, cardiogenic and vasogenic – the causes of which are summarized in Table 4.1.

In hypovolaemic shock, the problem is that there is a loss of fluid from the circulation. In cardiogenic shock, there is a failure of the pump, although the blood volume is not affected. While in vasogenic shock, the blood volume is again not affected but rather the arterioles and capillaries dilate, leading to diminished venous return and hence diminished cardiac output, which in turn leads to decreased tissue perfusion, i.e. shock.

The body has compensating mechanisms against shock which come into operation after injury, and which can give rise to misleadingly normal blood pressures in the A & E patient. The main result of these mechanisms is vasoconstriction.

Decreased renal perfusion leads to the release of renin which, in turn, leads, via the plasma protein angiotensinogen, to angiotensin, a powerful vasoconstrictor at the microcirculatory level. In addition, there is adrenaline and noradrenaline release, both of which are vasoconstrictors. This may allow patients to compensate for circulatory loss for some time with a normal blood pressure, especially if they are young and have, therefore,

more elastic walls to their blood vessels.

Significant changes will occur in the urine output of the shocked patient. The reduction in circulating volume will reduce glomerular filtration and hence urine formation. Furthermore, the hormone aldosterone and the antidiuretic hormone will be released as part of the compensatory effect, both of which will diminish urine output. In hypovolaemic shock, urine output may be less than 30 ml/h. This is a critical level since output below this value is indicative of renal failure. Hypovolaemic shock is therefore the major cause of acute renal failure.

Assessment

In assessing the patient's circulation, we first of all need to know if the heart is beating and, if it is, whether it is producing an effective circulation. You therefore need to take the patient's pulse manually to record *accurately* both rate *and rhythm*. If the patient is unresponsive and making no apparent respiratory effort, the carotid pulse should be palpated and, if absent, a state of cardiac arrest assumed. The alarm should be raised first and then CPR initiated (see p. 61).

If the patient has a cardiac output, the next step is to assess the risk of shock. Continual monitoring of blood pressure is required, and the nurse should bear in mind the possibility of

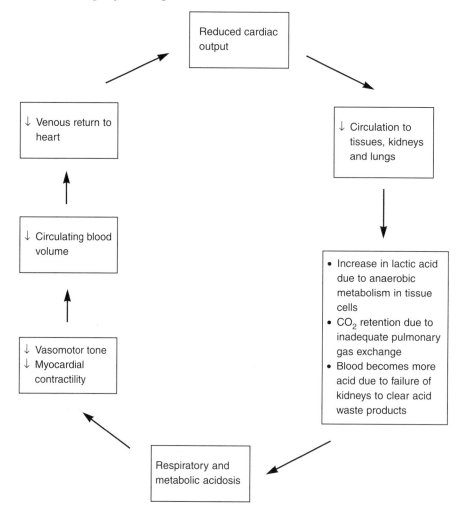

Once this vicious circle has become established it is very difficult to break.
NB: ↓ indicates reduction in.

Fig. 4.6 Irreversible shock

compensated shock as outlined above. Respiratory rate must also be monitored, as when increasing, this is one of the most sensitive indicators of shock. Both the respiratory rate and the pulse rate will rise in shock, the respiratory rate in response to the body's need to try to increase tissue oxygenation and the pulse in response to the falling blood pressure. The condition of the skin should be noted as the increased production of adrenaline and the resulting vasoconstriction will lead to a cool, pale and moist skin. The time for capillary refill to occur after blanching a digit by momentarily squeezing the extremity should be less than 2 seconds. A longer time is an indication of likely shock (Budassi-Sheehy, 1990). If the patient is conscious or if witnesses are present, a history of the accident is required. The history will often indicate the risk of injuries that may produce hypovolaemia, e.g. trauma to the right upper quadrant of the abdomen will alert the nurse to the risk of liver damage.

The patient's mental state should also be

assessed as psychological support is very important.

Intervention

The most common cause of shock in the A & E department is hypovolaemia. Immediate nursing interventions should be to elevate the foot of the trolley to try to increase the volume of blood in the vital heart–lung–brain circulation, to administer high concentration oxygen to assist tissue oxygenation, to control any obvious bleeding with pressure dressings and to offer psychological support to the patient.

As hypovolaemic shock is the type of shock most commonly seen in A & E, and as it requires large-scale circulating volume replacement therapy, the nurse must be prepared to offer support to the medical staff in carrying out such potentially life-saving measures. Cannulation of the ante-cubital fossa is the first measure when attempting to establish an intravenous line. Most nurses now cannulate, however, you also need to assist the medical staff to establish an internal jugular or sub-clavian vein with a wide bore cannula. Accurate fluid balance charts are required as there may be three drips running at once, together with other central monitoring. Clear fluids alone, such as normal saline, are not satisfactory as they are easily excreted by the kidneys and can leak from damaged capillaries. Therefore, in resuscitating the hypovolaemic patient, crystalloid solutions such as Ringer's lactate may also be used to restore interstitial fluid loss. Colloid solutions such as Haemaccel or Gelofusin are used as a temporary measure until whole blood is grouped and cross-matched. These IV solutions have such large molecules that they are not readily filtered out by the kidneys, and due to the osmotic pressure they exert, fluid is moved from the intracellular compartment into the circulation. All intravenous fluids should be warmed by the most appropriate methods.

A supply of O Rhesus negative blood should be available for emergency transfusion if one is needed while the patient's blood is being grouped and cross-matched. Catheterization of the patient may be required in order to monitor urine output accurately on an hourly basis (see p. 39).

The principles discussed above are all applicable to patients who have suffered injuries such as fractures, major wounds and chest trauma. The second section of this chapter will now look at three specific types of trauma – abdominal trauma, head injury and burns – showing how the basic principles discussed above are applied in practice to patients with such serious problems as these.

Abdominal trauma

Pathology

The seriously injured patient can have an almost infinite variety of abdominal lesions. They can be due to blunt trauma such as a severe blow, to crushing, or to deceleration forces associated with high velocity road accidents. Alternatively, there can be a penetrating injury due to stabbing, impalement or bullet or shrapnel wounds.

The major life-threatening pathology associated with abdominal injury is hypovolaemia, due to either a leaking major blood vessel or the rupture or laceration of a vascular organ such as the spleen or liver. A correctly restrained car occupant in a high velocity collision may sustain a tear of the aorta due to the deceleration forces involved; a person falling from a ladder or a motorbike may take the brunt of the fall with their abdomen, leading to the rupture of the spleen. Penetrating injuries may lacerate major blood vessels as well as the viscera.

A second major area for concern is peritonitis, caused by the rupture of an organ such as the bowel or gall bladder. It can be either an infective or a chemical peritonitis.

Damage to the diaphragm is a serious problem due to the interference that will occur with respiration, and it should always be considered as a possibility in abdominal trauma.

Assessment

In undressing the patient, the abdomen should be carefully examined for external evidence of trauma such as bruising, wounds or 'tattooing'. The phenomenon of tattooing is found where a very high pressure has been applied to the skin through clothing, resulting in the pattern of clothing being transferred to the skin. Examples are commonly found on the chest and abdomen due to seat belts restraining a patient in a high velocity accident, or in victims of assault who have been kicked or struck with an object such as a baseball bat. The relationship of such external markings to the organs of the abdomen should be considered in assessing possible injury.

Small puncture wounds may conceal very serious damage in cases of stabbing. It is very important to try to obtain an estimate of the depth of the wound and the direction of entry in order to assess the seriousness of the injury. Contrary to common belief, the entry and exit wounds of bullets are usually both small, even with high velocity bullets, yet they may conceal catastrophic damage, especially in the case of high energy missiles due to the shock wave and cavitation effects of supersonic projectiles. Bullets which explode on impact, such as those used by Ryan in the Hungerford Massacre of 1987, or a short-range shotgun blast, can produce huge and grossly contaminated wounds.

Close monitoring of the vital signs is required in order to detect signs of hypovolaemia as early as possible. Abdominal girth may be expected to increase with haemorrhage. However, its measurement is so unreliable that it is of no value.

The appearance of one or two drops of blood at the external urinary meatus is evidence of rupture of the urethra. Patients who are suspected of having urethral damage should be asked to try to avoid passing urine, while the advice of a urologist is sought. All other patients, however, should be asked to provide a specimen of urine to test for haematuria, which may indicate trauma to the kidney. It is unusual for the bladder to rupture unless it is full, which unfortunately it often is in the case of late night road accidents.

Vaginal bleeding (other than menstrual) indicates that significant gynaecological trauma may be expected.

The A & E nurse should be able to recognize bowel sounds, or their absence which indicates paralytic ileus. Nurses should also be able to recognize the guarding sign associated with peritonitis; the patient holds the abdomen tense, lying flat on the trolley, unwilling to sit or bend at the waist as it is too painful. The recognition of such signs is essential in the initial nursing assessment if the patient is to be correctly prioritized by the nursing staff.

Intervention

Prompt surgical intervention is required after stabilization of the patient's circulatory status. Nursing staff will be fully involved in IVI and vital sign monitoring, in ensuring that the patient is kept nil by mouth, and possibly in passing a nasogastric tube. The usual hospital protocols concerning any patient going to theatre must be observed as far as is possible.

If there is an impaling object *in situ*, it is best left there until it can be removed under controlled conditions in theatre while the wound is carefully explored. It is conventional surgical wisdom that the track of any penetrating injury must be fully explored.

All patients who are to undergo surgery need psychological support and explanations of what to expect, both before and after surgery. This applies especially to the patient who is to be operated upon in this kind of emergency situation.

Although peritoneal lavage is no longer high on the diagnostic list, it may still be used as a secondary choice. More often an ultrasound scan is carried out. A peritoneal lavage will indicate if there is blood in the peritoneum, which is a strong indication of the need for laparotomy. The test consists of running 10 ml/kg of Ringer's lactate or normal saline via a peritoneal dialysis catheter and an ordinary IVI giving set into the patient's peritoneum, allowing it to drain off by syphonage and, most importantly, assessing the fluid that returns. If there is no trauma, it should be clear. Frank blood or evidence of 100 000 red cells per mm^2 is taken as evidence of intra-abdominal bleeding (Baskett, 1993). Research by Driscoll *et al.* (1992a) suggests that qualitative 'rule-of-thumb' estimates are unreliable and the only way of determining the concentration of red cells is by quantitative measurement. Strict asepsis should be followed, and the skin should be prepared with iodine in spirit. The procedure is carried out under local anaesthetic and the small incision is made with a scalpel.

The blood loss may be so severe in some cases that circulatory resuscitation in A & E is not possible and immediate surgical intervention is needed as a life-saving measure. In such extreme cases, the A & E team should be able to get a patient, if necessary, from the resuscitation room onto the operating table within 15 minutes.

Evaluation

It is now recognized that stabilization both in the pre-hospital and A & E department may not be possible when dealing with the trauma patient. The term resuscitation is more appropriate. It is imperative that the surgical team is involved from an early stage of the resuscitation process, so that an early assessment can be made on the patient's appropriateness for surgery, or observation.

It is essential to evaluate whether the patient understands what is being explained – both explanations about what is happening in A & E and those concerning what will happen in theatre subsequently. Psychological support revolves around patient understanding.

In dealing with hypovolaemia, steps such as elevating the foot of the trolley, IVI administration and stopping any external bleeding can be evaluated by monitoring BP, pulse and respiration.

Abdominal trauma may be very painful, therefore effective intravenous analgesia should be given promptly and its effectiveness in relieving pain evaluated. (See Fig. 4.7 for Critical pathway example: the patient with multiple trauma.)

Head injury

Pathology

The brain consists of relatively incompressible tissue. Therefore any force applied to it will be immediately transmitted through the tissue. This means that a blow delivered to one side of the head can produce brain injury on the opposite side, as the brain, which is independent of the skull, impinges on the inner surface of the skull.

The skull forms a closed box. The clinical implication of this is that if any bleeding occurs within the skull, raised intracranial pressure will result as there is nowhere for the haematoma to expand, other than to force the brainstem through the tentorial notch or foramen magnum. This condition is known as brainstem herniation.

Around one million people attend hospital with some form of head injury every year in the UK of whom half are under 16 (Royal College of Surgeons, 1999). The most common mechanisms of injury are falls 41%, assaults 20% and RTAs 13%. Road traffic accidents produce the most serious injuries. Despite this, the majority of head injuries seen in A & E are simple concussions. In concussion, after impacting on the inner surface of the skull, the brain suffers a brief interruption to the reticular activating system. This causes a short period of unconsciousness and amnesia. Bruising or contusion of the brain surface leads to more significant injury and neurological disturbance.

A much more serious injury occurs when a blood vessel is torn, leading to haemorrhage and haematoma formation in either an epidural (between dura and skull) or subdural (below the dura) location, or within the brain itself. North American studies have shown mortality rates for epidural haematoma of 25–50% and for subdural haematoma 70%, indicating the seriousness of these injuries (Budassi-Sheehy, 1990).

In such major injuries, there may be a period of unconsciousness after which the patient regains consciousness. During this period of consciousness, the haematoma associated with the bleeding blood vessel develops, leading to a rise in intracranial pressure which will cause a gradual diminishing in the level of consciousness. This period of consciousness is known as the 'lucid interval', and the reason for observation of head injury patients is to try to detect evidence of a diminishing level of consciousness, associated with rising intracranial pressure, as early as possible so that surgical intervention might relieve the pressure and improve the outcome.

Raised intracranial pressure or haematoma formation may manifest itself by compression of the third cranial nerve (oculomotor) which controls the iris and hence the size of the pupil. A sluggishly reacting or dilated pupil is evidence of compression of the oculomotor nerve if it is associated with diminished level of consciousness. There are a variety of other causes of unequal or non-reactive pupils unassociated with head injury. It must be emphasized that this is a late sign that will develop *after* a fall in the level of consciousness.

Skull fracture is not a very reliable guide to the seriousness of the injury, as many patients with a fractured skull have no significant

	0–5 min	6–15 min	16–60 min
Documentation	Registration as A & E patient	Notes ready for writing in. ID tag applied to patient	Completed for admission to ITU
Assessment	Triage as top priority with multiple trauma. Primary survey of life-threatening problems (ABC)	BP P RR T ECG PaO$_2$ GCS commenced. Secondary survey obtained history from patient. Take bloods. Monitor peripheral circulation in injured limbs. Pain	Continue vital signs monitoring. Peritoneal lavage XR: comes after resuscitation
Medication	–	Analgesia for pain. Other urgent drug therapy as required (e.g. in CPR)	Analgesia. Adsorbed Tet Tox. Other drug therapy as required
Treatment	Commence CPR if needed, secure airway, ventilate	Commence therapy as soon as need for intubation, ventilation, circulatory support identified. O$_2$ therapy MAST	Catheterize. Chest drains if needed, IV therapy continues for low BP. Resusc. Continues until VS stable, consider urgent surgery
Nursing care	Begin undressing patient. Obtain history from ambulance crew	Undress patient. Give psychological support, assist medical team in resusc. Dress wounds (NB Universal Precautions apply). Immobilize injured limbs/neck. Prevent harm to patient e.g. cot sides	Maintain psychological support, be with patient at all times. Maintain IV document fluid balance
Referrals	–	Senior medics see patient in A & E	Arrange transfer to theatre/ITU
Family	Direct to private waiting room	Offer use of phone psych. support, try to obtain history	Keep informed of progress, allow to see patient
Discharge	–	–	Transfer ITU, theatres or specialist unit

Fig. 4.7 Critical pathway example: the patient with multiple trauma

neurological deficit, while other patients sustain serious brain damage without a fracture. Head injury, for example, is the leading cause of death in motor vehicle accidents; 2390 out of 4898 RTA deaths in England and Wales in 1990 were due to head injury. However, in 28% of cases there was no skull fracture (OPCS, 1991).

Two types of skull fracture are important,

however. First, if the fracture is an open one, there is the risk of infection, which may involve the skull itself (osteomyelitis), or the meninges surrounding the brain leading to meningitis. For an open fracture of the skull, there does not need to be a scalp wound as the fracture may be through the base of the skull, communication with the fracture occurring via one of the eustachian tubes, the mouth or one of the ears. Secondly, if the skull fracture is depressed, the piece of bone pressing on the brain may act as an irritable focus and may cause fitting. A CSF leak may occur due to a tear in the meninges and as a consequence there is the risk of intracranial infection.

Assessment

After assessing airway, cervical spine, breathing and circulation, the next parameter to measure is level of consciousness and changes that occur in that level, as this will give the first warning of rising intracranial pressure. It is essential to establish a baseline level of consciousness, and the nearer that baseline is to the time of the accident the better. Witnesses, relatives, ambulance crew and police officers are all key personnel who can help nurses to estimate what the patient's level of consciousness was before arrival in A & E. The importance of level of consciousness as a guide to head injury progress cannot be over-emphasized.

Such an assessment must avoid subjective terms like 'semiconscious' or 'drowsy' which mean different things to different people. The objective Glasgow Coma Scale is, therefore, recommended. On this scale, consciousness is assessed in terms of motor response, verbal response and minimum stimulus required to produce eye opening. Fig. 4.8 shows a coma scale. Alternatively, points can be allocated for each response on the scale starting from zero

for no response up to 4 or 5 for the maximum response, the scores for each part of the scale being added together to produce a total known as the Glasgow Coma Score (GCS). Proehl (1992) stresses the need for nurses to base their score on the patient's *best* responses in each category, while remembering that factors such as paralysis, intubation or periorbital swelling can invalidate all or part of the GCS assessment.

In assessing motor response to painful stimuli, the nurse is recommended to apply pressure to the nail bed of one of the patient's fingers with a pen or similar object and his/her own thumb (Proehl, 1992). Note whether the arm is withdrawn towards the patient's body (flexion to pain) or extended away from the body (extension to pain). This latter extensor response indicates brainstem compression, a very serious condition.

Orientation should be assessed in time and space with simple questions such as 'Where are you?' and 'What day is it?' and 'What time of day is it roughly?' Questions such as 'Do you know that you are in the Royal Infirmary and it is Wednesday afternoon?' are not helpful. An answer 'Yes' to this type of question is not proof of anything! The importance of objective observations is highlighted by Morris (1993), who found that, in a sample of 100 head injury referrals by casualty officers to a regional neurosurgical unit, only 30% correctly used the Glasgow coma scale. Eighteen per cent of doctors were completely unable to use the

Fig. 4.8 Coma scale

scale. The biggest problem area was incorrect assessment of the response to painful stimulus; 56% of patients had an inappropriate technique used.

In order to determine if the patient lost consciousness, in the absence of witnesses, the nurse should ask the patient to recall the accident. A gap in recall indicates the strong likelihood of unconsciousness, although this period may not be as long as the period of amnesia. Retrograde amnesia refers to a period of amnesia before the accident, while post-traumatic amnesia refers to amnesia after the accident.

In assessing pupil size and response, light of the same intensity should be used in each eye. The nurse should also be checking that when light is shone in one eye, the other responds as well. Unequal pupils in an alert, orientated patient are highly unlikely to indicate any head injury pathology as unequal pupils are a late sign following diminished level of consciousness due to raised intracranial pressure.

Physical signs that should be looked for include scalp wounds. Scalp wounds should alert the A & E team to the possibility of open fractures of the skull and of hypovolaemic shock which can be greatly exacerbated by profusely bleeding scalp wounds, if not primarily caused by such wounds, especially in the elderly. An important sign to look out for is bruising around the eyes (periorbital ecchymosis), often called 'raccoon eyes'; this indicates an intraorbital fracture or basilar skull fracture. Bruising appearing 12–24 hours after injury, behind the ears in the mastoid area, is known as Battle's sign and also indicates basilar skull fracture.

Further evidence of a fracture of the base of the skull is provided by CSF leakage from the nose (rhinorrhoea) or the ear (otorrhoea). Bleeding from within the ear also indicates a fracture of the base of the skull. If there is fluid leaking from the nose, the patient should not be allowed to blow the nose as this could cause contamination of the meninges.

The development of any obvious limb weakness should be reported as this suggests damage to the motor centres in the brain. The nature and duration of any fits must be carefully documented, and medical attention drawn to their presence immediately.

In monitoring the vital signs, respiratory rate is vital, as brain damage may involve the respiratory centre leading to disturbance of both depth and rate of breathing. Respirations may become progressively more shallow and gradually fade away. The temperature regulating centre is thought to be adjacent to the hypothalamus and damage in this region can lead to hyperthermia (temperatures over 40°C). The patient may, however, be hypothermic as a result of lying still for a period of time after the injury in a cold environment. An accurate baseline temperature is therefore required.

A late sign of serious head injury is a rising BP and a slowing pulse. This is explained in terms of the raised intracranial pressure making the heart beat more strongly as blood has to be forced into the brain in order to overcome capillary resistance. Baroreceptors that are situated in the carotid arteries monitor blood pressure and in response to a rising blood pressure act via the cardiac centre in the brain to slow the heart rate. This is the same mechanism responsible for increasing the heart rate when the blood pressure falls.

Assessment of children after head injury requires the nurse to allow for the varying stages of cognitive development. Information from the parent about normal behaviour is invaluable if the nurse is to observe abnormal behaviour. As Harrison (1991) states, the normal observation of adult head-injured patients requires adaptation to suit the needs of children and her paper gives a good account of such procedure.

Intervention

Airway and breathing must be main priorities in intervention. Administration of high concentration oxygen to head injury patients is beneficial because it reduces cerebral CO_2 levels, and high levels of CO_2 in the brain cause cerebral oedema, thereby raising intracranial pressure further.

In handling and moving head injury patients, the nurse must realize the possibility of spinal injury. Unconscious patients must be assumed to have a spinal injury until proven otherwise, and great care should be taken even if the patient is conscious.

The absolutely vital role of the nurse is the scrupulous monitoring of the level of consciousness, and the maintenance of the patient's airway and respiration.

Medical interventions that will require nursing support include: intubation and ventilation of the patient in order to ensure adequate oxygenation of the brain and airway management; a detailed neurological exam; X-rays; possibly CAT (computerized axial tomography) scanning to define areas of bleeding in the brain accurately (this may be done under general anaesthetic); anticonvulsant or antibiotic therapy as required. An osmotic diuretic, mannitol, may be given to try to shrink the brain by reducing oedema. This requires catheterization but may help as a temporary measure pending transfer to specialist neurosurgical care (Sinclair, 1991).

The vast majority of patients seen in A & E will fortunately have only suffered minor head injury and will be discharged home. Symptoms such as dizziness, headaches, irritability, poor concentration and memory loss may last for days afterwards and a study by Lowdon *et al.* (1989) reported that among a sample of 114 such patients, 90% reported these symptoms lasting up to two weeks after injury. It is important that the nurse discuss these symptoms with the patient and a friend or relative, and also stress the need for the patient to be brought back to hospital if they persist or worsen.

Evaluation

It is essential that senior nursing staff ensure that junior staff understand fully the reasons why they are performing the repeated observations that they are carrying out on the head injury patient. If junior staff do not understand fully, the observations will not be performed accurately and the significance of some vital change will go unreported. Senior staff should monitor the accuracy of their juniors' observations, doing so discreetly and using such a process as a teaching tool.

The patient with burns

Pathology

The key factors in burn pathology are the area of the burn, the depth of the burn, and any special areas of the body, such as the respiratory tract, that are involved.

Area

The burnt area will almost immediately begin to lose fluid which is very similar to plasma in its composition. If sufficient fluid is lost from the burn, hypovolaemic shock will develop. The area of the burn is, therefore, crucial as it determines the volume of fluid lost. Area may be estimated using Wallace's Rule of 9 (Fig. 4.9).

As a rule of thumb it may be assumed that in burns of 15% of surface area or greater in adults, and 10% or greater in children, hypovolaemia will develop. In these cases, therefore, the patient will need an IVI. If such an infusion is not commenced and the hypovolaemia not vigorously treated, the outcome may be fatal.

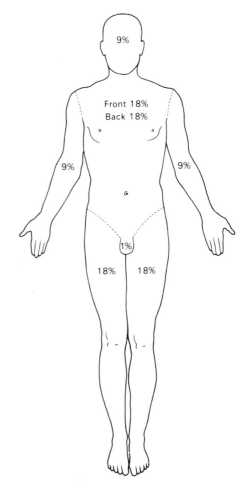

Fig. 4.9 Wallace's Rule of 9 for estimating area of burns

In reading about burns, the nurse may be confused by the different statements that are made about the type of fluid that should be used to correct hypovolaemia from burns. This is because there is a marked difference of opinion among the various specialists in the field. The basic requirements in the burn patient are protein, salt and water in such a form as will stay in the circulation. Sodium chloride is lost in great quantities in the burn exudate, along with protein, and therefore must be replaced. However, the hypovolaemic patient also needs fluids that will stay in the circulation rather than those which rapidly escape into the various other fluid compartments of the body. Thus, although normal saline contains the sodium chloride required, it will not effectively expand the circulation and, although Haemaccel is a plasma expander, it does not contain sodium chloride. Solutions such as Dextran 70 and plasma protein faction (PPF), however, have both properties.

Fluid loss from a burn continues for over 24 hours after injury. This is of significance in planning dressings for patients who are to be discharged home with relatively minor burns. For the major burn requiring inpatient treatment, the continual fluid loss has to be taken into account in working out an IVI regimen. Various formulae are used in this connection, one of the best known being the Mount Vernon formula (Wardrope and Smith, 1992), which calculates a unit volume of fluid from the patient's size and the area burnt.

Unit volume = Area burnt (%) × Patient's weight (kg)/2.

This unit volume of fluid is then administered in blocks of 4 hours, two blocks of 6 hours and one block of 12 hours, measured from the time of the burn and subject to adjustment in the light of the patient's condition.

Depth

Burns are classified by their depth as either full thickness, partial thickness or superficial.

A full thickness burn is one in which the full thickness of the skin has been destroyed (Fig. 4.10). The appearance is a typically dull grey area or, in flame burns, a dark brown or black. Because the nerve endings have been destroyed, there is usually a loss of sensation. The remaining tissue is hard and leathery. This poses a special problem in circumferential burns because the inelastic surface tissue will act as a tourniquet around the limb, within which there will be swelling due to the burn oedema. The result is occlusion of the circulation, gangrene and loss of the limb, unless the limb is excised longitudinally through the eschar tissue to allow room for expansion and for the release of pressure. This is known as escharotomy.

Healing of a full thickness burn occurs by

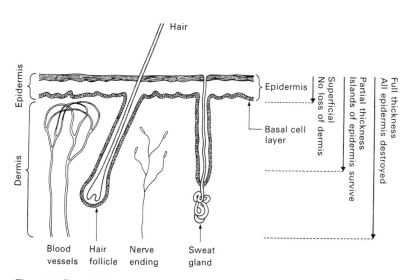

Fig. 4.10 Depth of burns

the formation of scar tissue, which is both unsightly and inelastic. The inelasticity will give rise to loss of function and severe contractures. The need, therefore, is to treat full thickness burns by skin grafting in order to retain maximum function and avoid contracture formation.

If the burn is only partial thickness, then areas of epithelium survive around hair follicles and sweat glands. This permits the re-epithelialization of the burnt area, provided that it is kept free from infection. Skin grafting is, therefore, not usually required and healing should occur with a full range of movement. Partial thickness burns usually leave the nerve endings intact; therefore, they may be differentiated from full thickness burns by a pin prick sensation test. Scalds and flash burns are typically partial thickness.

Superficial burns involve a reddening only of the most superficial layers. This is known as erythema and is of minor importance compared to the other two types so far discussed. In estimating burn areas, erythema should be excluded.

One final type of burn that should be mentioned is the burn due to electricity. It is characterized by a small surface wound where the current entered the body, but within there may be major damage with burns extending down to the bone and involving structures such as tendons, muscles and nerves. The potential effect of the electric current on the heart should be considered during treatment.

Special areas affected by burns

Oedema of the face and neck can have serious implications for the airway. Inhalation of flames or hot gases will cause burn oedema in the respiratory tract itself. The threat of an occluded airway is very real in such cases and an early tracheotomy or intubation, if possible, is indicated. Facial oedema will quickly make it impossible for the patient to open their eyes. This has two implications; first, if the eyes are to be examined properly, they must be examined immediately, and second, the patient may fear that their sight has been lost altogether, when the problem is simply that they cannot open their eyes.

Psychological effects

The nurse should realize that there are profound psychological effects from a burn which affect not only the patient but also their relatives. There is the fear of disfigurement and altered body image on the one hand, and on the other, there are the inevitable feelings of guilt associated with the parent of a young child that has been burnt.

From the nurse's very first encounter with the patient, psychological support will be essential. Reference has already been made to the likely guilt feelings that parents of young children will be experiencing. In addition, adults will be fearing disfigurement as a result of their injuries.

It is very difficult at this early stage in A & E to deal with a straight 'Will I be scarred for life?' question. But this is precisely what is in the mind of the burn victim, and may even be on their lips. If asked, the nurse should try to answer the question fairly and frankly, pointing out that at this early stage it is very difficult to say with any degree of certainty what the outcome will be. Such an answer is better than bland reassurances about the wonders of modern plastic surgery. On the other hand, the question may remain unasked; if this is the case, the nurse should try to get the patient to verbalize their fears and to get the matter out in the open for realistic discussion.

The degree of distress displayed by the patient may be markedly reduced by simply talking about the problem and offering support as appropriate.

Later effects

After the patient has moved to the ward, complications can develop. These include renal failure, toxaemia, anaemia, paralytic ileus and, in the case of children, 'burn encephalopathy'. These complications can combine to make the burns victim an extremely challenging person to care for.

Assessment

Assessment of the burns victim commences with the normal template of the ABCs. The nurse should note whether the burns involve the face and neck areas, and whether there is any evidence of the patient having inhaled flames or hot gas. Such evidence would include soot in the nasal passages or blistering around the mouth and lips.

It is important to obtain a history of the accident – what caused the burn, the time the burn occurred and what, if any, first aid has been applied. The next point to determine is how much pain the patient is feeling. Some burns cause remarkably little pain; ironically they are usually the more severe full thickness burns as the actual nerve endings have been destroyed, but other burns can be extremely painful.

The area of the burn should be estimated, using Wallace's Rule of 9 (see Fig. 4.9). This rule divides the body area up into multiples of 9%. For small areas, the area of the patient's hand can be taken as 1% of the body area. Areas of superficial erythema and redness should *not* be included in this calculation. Alternatively, detailed charts of the body showing the percentage area of different parts may be used for estimating the area of the burn. These are known as Lund and Browder charts .

The last point to estimate is the depth of the burn. The appearance will give some clue: a full thickness burn is typically a dull grey colour with tough leathery eschar tissue; a partial thickness burn is usually red or pink in colour. Sensation is absent in the full thickness burn but present in a partial thickness burn. This may be tested for with the pin prick method.

A sketch of the burn is a useful means of recording its extent; areas of suspected full thickness burn can be shaded in and labelled as such.

Baseline observations are important to monitor the circulatory status of the patient and to detect any signs of hypovolaemic shock at the earliest stage. They should be repeated as frequently as the patient's condition indicates.

The psychological effects of the burn on the patient and on the family should be assessed, especially where young children are involved. Is the mother hostile and defensive, or anxious and expressing feelings of guilt? One important aspect that has to be assessed is whether the child's injuries match the story of the parent, as burns constitute a common form of child abuse.

In electrical burns, it is important to take an ECG. Continuous cardiac monitoring should be instituted if there is a history of collapse, electrical current is suspected of having passed through the thorax, voltages in excess of 1000 V were involved or if the 12-lead ECG shows

abnormalities (Burn, 1999). Function should be assessed together with sensation in view of the risk of damage to deep structures such as tendons and nerves.

First aid

Many products are available for immediate care of burns. Many fire services now use dressings made with tree oil that allows heat evaporation but prevents hypothermia, one example is 'Burnshield'. If only small areas are burnt such as a hand, then copious amounts of water can be used to restrict the burning and prevent airflow over the limb which is one of the major causes of pain. In severe burns the use of water should not go on for longer than ten minutes as vasoconstriction and hypothermia may be caused by prolonged and extensive immersion.

Airway

The first priority for the burns patient is to safeguard the airway, and if assessment reveals problems due to oedema, tracheotomy or intubation will be considered. The A & E nursing team must be able to respond at once to the need for emergency tracheotomy or intubation in such a situation. Upper airway oedema peaks at 24–48 hours after injury. Treatment in less severe cases consists of administering humidified oxygen, maintaining close observation, an upright position and chest physiotherapy aimed at preventing atelectasis.

Pain relief

The application of cold soaks (gauze dressing pads and sterile water for irrigation) to the burnt area will usually reduce the pain felt by the patient though the risk of hypothermia should not be overlooked. The immediate generous administration of Entonox gas will further relieve pain.

In many burns, the administration of intravenous morphine is recommended. The best method is to dilute 10 mg of morphine in 10 ml of water for injection, and then to give, slowly, sufficient of the drug to achieve the desired degree of sedation and pain relief.

In dealing with young children, sedation is very important as it is impossible to dress properly limbs that are flailing in all directions at once. Furthermore, the more distressed the child, the more distressed will be the parents who are already probably feeling desperately guilty and blaming themselves for their young child's misfortune. A child may be sedated with oral trimeprazine syrup, but it must be remembered that the child can still feel the pain and that therefore some other analgesic agent is required in addition. When dressing burns on young children, the parents should be encouraged to give analgesia prior to them attending the department. This will allow the child to attend the department in a more relaxed state. Nurses should allow them to sit on their parent's lap as being held by a parent will be a source of comfort in what the child is currently experiencing as a very frightening experience. Play and distraction therapy will also help the child with the dressing change.

The IVI and fluid balance

If the burn is over 15% of the body surface area, an IVI will be required to prevent hypovolaemia. Apart from nursing assistance in siting the infusion, it will be a key part of the resuscitation effort that an accurate fluid balance be kept. Catheterization, with hourly urine measurements, is essential due to the risk of renal failure. The kidneys should be able to produce a minimum of 0.5 ml of urine per kg body weight per hour; failure to do so indicates that they are being underperfused and that, therefore, inadequate IV fluids are being given to deal with the burn shock. For an average adult, the hourly urine output should not drop below about 30–35 ml (Hudak and Gallo, 1994).

Transfer

Most hospitals do not have a burns unit, therefore patients who are suffering from major burns will be transferred to your local regional centre. It is important that liaison occurs so that local guidelines are followed. This will ensure continuity of care for the patient. Minor burns patients may need a secondary referral if plastic surgery is needed or infection becomes a problem.

Trauma scoring systems

Such are the complex possible permutations of injuries in multiply-injured patients, attempts have been made to devise simple scoring systems which will indicate those patients at most risk of death in order to prioritize treatment. Much of this work originated in the USA and has now become common practice in the UK. Davies (1993) has provided good introduction to this subject and shows that the Revised Trauma Scoring system, based upon the systolic BP, respiratory rate and GCS, correlates well with the probability of survival. There are drawbacks with this approach, not least of which, as Davies points out, is the validity of importing a North American system with its very different patterns of trauma to the UK.

References and further reading

Armstrong R, Bullen C, Cohen S, Singer M, Webb A (1991) *Critical Care Algorithms.* Oxford: Oxford Medical Publications.

Baskett P (1991) Management of hypovolaemic shock. In Skinner D, Driscoll D, Earlam R (eds) *ABC of Major Trauma.* London: BMJ.

Baskett P (1993) *Resuscitation Handbook* 2nd edn. London: Wolfe.

Budassi-Sheehy S (1990) *Manual of Emergency Care.* St Louis: C.V. Mosby.

Bullock R, Teasdale G (1991) Head injuries. In Driscoll P, Skinner D, Earlam R (eds) *ABC of Major Trauma.* London: BMJ.

Burn D (1999) Electrical burns. *Emergency Nurse,* 7:2, 27–32.

Chamberlain D (1990) Ventricular fibrillation. In Evans TR (ed.) *ABC of Resuscitation.* London: BMJ.

Davies S (1993) Trauma scoring. *Accident and Emergency Nursing,* 1:125–31.

Driscoll P, Skinner D (1991) Initial assessment and management. In Skinner D, Driscoll P, Earlam R (eds) *ABC of Major Trauma.* London: BMJ.

Driscoll F, Hodgkinson D, Mackway-Jones K (1992a) Diagnostic peritoneal lavage: it's red but is it positive? *Injury,* 23:4, 267–9.

Driscoll P et al. (1992b) Organising an efficient trauma team. *Injury,* 23:2, 107–10.

Durren M (1992) Getting the most from pulse oximetry. *Journal of Emergency Nursing,* 18:4, 340–2.

European Resuscitation Council Working Party (1997) Adult advanced cardiac life support: the European Resuscitation Council guidelines 1997. *BMJ,* 306:1589–93.

Ferguson J, Mardel S, Beattie T, Wytch R (1993) Cervical collars: a potential risk to the head-injured patient. *Injury,* 24:7, 454–6.

Folman Y, Masri W (1989) Spinal cord injury: prognostic indicators. *In jury*, **20**:4, 92–3.

Galasko C (1993) Neck sprains after RTA: a modern epidemic injury. *Injury*, **24**:3, 155–7.

Harrison M (1991) The minor head injury. *Paediatric Nursing*, Dec 1991,15–19.

Haughton L, Driscoll P (1999) Cervical immobilisation – are we achieving it? *Pre-hospital immediate care*, **3**:17–21.

Hudak C, Gallo B (1994) *Critical Care Nursing.* Philadelphia: B. Lippincott Co.

Lowdon I, Briggs M, Cockin J (1989) Head injury. *Injury*, **20**:4, 193–4.

Morris K (1993) Assessment and communication of conscious level: an audit of neurosurgical referrals. *Injury*, **24**:6, 369–72.

OPCS (1991) *Mortality Statistics England and Wales.* London: Government Statistical Service.

Proehl J (1992) The Glasgow Coma Scale; do it and do it right. *Journal of Emergency Nursing*, **18**:5, 421–3.

Randall PE (1986) MAST: a review. *Injury*, **17**:6.

Robinson D, Cassar-Pullicino VN (1993) Acute neck sprain after RTA: a long term clinical and radiological review. *Injury*, **24**:2, 79–82.

Royal College of Surgeons England Working Party (1999) *The Management of Head Injuries.* London: Royal College of Surgeons.

Royal College of Surgeons England (1988) Report of the Working Party on the Management of Patients with Major Injuries. London: Royal College of Surgeons.

Sexton J (1999) Can nurses remove spinal boards and cervical collars safely? *Emergency Nurse*; **6**:9, 8–12.

Sinclair M (1991) *Nursing the Neurosurgical Patient.* Oxford: Butterworth-Heinemann.

Walsh M, Ford P (1989) *Nursing Rituals: Research and Rational Action.* Oxford: Butterworth-Heinemann.

Wardrope J, Smith J (1992) *The Management of Wounds and Burns.* Oxford: Oxford University Press.

Watson D (1991) Management of the upper airway. In Skinner D, Driscoll P, Earlam R (eds) *ABC of Major Trauma.* London: BMJ.

Chapter 5

NURSING CARE OF THE EMERGENCY PATIENT

Care of the patient with chest pain

Pathology

Ischaemic heart disease (IHD) is the most common serious cause of chest pain seen in A & E departments. In 1997 122 422 people died as a result of ischaemic heart disease in England and Wales alone (National Statistics Office, 1998). The causes of IHD are many, involving social and psychological factors. For example, in 1996, the prevalence of treated coronary heart disease per 1000 patients in men was 34.7 compared to 20.8 for women (Social Trends, 1999). The class gradient discussed on p. 3 is found in IHD mortality, ranging from a standardized mortality rate of 63 in class I to 182 in class V (SMR for whole all social classes =100), in other words it is three times higher in class V compared to class I (Drever and Whitehead, 1995). There is a marked regional variation within the UK as shown in Table 5.1.

Table 5.1 Regional variation in UK mortality rates for IHD 1996

Region	Mortality rate per 100 000 pop.
Scotland	294
N. Ireland	288
North West England	270
Northern & Yorkshire	268
Wales	259
West Midlands	253
Trent	251
N. Thames	224
Anglia & Oxford	218
South and West	216
South Thames	205

Source: Regional Trends no. 33 (1998)

IHD is a disease of late middle age to old age. The prevalence rate of coronary heart disease in men aged 44–54 was 27.1 per 1000 in 1996 but, in the age group 65–74, it was 170.4; for women the figures were 12.2 and 106.9 respectively (Social Trends, 1999).

The majority of deaths from IHD occur soon after the onset of pain. Thompson and Webster (1992) cite a typical figure of 60% of deaths occurring within one hour of infarct.

It is important to differentiate between angina and a myocardial infarction (MI). If the diseased coronary artery circulation is unable to meet an increased oxygen demand from the myocardium (usually due to exercise), metabolic changes occur in the hypoxic myocardium which produce the classic pain of angina pectoris – a diffuse, retrosternal pain which will usually disappear with rest or GTN medication.

If, instead of an inadequate blood supply (angina), there is a complete occlusion of the blood supply to a portion of the myocardium, that part will die, and a myocardial infarction will have occurred. The pain is localized in the centre of the chest. It is usually severe and crushing in nature, radiates into the left arm and possibly into the jaw, and it is not relieved by rest. The pain may be atypical, however, and in the elderly in particular, pain may be absent or at least not reported by the patient.

Assessment

The initial step is to obtain a history from the patient in order that other possible causes of chest pain may be eliminated (see Table 5.2) A useful tool to guide analysis of the presenting symptom is the PQRST approach which can be applied to any symptom, not just pain.

- P: Provocation/Palliation. What brings on the pain? What relieves the pain?
- Q: Quality. Describe the nature of the pain.

Table 5.2 Differential diagnosis: causes of chest pain

	Angina	Gastrointestinal	Musculoskeletal	Respiratory
Provocation	Exercise Emotional upset	Related to food consumption	Related to trauma, physical effort	Increases with inspiration or trunk movement
Palliation	Rest GTN	Antacids	Mild analgesics, heat, rest	Little relief
Quality	Tightness	Burning, discomfort, wind	Ache	Sharp, grabbing (pleurisy, pneumothorax or pulmonary embolism) or dull, aching in pneumonia
	Stops patient activity	Patient carries on activity	Patient carries on activity	Lower chest, sometimes bilateral
Region	Retrosternal	Epigastric/retrosternal	Intercostal	Pneumothorax on entire side of chest
Radiation	Arm, wrist, hand, jaw	Unlikely, though possibly through to back	Backache	Pneumothorax radiates to back
Severity	Moderate	Variable	Moderate, though variable	Moderate to severe
Timing	Recent specific onset	Vague onset, though may waken patient from sleep	Shortly after physical effort	Sudden onset and then continual pain

- R: Region/Radiation. Where is the pain and does it radiate anywhere?
- S: Severity. Ask to rate the pain on a score of 0–5.
- T: Time. How long has the patient had the pain?

If the patient is experiencing a myocardial infarction (MI) rather than angina, the patient is often unable to point to any particular thing that brought the pain on nor can they relieve the pain (P). The pain is often described as constant, gripping or crushing in nature (Q) and while it is classically central chest pain with radiation into the left arm and/or jaw, the presentation may be atypical with pain absent altogether, especially in older people (R). The pain is very severe (S). The angina symptom analysis presented in Table 5.2 should be compared with the description of MI pain presented above.

It is important to check whether there is any previous cardiac history and what medication the patient is taking. Mental state should be assessed as chest pain is a very frightening experience, and fear and anxiety can make the condition worse.

The general appearance of the patient should be noted as pallor and a cold clammy skin suggests shock, indicating that the patient is seriously ill. Vital signs should be recorded. A rapid respiratory rate is usually seen in cardiac pain, associated with pulmonary congestion and/or the effects of anxiety. The pulse must be assessed for both rate and rhythm. A bradycardia carries a poor prognosis in acute MI. A systolic BP below 90 mmHg usually indicates shock, and if the patient is indeed suffering from an acute MI, then the presence of cardiogenic shock also indicates a poor chance of survival. An accurate temperature reading is essential to help to eliminate chest infection as an alternative possible cause of the pain.

The next step in assessment is to carry out a 12-lead ECG in order to discover any arrhythmia and evidence of MI or ischaemia. Before performing an ECG, the nurse should explain *in language the patient understands* exactly what is to be done and why, e.g. 'This machine will take a recording of your pulse rate which will help us find out what is causing your pain.'

The initial history taking and physical assessment is crucial for correct triage and management. Quinn (1997) cites evidence

ECG Report

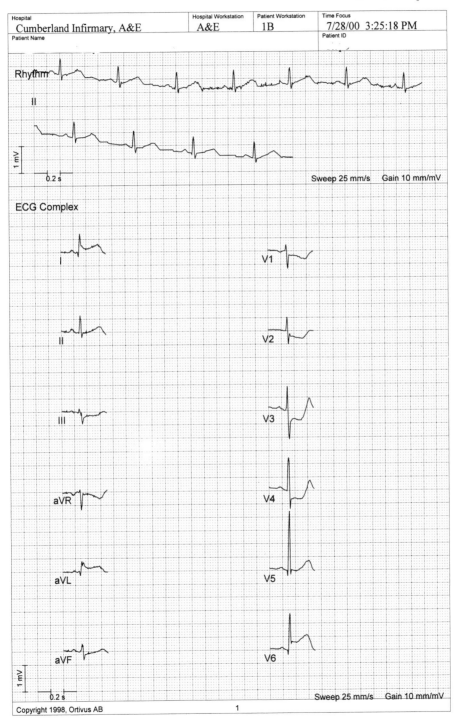

Fig. 5.1 ECG report

indicating that less than half the patients admitted to coronary care units have had an MI and not surprisingly therefore, only a small proportion of patients presenting at A & E with chest pain have actually had an MI. It is crucial therefore to prioritize those patients at high risk of having had an MI ahead of others. In reviewing the literature, Quinn lists the following as key indicators of a serious prognosis: acute ECG changes (see below), systolic BP<100, a previous history of IHD, arrhythmia, diabetes mellitus, increasing age, breathlessness and signs of acute heart failure.

If nurses are to perform ECGs in A & E, they must understand what they are doing. In brief, they are recording the electrical activity of the heart with a delicate and sensitive machine. The machine should be handled with respect, and every effort should be made to obtain good electrical contact. Electrodes are now usually pre-gelled for good contact and should not therefore be positioned on hairy parts of the body. The inside of the wrists and ankles should be used and any chest hair removed with a razor. Patient movement, muscle tremor, and simple mains electric background hum will all cause interference.

Of the leads that are attached to the limbs, the right leg lead is an earth and plays no active part in the recording. There are, therefore, three limb leads which the machine uses to record the heart's electrical activity in six different combinations. Each of these leads gives a different view of the heart, together with the chest lead which is also used in six different positions. The result is 12 different views of the heart (see Fig. 5.1) which make it possible to localize the damaged part of the myocardium depending upon which leads show evidence of infarction. If, for example, leads II, III and aVf show the characteristic changes of an MI, it can be deduced that it is the inferior part of the heart that is damaged.

The basic components of an ECG are the:

P wave	Spread of electrical activity through the atria.
P–Q interval	Conduction of electrical impulse via the bundle of His to the ventricles.
QRS complex	Spread of electrical activity through the ventricles. The Q wave represents the first electrical activity away from the bundle of His in the intraventricular septum.
T wave	Repolarization of cells ready for next contraction.

Figure 5.2 shows how the heart's conducting mechanism is related to the ECG. The machine is set to record a current towards the electrode as an upwards deflection.

The following key ECG changes are associated with an MI or ischaemia (see Fig. 5.3).

1. *Pathological Q wave.* An exaggerated Q

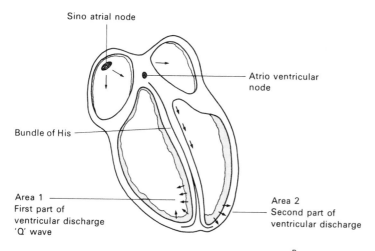

Fig. 5.2 Conducting mechanism of the heart and the ECG

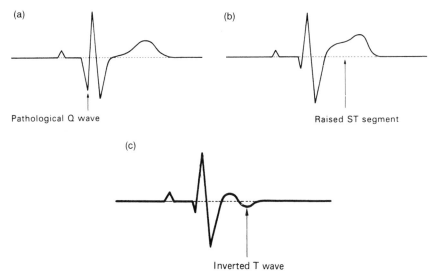

Fig. 5.3 ECG changes associated with IHD (a) Dead myocardium: pathological Q wave; (b) Damaged myocardium: raised ST section; (c) Ischaemic myocardium: inverted T wave

wave indicates an area of dead myocardium, i.e. an MI has occurred at some time. However, as this is a permanent change in the ECG, it could relate to an episode that happened a year or more ago. Therefore, on its own, a pathological Q wave does not indicate an acute MI. Consideration of Fig. 5.2 shows that the Q wave is normally lost in the electrical activity of area 2. However, if area 2 is dead myocardium, there will be no electrical activity present and the whole of the normal activity in area 1 will be recorded, producing an exaggerated Q wave. The dead area of myocardium acts as an 'electrical window', allowing us to record activity normally swamped by healthy myocardium.

2. *Elevated ST segment.* This indicates acutely damaged myocardium and may be thought of as being due to the damaged cells leaking potassium ions (K) after each contraction. This leads to an excess of positive charges and hence the ST section is elevated above the normal baseline of the EGG (the isoelectric state).

3. *T wave inversion.* This may indicate myocardial ischaemia, but not an actual MI. Depression of the ST segment may occur during an actual anginal attack.

It is possible sometimes that the ECG does not initially reveal the tell-tale signs of an MI.

A normal ECG alone does not mean the patient can be safely sent home, and if a history suggestive of MI is obtained, great caution should be exercised. Usually blood samples will be taken for cardiac enzymes and the patient admitted for a short period of observation, even if a normal ECG is obtained. In addition to evidence of MI, the ECG will reveal if there is any serious arrhythmia present. Therefore, the rhythm strip automatically recorded from lead II should be noted carefully. The patient should be attached to a cardiac monitor which should be readily visible to nursing staff. The patient should be reassured and a careful explanation given about the cardiac monitor.

To read an ECG it is essential to be methodical. Examine the trace first of all for P waves, noting whether they are present and if so whether they are followed by a QRS complex. The QRS complex should then be examined to check whether it is of normal shape and size and finally look at the T wave to see whether it is normal or inverted. With this systematic approach it becomes easier to spot the following major life-threatening arrhythmias which the nurse should be able to recognize on a monitor (see Fig. 5.4).

1. *Asystole.* No cardiac activity, cardiac arrest. It is essential to check the patient before

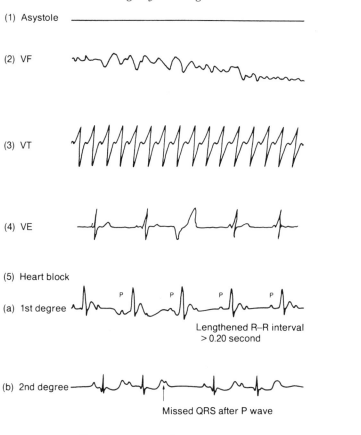

(1) Asystole

(2) VF

(3) VT

(4) VE

(5) Heart block

(a) 1st degree

Lengthened R–R interval
> 0.20 second

(b) 2nd degree

Missed QRS after P wave

(c) Complete

Fig. 5.4 Serious arrhythmias

instituting CPR as disconnected electrodes can produce a trace very similar to that of asystole.

2. *Ventricular fibrillation (VF)*. Rapid quivering of the ventricles associated with a rapid, disorganized pattern of electrical activity. There are therefore no recognizable QRS complexes or P waves. No output is produced. Effectively VF is cardiac arrest. This requires immediate defibrillation and full CPR. Check first the patient's condition and responsiveness as electronic gremlins such as loose leads may be responsible!

3. *Ventricular tachycardia (VT)*. Caused by a ventricular pacemaker taking over pacing the heart and firing at a very rapid rate, 15–250 beats per minute. There are no P waves, only regular, bizarre ventricular complexes. Cardiac output falls to very low levels. There is insufficient time for the ventricles to fill between each beat. The patient loses consciousness and

proceeds to VF unless spontaneous remission occurs.

4. *Ventricular ectopics (VEs)*. If there is an irritable focus in one of the ventricles, it may begin firing off pacing impulses itself, leading to premature ventricular contractions or VEs. No P wave is seen, the beat comes early, and the shape of the QRS complex is different from normal as it represents an atypical conduction of electricity through the myocardium. Occasional VEs are not a cause for concern, but if they start to occur in runs, there is the possibility of a VT developing. Bigeminy is the coupling of a normal beat with a VE immediately afterwards. Trigeminy occurs when every third beat is a VE.

5. *Heart block*. First degree block involves a delay in the conduction of the electrical impulse through the AV node. The P–R interval is, therefore, lengthened and if it is

greater than 0.2 seconds, first degree block exists. This condition usually does not produce any clinically significant effects but may worsen until some of the impulses are not conducted at all. In this case, P waves may be seen with no QRS complexes to follow and a ventricular beat is dropped as a result. This is second degree block and may progress into a complete heart block (CHB) where the AV node fails to conduct any impulses at all. A ventricular pacemaker may take over to produce a slow rhythm (approximately 20–30 impulses per minute) which bears no linkage to the regular pattern of P waves which may still be seen. Such a slow rate leads to heart failure, and if the ventricular pacemaker fails to fire, the patient collapses with no cardiac output (Stokes-Adams attack) which will be a terminal event unless the ventricular pacemaker picks up again very quickly.

The key steps therefore in assessing the patient with chest pain are to obtain a history of the pain, previous medical history and medication, assess the patient's appearance and mental state, record vital signs, and perform and interpret an ECG.

Intervention

In the case of patients with chest pain, prioritization is the vital first step in nursing intervention. This is because of the close relationship between the time of death and the onset of symptoms (see p. 53). If the assessment described in the previous section is carried out accurately by the nurse, the patient may be assigned the correct priority and triage will have been correctly carried out.

One of the main thrusts of intervention is to limit the area of damage to the myocardium. To this end, high concentration oxygen should be administered at once. The patient should be cared for sitting upright to assist respiration. Unrelieved pain will contribute to higher levels of anxiety, stimulation of the sympathetic nervous system and hence increased cardiac activity, the result of which is that myocardial oxygenation is seriously compromised. Pain relief is, therefore, an urgent priority. Pain may be effectively relieved by the use of Entonox gas, which has the advantage of being 50% oxygen. Intravenous access should be secured immediately if it has not been done so already

as opioid analgesia, such as diamorphine, is required via the IV route at once, for effective pain relief. It is usually given in small increments up to a dose of 5.0 mg until pain relief is achieved. An antiemetic drug, such as prochlorperazine (12.5 mg), should also be given prophylactically, and naloxone, the specific antidote to opioids should be immediately available in case of accidental overdose.

The relief of fear and anxiety will also assist in pain reduction. Psychological support is therefore essential. The patient should be cared for in a special cardiac cubicle removed from the noise and bustle of the busy department, where monitoring can be carried out unobtrusively, i.e. with the monitor volume control on zero, and with the monitor invisible to the patient (but visible to staff). Explanations of what is happening together with the nurse's own attitude will reduce tension and fear, as will relief of pain, and the presence of family/friends.

The admission procedure to CCU should be expedited as much as possible, remembering the high risk of cardiac arrest in the immediate post-infarction period.

Thrombolytic therapy aimed at dissolving the clot should be instituted at the earliest opportunity as it is more effective if given within 6 hours of symptom onset and even more effective if given within 2 hours (Quinn, 1999). Agents used include streptokinase, urokinase and rtPA (recombinant tissue-type plasminogen activator). It is alarming, however, to read that Hood *et al.* (1998) report thrombolytic therapy was not available in 35% of A & E departments. Quinn cites national guidelines requiring thrombolytic therapy to begin within 30 minutes of arrival at hospital (door to needle time), yet is able to show how resistance to change and cumbersome hospital procedures mean this is rarely achieved. As the evidence shows that the success of thrombolytic therapy in reducing mortality from MI is highly time dependent, every effort must be made in A & E to ensure this 30-minute guideline is achieved. X-rays should not be obtained in A & E as this delays transfer to CCU.

It should be the aim of an A & E unit to be able to transfer a patient with chest pain to CCU within 15–20 minutes of arrival. The transfer should always be undertaken with two porters and a qualified nurse and with necessary resuscitation equipment. It is not a good idea to take relatives over to the CCU with the patient in case an emergency should develop in transit. It is better to take them over a few minutes later when the patient has been safely bedded down. It is important to prepare both patient and relatives so that they know what to expect in CCU; the array of monitors and other high-tech equipment can be very frightening and anxiety provoking.

Cardiac arrest

Cardiac arrest may have occurred outside hospital or despite our best efforts, within the department. A patient in cardiac arrest may be defined clinically as being unrousable and having no detectable carotid pulse. It is common for the individual to have received no basic life support while waiting for the ambulance. Response times even at best can be eight minutes or more, therefore, it is not surprising that these patients have a poor short-term and long-term outcome. The rhythm on arrival is often a non-ventricular fibrillation or tachycardia event. However, if a patient arrests within the department the prognosis is good if it is a shockable rhythm and defibrillation can be performed within 90 seconds.

If there is no cardiac output, you must follow the BLS algorithm outlined in Fig. 5.5, calling for assistance immediately before commencing resuscitation. After clearing the airway, the patient's lungs should be slowly inflated twice with oxygen using a bag/mask device. The best indicator is that you can see the chest wall gently rise, before chest compressions are commenced to produce an effective circulation. If a bag/mask is not available, 'mouth-to-mouth' expired air respiration should be commenced with two slow breaths. It should be remembered that there has been no demonstrated case of HIV transmission by this route and Zideman (1990) considers there is no realistic risk of AIDS infection as a result of mouth-to-mouth resuscitation, so long as blood is not present in the saliva. This view is supported by Baskett (1993).

The nurse should place both hands together on the sternum at a point some two fingers' width up from its lower end (xiphisternum). The fingers should be interlocked and the arms held straight, the aim being to use about half the nurse's body weight to compress the sternum by 4–5 cm. A rate of about 100 compressions per minute carried out correctly will give a cardiac output of between 33% and 50% of normal, sufficient to prevent cerebral damage and give Advanced Life Support (ALS) techniques a chance to be successful.

A 5:1 ratio of compressions to ventilations is required in two-person life support, or 15:2 in single person CPR.

The patient should be connected to an ECG monitor as soon as possible in order that cardiac activity may be monitored. The ECG and the presence or absence of cardiac output,

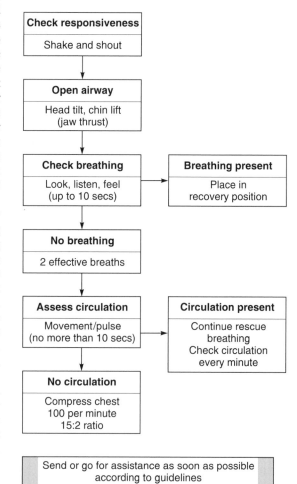

(a)

Fig. 5.5a, b Adult basic and advanced life support (European Resuscitation Council Guidelines, 1997)

as measured by a carotid or femoral pulse, will determine the medical treatment that follows in accordance with ALS guidelines (Fig. 5.5). Effective CPR must be maintained at all times to ensure an oxygenated blood supply continuously reaches the patient's brain. Intubation greatly assists airway management but an oropharyngeal airway used with a bag and mask device can effectively keep the patient ventilated in the meanwhile.

In a cardiac arrest the three most likely cardiac arrhythmias to be found are ventricular

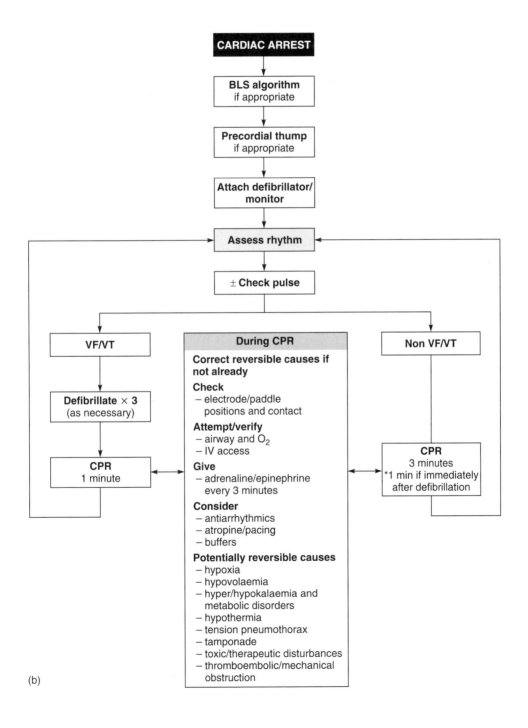

(b)

fibrillation, asystole, or electromechanical dissociation. Other arrhythmias are discussed on p. 58. In asystole there is no cardiac electrical activity (straight line on the ECG), while in electromechanical dissociation the ECG looks normal except that unfortunately the heart is not responding and producing any contractions; cardiac output is therefore nil. Ventricular fibrillation is a condition where there is uncoordinated electrical discharge throughout the ventricles. While it is the most common cause of cardiac arrest it is also the condition with the best survival rate due to the efficacy of prompt defibrillation. The result is that the myocardial muscle only quivers instead of carrying out its normal coordinated contraction and cardiac output effectively ceases. Giving an electrical shock, defibrillation, aims to produce a simultaneous depolarization of all the myocardial cells, thus allowing them to repolarize at the same time and hopefully restore normal coordinated electrical and muscular activity. Resuscitation guidelines are aimed at ensuring defibrillation occurs at the earliest possible opportunity as prospects for success decrease rapidly with time, consequently A & E nurses should all be trained in defibrillation as they are the most likely staff to witness an arrest

Effective ventilation and chest compression must be maintained throughout, except during defibrillation since the nurse would also receive the electrical shock!

In young children a different approach is required – the heel of one hand only for a small child, and two thumbs for a baby. The rate needs to be again 100 compressions per minute, and the respiration rate correspondingly quicker but also more shallow.

The nurse will usually be responsible for drawing up and administering various drugs in a CPR attempt. It will greatly expedite the proceedings if nursing staff know what is likely to be asked for and have the drugs to hand. Some of these drugs may be given via an endotracheal tube in a cardiac arrest. Lignocaine, atropine, naloxone and epinephrine are readily absorbed through the lungs, and this route should therefore be considered where an IV line cannot be readily established (e.g. in children). Doses should be doubled for administration via an ET tube. There is, however, little evidence to show these drugs

have a positive effect upon outcomes. Kloech (1997) showed that the only interventions which are truly beneficial to a patient in cardiac arrest are basic life support, defibrillation and tracheal intubation.

The nurse needs to know how to charge the defibrillator and to apply conducting pads to the chest in the correct positions (sternum and apex of the heart). If necessary, the nurse should be prepared to defibrillate if the nursing and medical staff have agreed to that being part of the nurse's role. The golden rule is to make sure that nobody is touching the trolley or else they too will receive a shock (200–360 Joules). The advent of semi-automatic defibrillators is allowing quicker and successful defibrillation. Although common in public areas, and used by lay professionals, e.g. airline cabin staff, they have not as yet pushed into both the hospital and A & E departments. These machines, however, are ideal for personnel within the hospital setting.

If CPR is successful in re-establishing cardiac output, continual ECG monitoring is required, and further drug therapy may be needed to stabilize the patient's rhythm.

Asystole does not respond to defibrillation, however, it is essential to be sure asystole is correctly diagnosed and is not misread from the monitor as it may actually be very fine VF. If in doubt, defibrillation is recommended (ERC, 1997).

Evaluation

The use of critical pathways greatly aids evaluation of care and Fig. 5.6 consists of an example of what a critical pathway might look like for A & E care of a patient with chest pain of suspected cardiac origin. Effectiveness of pain relief must be assessed, and in the case of administration of opioid analgesia, respiratory effort must be closely watched due to the depressant effect of opioids on respiration. Periodic checks on oxygen administration are required. The patient may remove the mask, especially to answer questions from the doctor, and leave it off.

It is very important to note how the patient's emotional state is progressing, as a modification in the environment (e.g. noise) or in the nursing personnel looking after the patient may be required to reduce anxiety.

	0–5 min.	6–15 min.	16–30 min.
Documentation	Registration As A&E pt.	A&E notes ready to write in	Admissions complete Hosp. notes available
Assessment	Triage nurse VS 02 sats. Pain History of presenting complaint Mental state	12 lead ECG Continual ECG monitoring VS incl.Temp. Previous medical history Mental state 02 sats.	Continual ECG VS & pain Mental state 02 sats.
Medication	–	IV morphine titrated for pain relief Prochloperazine 12.5 mg Thrombolytic agent if indicated as per protocol	
Treatment	02 therapy	Insert and heparinize IV cannula 02 therapy	02 therapy
Nursing care	Sit upright Psychological support Close observation	Undress & make comfortable in upright position Psych. support Close observation	Continued as before
Referrals	A&E SHO	Medical on take team/CCU	Transfer to CCU
Family	Inform if not present	Allow to see pt Explain what is happening	Escort to CCU
Discharge	–	Arrange transfer to CCU	Transfer to CCU

VS = vital signs.
This pathway is only strictly applicable if the assessment indicates acute chest pain possibly/probably of cardiac origin

Fig. 5.6 Critical pathway for the care of a patient with chest pain of suspected cardiac origin

Care of the patient with respiratory distress

Pathology

The principal causes of respiratory distress (other than trauma) are:

1. *Pulmonary oedema.* This in itself is not a disease but rather it is a symptom. The most usual causes are heart failure, MI and other cardiac conditions, but there are many other possible diseases that give rise to pulmonary oedema. The usual picture is one of back pressure from the left side of a diseased heart into the pulmonary circulation. The increased pressure in the pulmonary capillaries interferes with the normal osmotic pressure gradient. This causes fluid to move from the cells into the capillaries. The result is fluid oozing into the alveolar spaces and interfering with oxygen exchange.

2. *Asthma.* A simple definition of asthma is that it is 'A disease characterised by wide variations over short periods of time in resistance to airflow in interpulmonary airways' (Rees and Price, 1995). The incidence of asthma appears to be increasing with 10% of children and 6% of the adult population having the disorder. There are approximately 2000 adult deaths per year in the UK, many of which

are thought to be preventable (Haslett *et al.*, 1999). Airflow resistance increases as a result of obstruction of the bronchial tree due to bronchospasm and inflammation. This leads to increasing mucosal oedema, and the formation of plugs of mucus within the bronchi, all of which obstruct the bronchi and lead to overdistension of the lungs (Corbin-West, 1992). A spontaneous pneumothorax can occur as a rare but serious complication. An asthmatic episode can be brought on by a range of factors, such as exposure to smoke and dust, exercise and cold air, pollen, spores, pets, house dust mites and in response to certain drugs (such as non-steroidal anti-inflammatory agents). The result is a reduced peak flow, breathlessness, the characteristic expiratory wheeze, hypoxia and understandable anxiety. Failure to respond to treatment leads to the severe condition of status asthmaticus.

3. *Anaphylaxis.* Although relatively rare, this condition is potentially fatal. It is a very complex phenomenon which is not yet fully understood, but can be simply described as an extreme over-reaction of the body's immune system to some provoking agent (antigen). The core of the process is the release of histamine and other chemical mediators as a result of degranulation of mast cells and basophils in the presence of newly formed antigen–antibody complexes (Henderson, 1998). A major study of anaphylaxis by the Project Team of the UK Resuscitation Council (1999) suggests that the term anaphylaxis be used to describe hypersensitivity reactions typically mediated by immunoglobulin E (IgE), while acknowledging that other serious reactions occur which do not depend upon hypersensitivity (anaphylactoid). In either case the presentation is similar, angio-oedema, urticaria, dyspnoea and hypotension. Cardiac collapse may occur leading to death. However, the Project Team points out that some patients may die from acute irreversible asthma or laryngeal oedema with few other symptoms.

4. *Acute on chronic bronchitis.* Acute infections in already chronically diseased lungs lead to very serious illness. The patient is often elderly and presents usually in winter.

5. *Pulmonary embolism (PE).* This occurs when a portion of thrombus in a systemic vein on the right side of the heart is dislodged into the circulation and lodges in either the main pulmonary artery (usually fatal) or a smaller artery. When a smaller artery is involved, a PE usually leads to an area of infarcted lung.

6. *Foreign body.* Small children are prone to inhaling all sorts of objects, some of which may lodge in the lower bronchial tree and cause serious chemical damage to lung tissue (e.g. a peanut) and/or areas of lung to collapse distally. Adults tend to come to A & E complaining of animal bones (e.g. fish or chicken bones) or other food being 'stuck in my throat'. Often they have swallowed the offending object but it has left a tear on the pharynx wall, which produces a sensation of an object being stuck.

7. *Smoke inhalation.* Modern synthetic materials contain substances which, when burnt, release toxic fumes (e.g. synthetic materials in carpets may release hydrogen cyanide and ammonia). This means that, in addition to possible burn injury, the patient may suffer serious respiratory impairment due to chemical lung damage or asphyxia from increased levels of carboxyhaemoglobin caused by carbon monoxide inhalation. During 1997 there were 749 deaths from CO poisoning, of which 108 were accidental (McParland, 1999). Although the large majority were suicides using car exhaust fumes, there is a real risk of accidental exposure, toxicity and death from defective household heating systems. Nobody may even suspect the nature of the problem as the patient presents in a drowsy, confused state with a history of nausea, vomiting, incoordination, dizziness, headaches and the signs of respiratory failure. Most victims of fires die as a result of inhalation injury rather than burns. Toxic fumes can also be inhaled in industrial accidents. Fumes can have systemic effects far beyond damage to the airways and lung tissues. For example, carbon monoxide, cyanide and hydrogen sulphide effect oxygen utilization throughout the body (Brownhill, 1997).

8. *Drowning.* Sea water is a hypertonic solution and therefore it exerts an osmotic pull, drawing fluid into the alveoli. Fresh water, on the other hand, is hypotonic and will readily diffuse into the blood through the alveolar wall. In doing so, however, the contaminants invariably contained in the water will destroy lung surfactant and the fluid will seep back into the alveoli. The result in either case is pulmonary oedema.

Of great significance in immersion injury victims is the time spent in the water and the temperature of the water. Hypothermia develops quickly leading to circulatory collapse. Immersion in cold water can produce serious cardiac arrhythmias, including bradycardia, which makes the patient appear lifeless upon rescue as there is no immediately palpable pulse or obvious respiratory effort. However, recovery is still possible. This is well documented in cases of persons falling through ice on frozen lakes.

9. *Hysterical hyperventilation.* Hysterical overbreathing disturbs the blood chemistry by blowing off large amounts of CO_2. This leads to an alkalosis and upsets the normal levels of serum calcium. The result is muscle spasm (tetany) which typically causes hyperextension of the fingers and abdominal pain (Fig. 5.7).

Assessment

Obtaining a history from a patient who is severely dyspnoeic is not easy. Those accompanying the patient, especially paramedics can often provide vital information concerning the person's previous medical history, such as whether they are a known asthmatic or have a severe allergy problem. If questions have to be asked of the patient, try to phrase them so that the answer is yes or no so that a nod of the head will suffice.

Assuming the primary survey reveals that the patient has a patent airway and is breath-ing, the rate and type of respiration should be observed together with the other vital signs.

A pulse oximeter probe should be attached to the patient's finger end as this provides vital information concerning the oxygen saturation of haemoglobin. Normal saturation levels are around 95–98%, but once this falls below 90% inadequate amounts of oxygen will be reaching body tissue and respiratory failure will be present (Woodrow, 1999). The pulse oximeter works by measuring the intensity of red and infrared light transmitted through the finger tip. It will only give meaningful and accurate readings in the absence of anything interfering with the passage of light, such as nail polish and if the patient has normal haemoglobin. When pulse oximeter readings are recorded, the nurse should also note whether the patient was on oxygen or not at the time and, if so, how much.

Wheezing indicates expiratory difficulty and is associated with asthma primarily, but may be found in other conditions, e.g. drowning and smoke inhalation. Stridor indicates difficulty on inspiration, often caused by a foreign body. The nurse should observe whether the breathing is easy or laboured and involving use of the accessory muscles of respiration (the shoulder girdle). As nurse practitioners develop in the A & E field, nurses are increasingly becoming competent in listening to breathing sounds with a stethoscope. The reader is referred to a more advanced text such as Walsh *et al.* (1999)

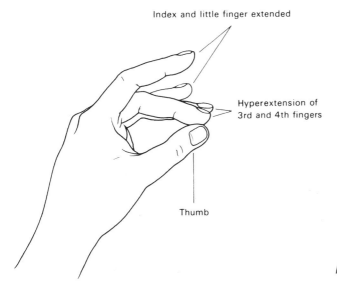

Index and little finger extended

Hyperextension of 3rd and 4th fingers

Thumb

Fig. 5.7 Carpo-pedal spasm

for details of this examination technique. A peak flow meter should be available as peak flows form a good guide to progress in treating asthmatic patients.

The following key points should be noted in assessing respiration:

• The longer the period of expiration the greater the degree of obstruction.
• A grey, sweating, dyspnoeic patient sitting upright is in grave danger of respiratory arrest.
• Respiratory rate does not equate with the degree of dyspnoea, it slows down as the patient becomes more tired with the effort of breathing.
• Dyspnoea in the elderly patient may be the only presenting sign of acute myocardial infarction (Corbin-West, 1992).

If the patient is Caucasian, observation of skin colour is a key step in assessment. A cold, clammy pale skin is frequently found in heart failure. Cyanosis, on the other hand, is a late sign and indicates severe respiratory failure. The pulse oximeter should have already alerted the nurse to the presence of respiratory failure. Inhalation of carbon monoxide (CO) allegedly produces a deceptively healthy pink skin due to the formation of large amounts of carboxyhaemoglobin, although McParland points out that in practice this is rarely seen (McParland, 1999).

Mental state must be assessed as respiratory distress is a very frightening experience and psychological support will be essential. Furthermore, confusion is an early sign of respiratory failure as it is due to cerebral hypoxia.

It is important to enquire if the patient has any pain and to obtain a description of it. Central chest pain requires treatment as for a cardiac problem, although it may be a pulmonary embolus that is causing the complaint. More generalized pain over one side of the chest, or extending around to the back, made worse by coughing or deep respiration, and of a sharp stabbing character, is caused by inflammation of the pleura and will be associated with acute infections such as pneumonia.

In examining the rest of the patient, the nurse should look for certain clues. The hands may reveal carpo-pedal spasm, typical of hysterical hyperventilation. Fingers may be nicotine-stained, indicating a heavy smoker who is prone to chronic chest infections. Alternatively, fingers may display the characteristic clubbing at the ends associated with long-standing pulmonary disease. Chronic obstructive airway disease produces a typical barrel-shaped or 'pigeon' chest. The legs should be examined for evidence of a deep vein thrombosis (DVT) that could have led to a pulmonary embolism. Are the calves the same size? Is there calf tenderness?

A specimen should be obtained of anything expectorated and whether it is blood stained or purulent should be noted.

The importance of a thorough assessment in cases of respiratory distress cannot be over-estimated. This is borne out by consideration of the following diagnostic criteria for severe and very severe life-threatening asthma, which are incorporated in best practice guidelines (Fig. 5.8).

Features of severe asthma

• Unable to speak a sentence in one breath
• Respiratory rate >25/minute
• Pulse rate >110/minute
• Peak flow <50% best known or predicted value, which can be determined from published tables based on gender, age and height.

Features of very severe life-threatening asthma

• Silent chest
• Cyanosis
• Poor respiratory effort
• Bradycardia or hypotension
• Exhaustion, confusion or coma
• Blood gases showing normal or high CO_2 tension (>5kPa), severe hypoxia despite O_2 therapy (<8kPa), low pH
• Peak flow <33% of normal or predicted value (Rees and Price, 1995).

Intervention

The patient should first be sat upright to help breathing and then high concentration oxygen should be administered. There is a theoretical problem if the patient has a long-standing history of respiratory disease. This relates to the fact that respiratory drive is normally stimulated by rising levels of CO_2 in the blood. However, in a patient with chronic respiratory

Asthma in accident and emergency departments

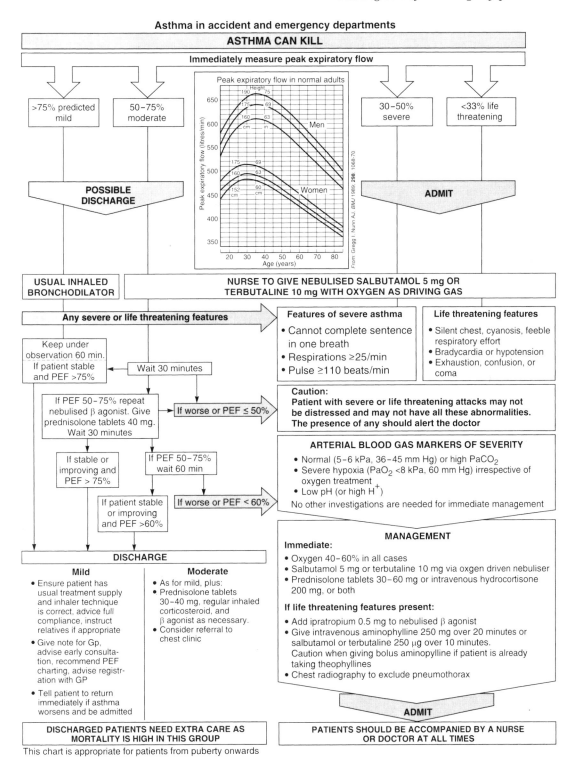

Fig. 5.8 Management of adult patient with asthma in A&E

disease, the body has adapted to high CO_2 levels and the respiratory drive, therefore, depends upon the secondary mechanism of low O_2 levels in the blood. Giving high concentration oxygen to such a patient may so increase arterial oxygen levels that the respiratory drive will be less effective and the patient's respiration become more shallow. Consequently, if assessment indicates the existence of a chronic respiratory disease, oxygen should only be administered in low concentrations such as 24% or 28%. This well-known theoretical risk is, however, of secondary importance if the patient is in severe respiratory distress with oxygen saturations of 90% or less. In such a serious situation (e.g. acute asthmatic) the patient is so hypoxic that only giving 24% oxygen will not be of any value. The lesser risk and greater benefit is to give the highest possible concentration of oxygen.

The patient who is confused because of cerebral hypoxia may not tolerate an oxygen mask. One solution is to use nasal oxygen cannulae or, as a temporary step, the nurse may hold the mask over the patient's face but without the mask touching the skin.

Psychological support is essential as the patient will be anxious and often very distressed. The nurse's own emotional behaviour will play a large part in determining the patient's (see p. 10). Particularly in conditions such as hyperventilation and to a lesser extent asthma, reducing anxiety will help to resolve the respiratory problem itself. The nurse always being visible and providing explanation of what is happening and why, will help the patient. Nothing could be worse than the acutely distressed patient, abandoned in a dark corridor, awaiting a chest X-ray, alone with the feeling that there is no way they can summon help if they need it. The presence of members of the family may have a beneficial effect on the patient's psychological status, and hence on the breathing. But it can also work the other way, especially when large numbers of people are involved or when certain key individuals are present with whom there is a relationship problem.

Frequent monitoring of vital signs is required, with the respirations deserving maximum attention. Pulse oximetry is essential in the management of patients in serious respiratory distress.

If confusion is present, precautions should be taken to prevent the patient from coming to harm; cot sides, close observation, and reality orientation, carried out at every opportunity, may all be necessary.

In cases of asthma the first line management, apart from high concentration oxygen and psychological support, is nebulized salbutamol 5 mg or terbutaline 10 mg given with oxygen as the driving gas. The minimum flow rate is 6 l/min as anything less than that will not produce droplets small enough to ensure rapid drug absorption through the lungs. If the nurse does not have access to a nebulizer, a combination of the patient's normal metered dose inhaler and a volumetric device will be a useful improvisation. The problem with the inhaler is that even with good technique only about 10% of a dose is actually absorbed, using a volumetric device can significantly increase this proportion. Recovery will be greatly expedited by a daily dose of 30–40 mg prednisolone and this should commence in A & E. The British Thoracic Society guidelines require oral steroids to be continued until the patient has no nocturnal disturbance, is able to carry out daily activities normally and has a peak flow measurement equal to their normal before the episode (Cross, 1997). This may take up to two weeks. Good communication between the A & E department and the patient's GP is essential for effective follow up. Intravenous hydrocortisone 200 mg may be given instead of or as well as, oral prednisolone. If the life-threatening features referred to above are present, ipratropium 0.5 mg should be added to the nebulizer and IV aminophylline, 250 mg administered over 20 minutes (see Fig. 5.8).

In cases of anaphylactic reaction, high concentration oxygen should also be given immediately without regard for any theoretical risks of chronic obstructive airways disease. The best position for the patient will be a compromise between lying flat with elevated legs for hypotension and sat upright to help breathing. Figs 5.9 and 5.10 show the recommended algorithms of the UK Resuscitation Council for managing anaphylaxis and attention is drawn to the intramuscular use of adrenaline, rather than IV.

Inhalation victims need particular attention to their airway because of the risk of mechanical occlusion due to oedema. High con-

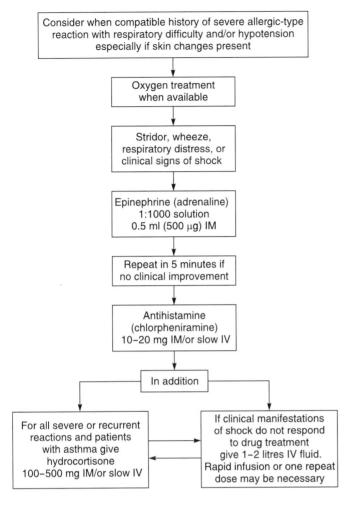

Consider when compatible history of severe allergic-type reaction with respiratory difficulty and/or hypotension especially if skin changes present

↓

Oxygen treatment when available

↓

Stridor, wheeze, respiratory distress, or clinical signs of shock

↓

Epinephrine (adrenaline) 1:1000 solution 0.5 ml (500 μg) IM

↓

Repeat in 5 minutes if no clinical improvement

↓

Antihistamine (chlorpheniramine) 10–20 mg IM/or slow IV

↓

In addition

For all severe or recurrent reactions and patients with asthma give hydrocortisone 100–500 mg IM/or slow IV

If clinical manifestations of shock do not respond to drug treatment give 1–2 litres IV fluid. Rapid infusion or one repeat dose may be necessary

Fig. 5.9 Anaphylactic reactions for adults; treatment by first medical responder. Source: Project Team of the UK Resuscitation Council (1999) Emergency treatment of anaphylactic reactions. Journal of Accident and Emergency Medicine*; **16**, 243–7*

centration oxygen is the key to their treatment in an attempt to restore normal blood gases and normalize their haemoglobin.

If a patient presents with hysterical hyperventilation, a useful approach is to ask the person to breathe in and out of a paper bag. The effect of this is to make them rebreathe their own CO_2 which will increase their CO_2 levels to normal, restore normal blood chemistry, and relieve the muscle spasm (tetany) that exacerbates the distressed state they are in. In many cases, it should be possible to have the patient breathing normally, without tetany, in 5–10 minutes.

Evaluation

Just because the patient is put in the correct position with the correct oxygen mask *in situ* does not mean that they are going to stay that way! They may remove the mask or slip down the trolley. Continual evaluation is essential to pick up these types of problems and to correct them. Some of the drugs given during respiratory distress are very potent, which makes it essential to watch patient progress closely; for example aminophylline and salbutamol can have cardiac side effects. ECG monitoring during the use of IV aminophylline is strongly recommended therefore. To take another example, if the patient has been given IV frusemide to combat pulmonary oedema, the nurse should think ahead to the likely diuresis that should ensue and record urinary output while being aware of the potential for acute urinary obstruction that might develop.

If a patient has been admitted with an acute asthmatic episode which has been successfully treated, it is important to talk with them about their asthma care. This is a good opportunity

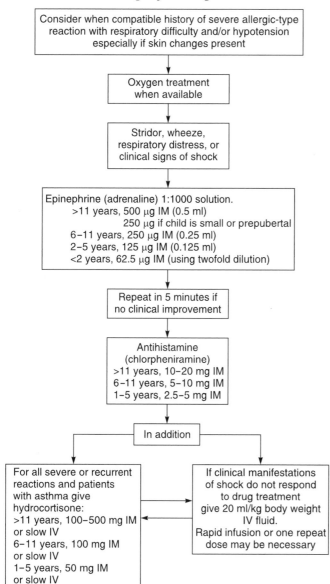

Fig. 5.10 Anaphylactic reactions for children; treatment by first medical responder. Source: Project Team of the UK Resuscitation Council (1999) Emergency treatment of anaphylactic reactions. Journal of Accident and Emergency Medicine; **16**, 243–7

to check their knowledge and assess their inhaler technique.

Care of the patient with impaired consciousness

Pathology

There are many reasons why a person's level of consciousness might be diminished. The following section concentrates on some of the more common causes of patients presenting at A & E with impaired consciousness with the exception of head injury and the effects of drugs and alcohol. Head injury has been dealt with already and drugs and alcohol will be discussed in Chapter 15. Neurological problems are the most obvious cause of an altered level of consciousness, although there are many metabolic disorders that can affect consciousness levels. An interesting perspective on the problem is offered in a survey carried out by Craig *et al.* (1997) who found that in one week at the Royal Victoria Hospital, Belfast, 8% of all patients presented with primary neurological symptoms (n=75). Most neurological presentations were 'out of hours' (75%). The three main symptoms were headaches (55%), altered level of consciousness (15%) and dizziness (10%). The key finding was that 27 of the patients were admitted, audit suggested, however, that only 17 of these patients should have been admitted. The researchers conclude that better training in neurology for A & E doctors or the provision of a neurological service in A & E, could make a significant reduction in inappropriate hospital admissions.

Common causes of presentation

1. *Cerebrovascular accident (CVA).* Stroke is the third most common cause of death in industrialized western countries and can be divided into two broad categories: ischaemic (70–80%) and haemorrhagic (approx 20%) stroke (Lott *et al.*, 1999). Ischaemic strokes are caused by occlusion of a cerebral artery due to embolism, thrombus formation and/or disease of the artery wall. The result is loss of blood to that part of the brain supplied by the blocked artery. A core of dead cerebral tissue results, which is surrounded by a damaged area of potentially salvageable tissue, the volume of which declines with the passage of time as more cells die. Haemorrhagic strokes are caused by rupture of a cerebral aneurysm or long-standing hypertension and are far more lethal, some 50% of patients die as a result of such an occurrence. Transient ischaemic attacks (TIA) are less serious events which produce a neurological deficit which resolves within 24 hours.

2. *Fits.* Fitting may be a sign of a range of pathological conditions, although there may also be no apparent cause of the fitting behaviour (idiopathic epilepsy). A fit is simply the manifestation of a paroxysmal electrical discharge within the brain. Fits may be focal, i.e. have a discrete point of origin within the brain or they may be generalized with the whole brain involved (Haslett *et al.*, 1999). The effect on the patient of either focal or generalized epilepsy may vary from a transient absence of awareness to full grand mal convulsion.

In grand mal epilepsy, the abnormal discharge of electricity first produces a characteristic aura if it is located near one of the sensory centres (e.g. smell, visual disturbance) and then proceeds to a tonic period of some 30 seconds or so when the musculature goes into spasm and the patient is, as a result, unable to breathe. This is followed by the clonic stage of convulsions which passes into a deep coma from which the patient gradually wakes up. At this stage, often referred to as the 'post-ictal stage', confusion is likely.

3. *Diabetes.* The most common presentation to A & E is hypoglycaemia. This is partly because it occurs more frequently than hyperglycaemia but also because it has a more rapid onset. However, diabetics who are maintained by oral hypoglycaemic medication alone (Type 2) tend to go 'hypo' more slowly than those who are insulin dependent (Type 1). Hyperglycaemia (diabetic ketoacidosis or DKA) often develops gradually over a 48-hour period in insulin-dependent patients. The other presentation to be aware of is the undiagnosed, non-insulin-dependent diabetic who presents in a non-ketotic hyperosmolar coma. Although rare, this carries a high mortality rate (Padmore, 1998).

The 'hypo' patient will have low blood glucose levels causing drowsiness, confusion or unconsciousness. As urine output has been normal, the patient will not be dehydrated or hypovolaemic. In hyperglycaemic states, the metabolism of fats leads to the formation of acid bodies known as ketones whose effects on the brain lead to unconsciousness and brain damage if this state (ketoacidosis) is not reversed. Ketoacidosis also causes nausea and vomiting. The body's efforts to excrete the excess glucose in the urine lead to dehydration, sodium depletion, hypovolaemic shock and electrolyte imbalance, all of which will be compounded by vomiting. The body seeks to correct the acidotic state by reducing CO_2 levels in the blood (CO_2 dissolves in water to form a weak acid). Hence the deep, sighing respirations characteristic of DKA. The usual cause of DKA is that for some reason the person has stopped taking their insulin. Patients must be advised to always keep taking their insulin, whatever else is wrong with them (Watkin, 1998).

4. *Acute infections and toxaemic states.* Any acute infection involving the brain, for example meningitis or encephalitis, will obviously affect the level of consciousness. Furthermore, any infection that leads to hypoxia (e.g. chest

infections) will diminish consciousness as will toxaemic states (e.g. uraemia).

Assessment

The first step must always be to assess airway, breathing and circulation, before moving on to assessing level of consciousness.

A history of the event, together with any relevant medical history, should be obtained. An epileptic fit may be described or the patient may be known as a diabetic. In undressing the patient, clues such as Medic-Alert bracelets, outpatient cards and injection sites should be searched for. Identification of the patient is essential, not only so that next of kin can be informed, but also so that hospital notes can be obtained.

Vital signs provide further information. The Type 1 diabetic in a DKA state is usually acidotic, dehydrated and hypovolaemic, therefore, deep sighing respirations, hypotension and tachycardia will be present. Capilliary blood glucose should be tested as this will reveal the presence of hypo- or hypergly-caemia. The stroke patient will often be hypertensive. Rapid respiratory rate will indicate hypoxia and pyrexia an infection. The patient may also be hypothermic if they have been in a cold environment for several hours with impaired consciousness. A core temperature below 35°C indicates hypothermia.

Limb weakness should be assessed for evidence of hemiplegia (or monoplegia). Plantar reflexes should be tested by stroking the outer soles of the feet with a sharp object. An abnormal upward curling of the toes indicates an upper motor neuron lesion such as a CVA or a post-epileptic state (Walsh *et al.*, 1999).

A urine specimen should be tested as the presence of glucose and ketones in the urine of a diabetic patient is strongly suggestive of ketoacidosis. A uraemic state will cause protein to appear in the urine.

Research by Ryan *et al.* (1998) suggests that many A & E departments are very poor at making and documenting vital signs and other key observations in patients with impaired consciousness. This study was based on an audit of 1200 sets of A & E notes and focused on epilepsy, but its conclusions about the need for accurate and standardized assessments may be extended to many other clinical conditions presenting as emergencies in A & E. Ryan *et al.* present a standardized pro forma document in their paper for the assessment of patients brought to A & E after a convulsion.

The medical assessment will include a detailed neurological exam, radiography and blood samples for culture and biochemistry. Recent developments in the treatment of ischaemic stroke with thrombolytic agents (recombinant tissue plasminogen activator (rt-PA) has recently been licensed for use in the USA) make it essential to discover as soon as possible whether the stroke is ischaemic or haemorrhagic in nature. Computed tomography scanning is the most reliable way to differentiate between the two possible causes at present (Roberts and Hughes, 1999). A good working relationship with the imaging department to allow rapid CT scanning is therefore essential to permit rapid diagnosis.

Intervention

The immediate interventions with regard to airway, breathing, circulation and unconsciousness have already been discussed. However, if the patient is conscious but confused, steps must be taken to protect the patient from potential harm. Cot sides should be set up and carefully checked. There should be continual nursing observation and, if necessary, the patient can be nursed on a mattress on the floor. Reality orientation is required with the nurse telling the patient what has happened, what time it is and where the patient is, in order that the patient may make some sense out of the situation. The information should be kept simple as consciousness is impaired.

By providing reality orientation, nurses can help the patient hang on to reality. Try to imagine waking up in totally unfamiliar surroundings, with complete strangers standing around, a gap of maybe several hours in your consciousness and your mental processes impaired by illness. You will then appreciate the importance of reality orientation as a nursing intervention.

Specific problems revealed by the assessment should be dealt with on their merits. Therefore, if the patient has had a fit, along with care of the patient in a confused post-ictal state, the possibility of the patient having a further fit should be considered. Observation is essential, with the aim of preventing accidental self-harm should a further fit occur. In such a situation, the patient is best left to get on with their fit, intervention being restricted to protecting the head if possible by using a blanket or pillow and by removing any objects that may harm the patient. The nurse should not attempt to restrain the patient or to force an airway into the mouth during either the tonic or clonic stages. This is dangerous and can lead to either the patient's teeth being knocked out or the nurse accidentally being bitten. Once the patient has stopped convulsing, he or she should be turned into the recovery position. The nurse should only then consider the use of an airway and then only if the patient tolerates it. Incontinence may occur due to relaxation of muscle sphincters at this stage. Therefore, the nurse must be prepared to clean the patient accordingly. If fitting is continuous and does not resolve after one attack, status epilepticus is said to be present. This serious condition requires urgent intervention to control the fitting and to prevent anoxic brain damage. This usually consists of intravenous diazepam. There is evidence of very wide variation in how A & E departments treat patients with admission rates varying from 34.6% to 91.7% for first seizures (Ryan *et al.*, 1998). This indicates the need for a more coordinated, evidence-based approach using clinical guidelines This need is emphasized by the fact that less than 1% of the cases reviewed by Ryan *et al.* showed any evidence of the question of driving being discussed with the patients.

The whole approach to stroke patients is undergoing a major change as it is being realized that vigorous early intervention and the introduction of stroke teams can greatly improve patient outcomes. The possibility of thrombolysis to treat ischaemic stroke is now being explored and in the USA where rt-PA therapy has been licensed, the aim is to have begun this treatment within 55 minutes of arrival at hospital and within 3 hours of the stroke beginning. Stroke teams and critical pathways have been developed by the emergency services (including ER) to identify those patients who might benefit from this therapy (Rapp, 1997). This work is based upon the NINDS trial which showed that patients treated with rt-PA were 30% more likely to have minimal or no deficit three months after their ischaemic stroke (NINDS, 1995). Health education campaigns aimed at increasing public awareness about the signs of stroke in order to cut the time lag between onset and admission should improve patient outcomes and could certainly be part of the A & E department's poster displays.

If assessment reveals that the patient is hypoglycaemic, and if the patient is able to drink, a glucose drink should be given immediately. As a guide, the following each contains 10 g of carbohydrate: 2 teaspoons of sugar, 60 ml of Lucozade, 90 ml of Coca Cola or 200 ml of milk (Watkin, 1998). A supply of Lucozade in the A & E fridge is therefore invaluable! If the patient cannot drink, IV dextrose 50% is given via a butterfly needle; 50 ml is usually sufficient to restore the patient to a normal level of consciousness. The cause of the 'hypo' should be discussed with the patient as prevention of future episodes should always be the goal. There are many complex reasons why a patient may have gone 'hypo', e.g. those who have had diabetes longest may have incurred neuropathic damage to the autonomic nervous system which means they are no longer aware of the early warning signs of a hypo (Padmore, 1998). Referral to a diabetic specialist nurse or the patient's own GP after a 'hypo' episode is an important step in ensuring good diabetic control for the future.

In a hyperglycaemic state, dehydration, acidosis and electrolyte imbalance need to be rapidly corrected with an IV infusion. A litre of 0.9% saline is usually given in the first hour with the aim being to give 2–2.5 l over the first 4 hours. Potassium supplements will be given depending upon serum potassium levels and 1.4% sodium bicarbonate may be administered IV if the patient is severely acidotic. Insulin is needed usually at 6 units/hour until blood glucose is within the 12–14 mmol/l range when a sliding scale is used, although by then the patient will have been admitted to a ward.

Hypothermia is best treated by gradual re-warming with warm drinks and the use of warmed blankets next to the skin. An extensive literature review by Chadwick and Gibson (1997) concluded that there was little convincing evidence in favour of continuing to use reflective metal space blankets for the treatment of hypothermia and recommended this practice cease. If a pyrexia of over 39°C is present, active steps, such as fanning must be taken to reduce the temperature. This is because if it rises to 40°C or above, fitting will often develop.

The possibility of an infection that could be transmitted to other patients in the department should be considered and the appropriate steps taken in line with hospital policy, paying particular attention to both careful hand washing and the use of universal precautions (e.g. disposal of waste and linen).

Care of the patient with abdominal pain

Pathology

The management of abdominal emergencies is described in surgical textbooks. It is, however, useful to present a brief table of the most common emergencies seen in A & E (Table 5.3). Patients who present with abdominal pain are usually self-referred, though some hospitals have a policy of seeing GP referrals in A & E. It is essential that the A & E nurse be able to prioritize such patients correctly.

Assessment

In order to decide upon the priority with which the patient will be seen, the nurse needs to determine the degree of pain the patient is in and the history of the illness and the associated pain. The vital signs are also essential in making this decision. Nurse practitioner training will equip the nurse with extra skills (such as the ability to palpate the abdomen correctly, listen for bowel sounds or carry out a rectal exam) which will make prioritization a more precise process. A rigid abdomen indicates peritonitis, a serious condition as perforation has occurred. A full bladder can readily be felt indicating retention of urine. A pulsatile mass in the midline is likely to be an aortic aneurysm.

In assessing the pain felt by the patient, nurses are in a very subjective area for, as already discussed, different people from different backgrounds interpret pain and illness in different ways. The PQRST approach to pain assessment referred to on p. 53 should be used. This will tell the nurse what provokes and/or palliates the pain, the quality of the pain (steady, gripping, or sharp), the region and where it radiates to, severity (rated on a 5-point scale) and how long the person has had the pain. Pains of an intermittent nature are

Table 5.3 Common causes of abdominal pain seen in A & E

System	Disease/disorder	Typical age	Comments
1. Gastro-intestinal	Indigestion	Young/middle age	Often presents as chest pain
	Alcoholic gastritis	Young/middle age	History of heavy alcohol intake
	Gastroenteritis	Young	Diarrhoea, risk of cross-infection
	Constipation	Any	Dietary advice needed
	Appendicitis	Young	Nausea and low grade pyrexia
	Peptic ulcer	Middle/elderly	Haematemesis and melaena. Peritonitis, rigid abdomen; shock if perforated
	Obstruction	Elderly	Possible cause of obstruction, cancer, adhesions, strangulated hernia
	Biliary colic	Young/middle age	Colic type of pain
2. Urinary	Renal/ureteric colic	Young/middle age	Colic type of pain, haematuria
	Cystitis	Young (female)	Need MSU and urinalysis
	Retention of urine	Elderly (male)	Palpable bladder, catheterize
3. Vascular	Aortic aneurysm	Elderly	Hypovolaemia, immediate surgery
	Saddle embolism	Elderly	Circulation to legs lost/impaired
	Mesenteric embolism	Any	Circulation to gut impaired

known as colic and indicate obstruction of the gut, ureter or bile duct (e.g. biliary or ureteric colic) while constant pain is typical of peritonitis and is generalized over the whole abdomen, indicating perforation has occurred. A more detailed discussion of the presentation of abdominal pain is found in Walsh *et al.* (1999).

In taking a history of the illness, the nurse should be checking for vomiting, the type of vomit – whether coffee grounds, fresh blood or bile – and any history of unusual bowel actions, such as diarrhoea, melaena or clay-coloured stools. Previous medical history should be noted as it may contain clues such as changing bowel habits and weight loss (carcinoma?), previous abdominal surgery (adhesions?), and episodes of similar pain relieved by eating (peptic ulceration?). Urine should be tested to exclude renal pathology.

The mental state of the patient, together with any social problems, should be assessed as urgent intervention may be needed. Sudden illness, pain and vomiting constitute a very stressful event for most people. Table 5.4 is not a rigid set of rules but rather a set of general guidelines. Each patient must be assessed in their own right as an individual.

Intervention

Pain relief is a major priority and this can initially be achieved with Entonox in many cases. Opioid analgesia should always be accompanied by antiemetic medication. An IV cannula should be sited as a precaution. Whatever the patient's pain levels, psychological support for both patient and family is required. The patient should be allowed to assume whatever position is the most comfortable for them.

Surgical intervention is frequently needed. Patients, therefore, should all be kept nil by mouth and, as far as possible, the correct hospital preoperative procedures with regard to matters such as consent, property and identification bands should be followed. Fear of surgery is to be expected and everything must be done to keep the patient and family informed of what is happening and why. This will help to reduce anxiety.

The surgical team will usually ask for IV fluids to be given and for plain abdominal radiographs. They may also ask for a nasogastric tube to be passed. Accurate fluid balance together with careful recording of stools is needed. The surgical emergency patient needs rapid admission to a ward and this, together with good pain relief, should be the aim of the A & E.

Evaluation

The degree of relief from pain and anxiety should be noted; further intervention may be needed. Continual monitoring of vital signs is needed to assess progress. It is important to check that the patient fully understands what has been said with regard to theatre, especially with elderly patients who will often nod in agreement to anything said by doctors without really understanding fully the implications. It is the responsibility of the nurse to check the degree of comprehension by the patient concerning future treatment plans.

Table 5.4 Nursing assessment of abdominal pain – important factors in prioritization

Medical Attention is Required		
Urgently	*Soon*	*Can wait*
BP less than 80 mmHg systolic	Coffee grounds vomit	BP 110 mmHg or more systolic
Severe constant abdominal pain	Melaena	Soft abdomen
Pulsatile abdominal mass	Palpable bladder	Normal stools
Cold leg(s)	Temperature over 38 °C	Constipation
No femoral pulse	Colicky pain	
Rigid abdomen	Haematuria	
No bowel sounds		
Haematemesis		

References

Baskett P (1993) *Resuscitation Handbook*, 2nd edn. London: Wolfe.

Brownhill R (1997) Toxic inhalation; nursing considerations. *Emergency Nurse*, 5: 2, 20–3.

Chadwick S, Gibson A (1997) Hypothermia and the use of space blankets: a literature review. *Accident and Emergency Nursing*, 5:122–5.

Corbin-West A (1992) The patient with bronchospasm: assessment, triage and teaching adjuncts. *Journal of Emergency Nursing*, **18**:6, 511–15.

Craig J, Patterson V, Rocke L, Jamison J (1997) Accident and emergency neurology; time for reappraisal? *Health Trends*, 29:3, 89–91.

Cross S (1997) The management of acute asthma. *Professional Nurse*, 12:7, 495–7.

Drever F, Whitehead M (1995) *Health Inequalities Decennial Supplement*. London: Office for National Statistics.

ERC – European Resuscitation Council Working Party (1997) Adult advanced cardiac life support: the European Resuscitation Council guidelines 1997. *BMJ*, **306**:1589–93.

Haslett C, Chilvers E, Hunter J, Boon N (1999) *Davidson's Principles and Practice of Medicine*, 18th edn. Edinburgh: Churchill Livingstone.

Henderson N (1998) Anaphylaxis. *Emergency Nurse*, **6**:3, 33–9.

Hood S, Birnie D, Swan L, Hillis W (1998) Questionnaire survey of thrombolytic treatment in A&E departments in the UK. *British Medical Journal*, **316**, 274.

Kloech W *et al*. The universal ALS algorithm. *Resuscitation*, 34:109–11.

Lott C, Hennes H, Dick W (1999) Stroke – a medical emergency. *Journal of Accident and Emergency Medicine*, 16:2–7.

McParland M (1999) Carbon monoxide poisoning. *Emergency Nurse*, 7: 6, 18–23.

National Statistical Office (1998a) *Mortality Statistics*. London: HMSO.

National Statistical Office (1998b) *Regional Trends 1998*, Vol 33. London: HMSO.

NINDS, The National Institute of Neurological Disorders and Stroke rt-PA Stroke Study Group (1995) Tissue plasminogen activator for acute ischaemic stroke. *New England Journal of Medicine*, 333: 1581–7.

Padmore E (1998) Predisposing factors in diabetic emergencies. *Accident and Emergency Nursing*, **6**:160–3.

Project Team of the UK Resuscitation Council (1999) Emergency medical treatment of anaphylactic reactions. *Journal of Accident and Emergency Medicine*, 16:243–7.

Quinn T (1999) Thrombolysis in Accident and Emergency; the exception not the rule. *Accident and Emergency Nursing*, 7:39–41.

Quinn T (1997) Assessment of the patient with chest pain in the A&E department. *Accident and Emergency Nursing*, 5:65–70.

Rapp K (1997) Code stroke: rapid transport, triage and treatment using rt-PA therapy. *Journal of Neuroscience Nursing*, 29:6, 361–6.

Rees J, Price J (1995) *ABC of Asthma*. London: BMJ.

Roberts M, Hughes G (1999) Recent advances in the acute management of ischaemic stroke. *Journal of Accident and Emergency Medicine*, **16**: 7–12.

Ryan J, Nash S, Lyndon J (1998) Epilepsy in the A&E department – developing a code of safe practice for adult patients. *Journal of Accident and Emergency Medicine*, 15:237–43.

Social Trends (1999) Vol 31. London: HMSO.

Thompson D, Webster P (1992) *Caring for the Coronary Patient*. Oxford: Butterworth-Heinemann.

Walsh M, Crumbie A, Reveley S (1999) *Nurse Practitioners; Clinical Skills and Professional Issues*. Oxford: Butterworth-Heinemann.

Watkin P (1998) *ABC of Diabetes*, 4th edn. London: BMJ.

Woodrow P (1999) Pulse oximetry. *Emergency Nurse*, 7:5, 34–9.

Zideman D (1990). AIDS, hepatitis and resuscitation. In Evans TR (ed.) *ABC of Resuscitation*. London: BMJ.

Nursing care of the injured patient

Chapter 6

FRACTURES AND DISLOCATIONS

Pathology – causes of fractures

Fractures are usually thought of as being due to trauma. This is not always the case, however, as repeated stress on a bone can lead to its fracture by a process similar to metal fatigue. Such a fracture is logically known as a stress fracture and is commonly seen in the foot (metatarsal) or the lower limb (fibula). Alternatively, bone can be so weakened by disease that it fails with little or no force involved. This is known as a pathological fracture and is seen, for example, where a tumour has led to secondary deposits in the bone (bony metastases).

Overall, however, the vast majority of fractures *are* due to trauma, and these are described as direct or indirect. In an indirect fracture, the break occurs at some point other than that where the force impacted against the bone; for example, a fall on an outstretched hand may lead to a fracture of the clavicle or wrist. Conversely, a direct fracture occurs when the bone breaks at the point of impact; thus, an over-the-ball-tackle in football leads to a fractured lower third of tibia and fibula.

Types of fracture

One very important distinction in considering fractures is whether or not the fracture is open or closed. If the fracture site is in direct contact with the outside environment, no matter how small the wound, it is an open fracture. The importance of this consideration stems from the risk of infection which can involve the bone, leading to the very serious condition of osteomyelitis.

Fracture types may be described according to the diagram in Fig. 6.1. Such a classification is important as the orthopaedic surgeon needs to know the mechanism of injury if the fracture is to be successfully reduced. This is because the logical way of reducing a fracture is to reverse the forces involved in the original injury.

Fractures and children

Children's bones have different properties that make fractures a special case when compared to fractures in adults. The much higher proportion of collagen fibres to calcium salts in children's bones means that the bones are less rigid. The result is the greenstick type of fracture where there is only an incomplete break and some cortical continuity remains. As bone growth is occurring at the epiphyseal cartilages located at either end of the bone, fractures involving this region are cause for special concern due to the risk of deformity from damage to the growing area. Such fractures are known as Salter's fractures and are graded I through V in order of seriousness.

Fracture healing

Fracture healing is a complex process that requires an infection-free environment, fracture immobilization and a good blood supply. Where possible the aim of management is to provide such a situation so that healing can occur conservatively. However, if it is felt that the nature of the fracture is such that this will not occur or that the hazards of lengthy immobilization are too great (e.g. in the cases of a pathological fracture or a fracture of the femur in an elderly person), then the surgeon may opt to fix the fracture internally by an operation.

The first step in healing is the formation of a haematoma at the fracture site (Fig. 6.2). The haematoma takes little active part in the

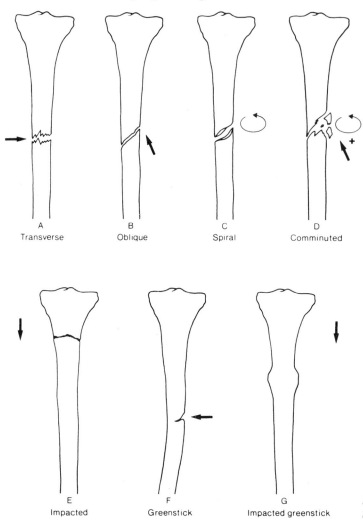

Fig. 6.1 Common patterns of fracture and associated forces

healing process and is quickly absorbed as cells from the deep surface of the periosteum divide and invade the haematoma. These cells are precursors of the osteoblasts, the cells that play an active part in the construction of new bone. The osteoblasts are responsible initially for the formation of callus, which is an immature matrix of collagen and polysaccharides that becomes impregnated with calcium salts and as a result is visible on X-rays. As the callus matures into bone, the final stage of healing occurs with another type of cell, the osteoclasts, helping to remodel the bone by stripping off the surplus bulge from around the fracture site and reopening the medullary canal.

Dislocations

When a joint is dislocated, by definition the two joint surfaces are so far displaced that there is no apposition between them. This dislocation also causes serious ligament and joint capsule damage. The term subluxation is used when there has been a partial dislocation, so that there is still some apposition of joint surfaces.

Complications of fractures and dislocations

If the fracture is open, the most feared complication is osteomyelitis. Gas gangrene

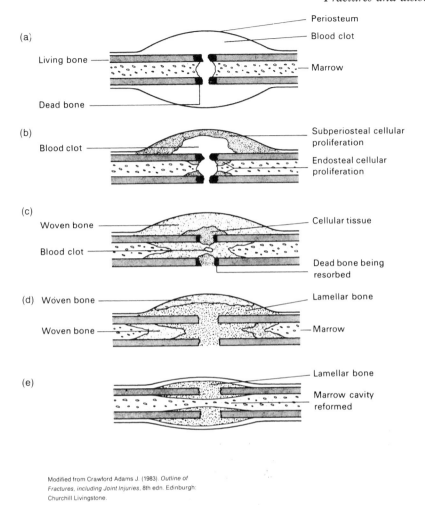

(a)
- Periosteum
- Blood clot
- Living bone
- Marrow
- Dead bone

(b)
- Blood clot
- Subperiosteal cellular proliferation
- Endosteal cellular proliferation

(c)
- Woven bone
- Cellular tissue
- Blood clot
- Dead bone being resorbed

(d) Woven bone
- Lamellar bone
- Woven bone
- Marrow

(e)
- Lamellar bone
- Marrow cavity reformed

Modified from Crawford Adams J. (1983). *Outline of Fractures, including Joint Injuries*, 8th edn. Edinburgh: Churchill Livingstone.

Fig. 6.2 Pathology of fractures and the healing of fractures. (a) Haematoma, with necrosis of the bone next to the fracture. (b) Subperiosteal and endosteal cell growth. The haematoma is absorbed. (c) Callus formation. The cells, osteoblasts, lay down intercellular substance which calcifies to form bone. (d) Consolidation. Osteoblasts lay down lamellar bone. The woven bone diminishes. (e) Remodelling. Along the lines of stress, the bone is strengthened. Elsewhere it is reabsorbed.

and tetanus are further major complications that are possible with a badly contaminated wound.

If there is pressure on a nerve or blood vessel due to the abnormal position of the bone or to tissue swelling, serious neurovascular complications can arise which, in extreme cases, can lead to the loss of the limb or to serious disability. Fracture above the humeral condyles can lead to the brachial artery being trapped, cutting off the blood supply to the forearm.

This is most often seen in children and leads to Volkmann's ischaemic contracture, a flexion deformity of the hand and wrist. Arterial damage in leg fractures can lead to amputation.

Bleeding from a fractured bone can cause hypovolaemic shock. One litre of blood may be lost from a mid-shaft fracture of the femur and two litres may be lost from fractures of the pelvis. In joint injuries, bleeding into a joint is called a haemarthrosis; such is the limited space within a joint capsule that the result can be a very tense painful joint indeed. If a fracture enters a joint, it is essential for the surgeon to seek as anatomically perfect a reduction as possible as any irregularity left in the joint will lead to the rapid development of osteoarthritis.

Assessment

The triage nurse will have to carry out a rapid assessment of the injured patient and should be looking for the cardinal sign of localized bony tenderness, i.e. pain upon palpating the fracture site. This sign is best elicited by gently feeling along the bone and watching the patient for discomfort associated with pressing a discrete area over a bone. Deformity of the limb may not be present if the fracture is undisplaced, therefore localized bony tenderness is *the* key sign.

Once the probability of a fracture being present has been assessed, the next step is to assess the amount of pain that the injury is causing the patient and the patient's understanding of the possible injury. Patient compliance with treatment will only be fully forthcoming if the patient understands fully the nature of the injury.

The neurovascular state of the limb should be assessed distal to the injury by feeling for a pulse, the location of which should be marked on the skin. Serious damage can occur if a blood vessel or nerve is involved in the fracture. Dykes (1993) recommends the 5 'P's of pain, pulses, paraesthesia, pallor and paralysis in assessing injured limbs. They should all be checked for distal to the fracture to ensure there are no signs of neurovascular damage. Any wound present should be examined with the possibility of an open fracture borne in mind.

Patient assessment should not be confined to the one limb where there may be an obvious fracture. If there has been sufficient force to break one bone, there may be other less obvious injuries as well, including fractures of other limbs. The type of accident therefore has a major role in determining the risk of further injuries. Vital signs should be recorded to give a baseline from which any deviation indicative of hypovolaemic shock may be detected. The blood loss from fractures alone may cause this condition, in addition to which there is the possible loss of blood from soft tissue injury. As a rule of thumb, an open fracture has twice the blood loss of a closed one. Once adequate analgesia has been given based on the patient's pain score, the affected limb should be immobilized in the best position possible. A range of splintage devices is available such as the box splint which may be used for a tibial fracture. Local anaesthetic blocks should also be thought of as a way to reduce the pain and discomfort.

The psychological and social status of the patient should not be overlooked. This is of great importance in dealing with the elderly because very often it is these factors rather than physical problems that determine management.

Similar considerations apply if the patient has a dislocated joint. Lack of normal joint movement, pain and deformity are the key signs that the nurse will find present upon assessment.

Intervention

Provided that there is no other life-threatening problem immediately identified, the first goal of intervention should be pain relief. The drug of choice is intravenous morphine dissolved in water for injection and titrated into the patient until adequate pain relief is obtained. Immobilization of the fracture will make a major contribution towards the goal of pain relief. Home-made or ambulance splints should be removed to allow adequate assessment of the limb (using Entonox as a supplement if required) and should be replaced with the most appropriate splint for the injury.

If there is a femoral shaft fracture, traction will be required. The traditional method was the use of the Thomas splint with skin traction to overcome the very strong pull of the thigh muscles and to immobilize the fracture. A more modern approach involves the use of traction splint systems (Donway or Hare splints) developed in the USA and Australia (Bache *et al.*, 1998). If these are correctly fitted by the pre-hospital personnel then they may need to stay *in situ* until the patient reaches the ward or theatre.

For fractures of the other long bones, traction is not required in A & E. Box splints are a convenient way of maintaining alignment of the limb. Other splints such as the vacuum splint can also be used to good effect. Such a system is far superior to old-fashioned methods involving bandaging the injured limb to a rigid splint. In the new system, the limb is surrounded by a bag containing plastic beads which, upon evacuation, collapses under atmospheric pressure to form a semi-rigid mould around the limb. The limb is not therefore under pressure, the splint is radiotranslucent and the limb is visible to allow continual observation of its vascular status. Furthermore, in application, the splints are far less painful for the patient (Greaves *et al.*, 1997).

The next step in relieving pain is to try to minimize swelling by elevation. Hand and wrist fractures should be in a high arm sling; fractures of the lower limb should be elevated by raising the foot of the trolley. Rings and other constricting jewelry should be removed at triage before swelling becomes a problem.

Movement of the injured limb should be minimized. The situation should not be allowed where successive doctors all want to look at the fracture, resulting in the splint being removed and reapplied several times. The use of an instant picture camera can be a good way of showing multiple personnel the injury without causing the patient further discomfort. Morphine should be given in acceptable doses via an intravenous cannula to reduce the pain.

Fear and anxiety will only increase the pain felt by the patient and tend to make for less cooperation. Clear explanation of what is happening and why, together with attention being paid to matters such as informing next of kin, will make a substantial contribution to pain control and the patient's well-being.

The pain of a dislocation may be partly relieved by supporting the limb, thereby removing any weight that the joint has to take. Psychological support and Entonox will also be useful for pain relief.

If the injury involves a wound, steps should be taken to wash out any gross contamination with a litre of normal saline immediately. A dressing should be applied, consisting of saline soaks and gauze pads soaked in iodine solution (e.g. Betadine). It may be assumed that the patient will be going to theatre soon; therefore, hospital protocols should be followed as for any patient going to theatre. Formal toilet and debridement in theatre is essential to prevent infection by washing out all traces of contamination and excising all dead or dubious tissue from the wound.

If a fracture is displaced or a joint dislocated, manipulation is required to restore the normal anatomical position of the bones involved. This is frequently undertaken in the A & E department. As nursing assistance will be required, the nurse needs to know something of the procedures which may be carried out.

Gross fracture dislocations of the ankle (e.g. the foot rotated at 90° relative to the tibia) require immediate reduction under morphine by disimpacting the fracture and rotating the foot back to the normal position. If reduction is not immediate, serious neurovascular damage will result. This is a first priority *before* X-ray. Severe injuries of the lower part of the leg in particular may require amputation and, as Clarke and Mollon (1994) have shown, primary amputation results in discharge home in half the time compared to patients where amputation is delayed (mean time in hospital of 24.3 and 49.8 days, respectively). Criteria for primary amputation are discussed by these authors and include complete disruption of the posterior tibial nerve, severe crush injury and serious associated multiple injuries.

The most commonly manipulated fracture in A & E is the Colles fracture using the Bier's block technique. A double cuff tourniquet is placed around the top of the arm which is then elevated to allow venous drainage before the cuff is pumped up to above arterial pressure as recorded by the attached pressure gauge. Local anaesthetic is then infiltrated into the arm via a butterfly, effectively anaesthetizing the whole forearm. The danger is that the anaesthetic drug may leak past the cuff if it deflates. If this occurs before the drug has been bound and rendered inert by plasma proteins, a serious and possibly fatal reaction may occur. For this reason lignocaine and Marcaine are no longer used, the safer prilocaine being preferred. Even with this safer drug, however, the cuff must remain inflated for at least 20 minutes. It is essential that a nurse stays with the patient throughout the manipulation and check X-ray stage, observing the cuff pressure gauge to ensure there is no leak, and observing the patient. Research has demonstrated that there is no difference in complication rates between units that fast patients prior to a Bier's block

	0–5 min	6–20/30 min	20/30–75 min
Documentation	Registration as A & E patient	A & E notes ready for CO	Admission referral form complete
Assessment	Triage nurse, check appearance and function, localized bony tenderness, pain, signs of neurovascular compromise	BP RR P CO exam patient Send to XR. Check for other injuries or medical conditions When did last eat or drink?	Is patient fit to be discharged? Check neuro-vascular status of limb distal to POP. Patient under-standing of POP care? Check XR if MUA
Medication	–	Opioid analgesia	Prn analgesia
Treatment	–	Consent for MUA if needed Set up IV if risk of hypovolaemia Dressing if open # Check Tet Tox status	MUA and/or POP or traction if # shaft femur
Nursing care	Remove splintage to allow exam. of limb. Psych support, NBM	Immobilize injury Monitor pain and neurovascular status of limb Remove constrictions such as rings. Cont. NBM, Psych support Explain procedures	Assist MUA/POP Teach POP/crutches care. Inform wd or make discharge arrangements. Role as patient advocate
Referrals	–	–	Orthopaedic-trauma team. Ward or follow up clinic, GP/ Dist. Nurse?
Family	Inform if not present	Stay with patient in cubicle, keep informed	Keep informed Can they cope if discharged?
Discharge	–	–	Wd/OPD

NB. Times are variable depending upon severity of injury and whether patient is to be admitted or discharged.
MUA = Manipulation Under Anaesthetic; POP = Plaster of Paris

Fig. 6.3 Example of critical pathway for patient with fracture or dislocation of limb

and those that do not and where complications did occur, they were unrelated to vomiting or the airway (O'Sullivan *et al.*, 1996). The practice of fasting patients as a precaution prior to Bier's block is unnecessary and therefore should be abandoned according to O'Sullivan *et al.* (1996).

Another common manipulation carried out in A & E is for dislocated shoulders. This technique involves the administration of an intravenous muscle relaxant and an opioid analgesic before manipulation. The patient is, therefore, not anaesthetized, but will be very drowsy. There is a significant hazard of respiratory depression so close nursing observation is required in the post-manipulation period.

See summary boxes (pp. 85–8) for brief descriptions of some of the more common fracture and dislocation injuries seen in A & E.

After the fracture has been successfully manipulated (if necessary) and immobilized in plaster of Paris (see Chapter 7), the nurse must consider the problems associated with discharge. These include transportation to home, a follow-up appointment (usually the following day to check the plaster), whether the patient fully understands how to use crutches and/or what precautions need to be taken with the plaster, and finally, whether the patient can cope. In dealing with the elderly, especially those who live alone, it is often the case that the fall that brought about the current injury was the final episode in a steadily deteriorating situation. The A & E nurse must therefore carefully assess the patient's ability to cope at home and if there is any doubt, discuss the matter further with the multidisciplinary team, in order to mobilize fully the community support or explore the possibility of admission to a care of the elderly ward.

If the patient is being admitted because of the fracture, preparation for theatre in accordance with local hospital procedures is required. In addition, an intravenous infusion is mandatory for fractures of the femoral shaft to prevent hypovolaemic shock. Fractures of the neck of femur, however, bleed very little and do not require an IVI to prevent hypovolaemia, although one may be erected to ensure adequate hydration of the patient in the preoperative phase.

Elderly patients with fractures of the femur have a very high risk of developing pressure sores. It seems that the causes are largely to be found outside trauma wards in the form of hard A & E, theatre or X-ray trolleys, where elderly patients lie immobile for hours on end. Turning such a patient in A & E is impractical. However, Spenco mattresses are available in sizes which fit trolleys and at least one such mattress should be available in A & E. Every effort should be made to transfer the patient to a ward bed where pressure area care may be instituted as rapidly as possible. This can be carried out by the use of nurse-led care pathways, sometimes referred to as fast tracks, which remove the need for patients to lie on trolleys in A & E for long periods of time.

Evaluation

The effectiveness of pain-relieving intervention should be continually checked, together with the neurovascular status of the limb. Although a limb has been elevated to reduce swelling, it should not be assumed that it will stay that way. Slings can slip and pillows can mysteriously vanish from under legs. Similarly, splinting should be checked at periodic intervals to ensure that it is still functioning effectively.

In evaluating the effectiveness of instructions given to the patient about either plaster of Paris or the use of crutches (see Chapter 7), it is important that the patient be asked to demonstrate that they have learnt what has been taught. Therefore, the patient should be asked to repeat the plaster instructions to ensure they know what to look for and the patient should be observed walking with crutches. It is not what has been taught that is important, but what has been learnt, and the only way to evaluate patient instruction is to assess what has been learnt.

If the patient is experiencing a minimum amount of pain and anxiety, if their injured limb is safely immobilized, and if its neurovascular status is secure, then the nursing intervention can be evaluated as successful.

Summary boxes for common injuries

Lower leg injury

Fractured lower tibia/fibula
Cause: Lateral force. Treatment: If it is displaced, manipulation under anaesthetic (MUA), POP cylinder, NWB will be called for. In an open fracture, wound debridement will be necessary. If undisplaced, a full-leg NWB, POP backslab will be necessary. Prone to non-union, usual risks if open.

Foot injuries

1. Fracture or dislocation of toes
Cause: 'Stubbed toe'. Treatment: Ring block and reduce if needed, strap to neighbouring digit for support with gauze padding. Watch out for swelling.

2. Metatarsal fractures
Cause: Heavy weight falls on foot or motorbike RTA. Treatment: Elevate foot, crutches, non-weight bearing (NWB), rest. Watch out for swelling and neurovascular damage.

3. Fractured calcaneum
Cause: Fall on to heel, usually from a height. Treatment: Immediate elevation, ice packs, NWB, rest. Watch out for associated injuries of the lower spine and swelling/neurovascular damage of the foot itself.

Wrist injuries

1. Fractured scaphoid
Cause: Fall on to palm of hand, usually in young adult. Treatment: Fracture often does not show on first X-ray, but if there is localized bony tenderness in 'snuff box', treat as fracture with POP to include base of thumb. Untreated, risk of osteoarthritis.

2. Fractured base of thumb (Bennett's fracture)
Cause: Longitudinal force, e.g. boxing. Treatment: Involves the joint, therefore, needs perfect reduction (possible internal fixation) to avoid osteoarthritis. POP to include interphalangeal joint.

Ankle injuries

1. Fractures of medial and/or lateral malleoli with or without ligament rupture with displacement of talus
Cause: Rotation and/or abduction or adduction, e.g. twisted foot while falling. Treatment: Simple fracture of malleolus requires a POP backslab, complete NWB for 24 hours, crutches. If ligaments are ruptured, internal fixation with screws will be necessary when swelling permits. Backslab and elevation meanwhile.

2. Trimalleolar fracture
Cause: Vertical compression, e.g. fall. Joint completely disrupted with posterior part of tibia fractured. Treatment: Internal fixation. Risk of osteoarthritis due to joint surface damage.

3. Fracture-dislocation of ankle (open)
Cause: Severe rotational force. Treatment: Immediate reduction under Entonox due to neurovascular compromise. Toilet/debridement, internal fixation. Risk of osteomyelitis, osteoarthritis, gas gangrene.

Forearm fractures

1. Fractured distal radius with posterior displacement (Colles fracture, see Fig. 6.4)
Cause: Fall on outstretched hand, elderly. Displacement requires correction by disimpaction, anterior manipulation and placing hand in ulnar deviation. POP backslab and sling, complete POP applied at 24 hours.

2. As above with anterior displacement (Smith's fracture)
Cause: Fall on hand in flexed position. Treatment: Manipulate as above with posterior manipulation. However, a POP which includes the elbow is necessary due to high risk of fracture re-displacing. Likely to need internal fixation.

3. Fractured mid-shaft radius and ulna (see Fig. 6.5)
Cause: High energy injury, often seen in children as a greenstick fracture. Treatment: Manipulation needed under GA for children, then POP. In adults, often internally fixed.

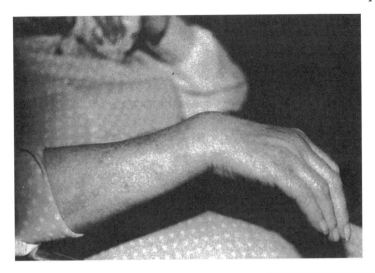

Fig. 6.4 Colles fracture

Injuries involving the shoulder

1. Dislocated shoulder
Cause: Fall on outstretched hand, usually anterior dislocation. Treatment: Reduce under IV muscle relaxant and opioid in A & E. Use Kocher method – apply traction along humerus with elbow bent at 90°, rotate arm laterally, carry elbow across body to midline, rotate arm so that hand falls to opposite side of chest. Alternatively pull along humerus with counter-traction in axilla.

2. Fractured clavicle
Cause: Fall on hand. Treatment: Conservative – with sling to support arm. Watch out for pressure on skin from bone ends.

Knee injuries

1. Fracture of the tibial plateau
Cause: Blow from the side, rotating femur on to lateral tibial condyle, e.g. car bumper hitting pedestrian. Treatment: After aspiration of haemarthrosis, POP, NWB. Osteoarthritis is long-term problem.

2. Fracture of patella
Cause: Direct blow. Treatment: If badly comminuted, patella is excised. If single fracture line, the two halves can be wired together.

3. Dislocation of patella
Cause: Flexion of knee. Patella always displaces laterally. The knee is held flexed. Treatment: Easily reduced under Entonox/IV diazepam. POP backslab.

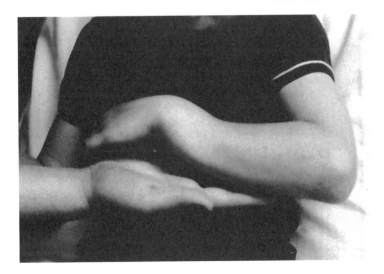

Fig. 6.5 Fracture of radius and ulna in 7-year-old boy

Hand injuries

1. Fracture or dislocation of digit
Cause: Direct blow. Treatment: Strap to neighbouring digit for support with gauze padding between. Encourage mobility. High arm sling for swelling.

2. Fractured metacarpal
Cause: Punching, usually fifth metacarpal. Treatment: If angulated, needs reduction and immobilization in volar slab in Edinburgh position, i.e. fingers extended and wrist cocked back. High arm sling.

Injuries to the thigh and hip

1. Fractured shaft of femur
Cause: High energy injury in young, pathological in elderly. Treatment: Traction to immobilize. IVI to prevent shock.
   Usually theatre for internal fixation.

2. Fractured neck of femur (or trochanteric region)
Cause: Usually in elderly to very elderly a minor fall, or pathological due to osteoporosis. Leg shortened and externally rotated. Treatment: Requires internal fixation within 24–48 hours. Major social and psychological problems.

3. Dislocation of hip
Cause: High energy injury. Leg shortened and internally rotated. May be driven through acetabulum in central dislocation leading to long-term problems with osteoarthritis. Treatment: Reduction under GA in theatre.

4. Fracture of pelvis
Cause: In the elderly, usually due to a fall causing fracture of pubic rami; in young people, due to a high energy injury with fracture of pubic ring in two places. Blood loss up to 2 litres. Treatment: IVI urgent, risk of ruptured bladder or torn urethra. In the elderly, should be treated with bed rest. Major injury – requires pelvic sling or external fixation.

References

Adams J C (1983) *Outline of Fractures*, 8th edn. Edinburgh: Churchill Livingstone.

Bache J, Armitt C, Gadd C (1998) *Practical Procedures in the Emergency Department*. London: CV Mosby.

Clarke P, Mollon R (1994) The criteria for amputation in severe lower limb injury. *Injury*, **25**:3, 139–43.

Dykes P (1993) Minding the 5ps of neurovascular assessment. *American Journal of Nursing*, June, 38–9.

Greaves I, Porter K, Burke D (1997) *Key Topics in Trauma*. Oxford: Bios Medical Press.

O'Sullivan I, Brooks S, Maryosh J (1996) Is fasting necessary before Bier's block? *Journal of Accident and Emergency Medicine*, **13**:105–7.

Chapter 7

PLASTER OF PARIS APPLICATION

Introduction

Plaster of Paris is the most convenient and cost effective way of immobilizing a fracture in A & E. The plaster of Paris cast (POP) is an old, tried-and-trusted, effective and relatively cheap option compared to the modern synthetic casts. Most injuries seen within A & E will need to be referred to a specialist clinic within 24 hours, therefore POP casts are applied to immobilize the fracture in a good position in the meanwhile. The cast will also give good pain relief by immobilizing the fracture. In more serious fractures which require definitive treatment at the first attendance, a POP may be applied to maintain a stable position while the patient is awaiting orthopaedic care. To prevent complications from the swelling of an affected limb, 'backslabs' are used within A & E. The cast is only half completed and then bandaged into place, allowing room for swelling to occur without the compression that would take place if the limb were contained within a complete cast (see p. 91). The patient will return to a clinic to have the cast completed when the risk of swelling is past, usually 24 hours later.

Basic principles

Plaster of Paris consists of hemihydrated calcium sulphate which is impregnated into bandage. Immersion in water causes an exothermic reaction to occur – heat is given off – as the hemihydrated calcium sulphate turns to hydrated calcium sulphate which sets to form the hard plaster cast. During the dry phase a small amount of constriction within the bandage occurs. If the limb also becomes swollen, a limb-threatening neurovascular problem can occur. Basic principles need to be observed when applying a plaster of Paris cast to avoid

this risk. The following considerations will allow the safe application of a cast.

Adequate padding of the limb

A POP is very hard both on the inside and on the outside, once dry. Therefore, unless it is well padded, there are potential problems for the skin. In particular, abrasion of the skin surface from the cast will cause the formation of broken areas leading to pressure sores or an infected wound. There should be a layer of an elasticated tubular bandage (stockinet) next to the skin, overlaid by one of the proprietary padded bandages that are available for this purpose. Particular attention should be paid to padding bony prominences such as the ulnar styloid and the head of the fibula. The padding should extend above and below the plaster so that it may be turned back over the ends of the POP, preventing skin friction by the plaster edges.

Water temperature

Water temperature determines setting time: the cooler the water, the longer the plaster takes to set. The nurse who is learning the techniques of plastering is, therefore, recommended always to use cold water, remembering to ensure that the bandage has been properly soaked through in the water, with some of the excess gently squeezed out before application. The most common errors that occur are to do with the water temperature and the soaking of the cast. Differing makes of plaster will need to be soaked in differing ways, so always refer to the manufacturer's guidelines.

Movement during application

If there is any movement of a joint during the application or the initial setting phase, cracks will form within the POP which will seriously weaken the plaster and lead to its failure in the long term. Joints must be held perfectly still during the initial stage of setting.

Moulding

The plaster must be moulded to the shape of the limb in order to maximize comfort and support for the fracture. This means that speed is of the essence in applying the plaster. There must be time before it starts to harden for gentle moulding to be carried out. Any moulding of a plaster needs to be carried out using the palmar aspect of the hand and not the fingers. If your fingers are used, indentations occur in the plaster leading to discomfort for the patient and possible skin breakdown.

Constriction

Tissue swelling accompanies most fractures and ligament injuries. If the limb is encased in a tight plaster, there will be no room for expansion to occur. This will cause compression of the soft tissues in the limb, leading to pain and a significant risk of neurovascular damage.

There are two main precautions that are taken to prevent this situation from occurring. First, in fresh injuries only a half plaster is applied, i.e. a backslab that covers only half the limb but that will still immobilize the injury while leaving room for tissue swelling to occur. Second, the limb must be elevated to encourage tissue fluid to move, under gravity, away from the injured region. Coupled with these two steps should be observation of the limb for any changes in colour, warmth or sensation, in order to detect signs of neurovascular compromise as soon as possible.

Because of the hazards of tissue swelling, it is essential in applying plaster not to make the POP too tight. The plaster bandage should be rolled onto the limb rather than a length of bandage unwound and then wrapped around the limb as shown in Fig. 7.1. This latter technique will make for a plaster that is too tight. This should also be remembered in applying the outer bandage to a backslab.

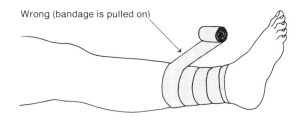

Wrong (bandage is pulled on)

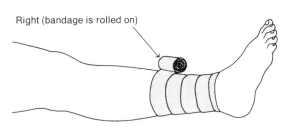

Right (bandage is rolled on)

Fig. 7.1 The incorrect and the correct method of application of plaster bandage

Limb positioning

Once plastered, joints will remain in the same position for up to several weeks. It is essential, therefore, that they be plastered in the correct position. In the lower limb, the ankle should be at a near perfect right angle as the patient's pain and discomfort will tolerate. There should always be some 10° of flexion in the knee. In the upper limb, the usual position for the elbow is at 90° with the palm of the hand facing the body if the whole arm is to be immobilized. If the hand is to be placed in plaster (usually for a fractured metacarpal that has been manipulated), the position that should be adopted is the one shown in Fig. 7.2. If you are unable to attain the correct anatomical position you should ensure clear documentation on the A & E card showing what angle you achieved.

Complete setting time

The plaster may seem very hard after some 5–10 minutes. However, it does take 24–48 hours to set fully, depending on the amount of plaster used. This must be explained to the patient. If it is a leg plaster, no weight must be

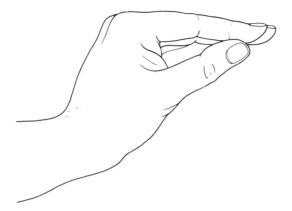

Fig. 7.2 Correct position for immobilization of the hand

allowed on the plaster until the patient has seen the specialist clinic. Crutches must be provided together with instruction and demonstration on how to use them (see end of chapter). Clothes should not be worn over a freshly applied POP as this will delay setting by interfering with the drying process. Nor should a patient try any artificial drying methods such as hair dryers or sitting in front of the fire. This will cause cracking of the plaster and potential burns due to radiation heat.

Patient education

It is important for the patient to understand and participate in the care of their plaster. Advice from the nurse on helping to live with a plaster needs to be given verbally and reinforced in writing. Elevation of any limb is paramount, as is rest. If the limb involved is an upper one, then a high arm or broad arm sling should be used for the first 24 hours to prevent swelling of the hand. If a lower limb, then the patient needs to be encouraged to elevate the limb as high as the hip so that venous return can occur. Simple ankle exercises if the ankle is not encased in plaster need to be encouraged every hour. If the ankle is involved then the toes should be moved with the same frequency. With lower limb injuries crutches should be encouraged to be used all the time so that the cast will not become damaged through weight bearing.

Plaster of Paris backslabs

In most injuries seen within A & E a backslab is usually applied to allow room for swelling and to facilitate easy removal of the plaster if required. It consists of a slab of several layers of plaster bandage, cut to the required length and shape, and applied over a well-padded limb. It is bandaged in place while still wet by an open-weave cotton conforming bandage. The end of the bandage is secured with a further piece of plaster sticking it down to the plaster underneath, but not to the open padding as this would effectively be completing the plaster.

Plaster casts for arm injuries
Colles cast

This type of cast will immobilize the wrist, but not the thumb. It is used for fractures of the distal radius. It should extend from just below the elbow to the metacarpophalangeal joints, leaving those joints free with a full range of movement. The thumb should be able to touch any of the fingers and the patient should have a reasonable grip. On the inner or palm-side of the wrist and hand (volar aspect), the plaster should extend no further than the proximal palmar crease. If the fracture has been manipulated, the position should be one of ulnar deviation and flexion. Differing ways of applying the cast exist and you should refer to your department guidelines.

Scaphoid cast

Scaphoid fractures are exceptions to the rule about swelling, for there is usually very little associated with this injury. They can, therefore, go directly into a complete cast. Scaphoid fractures are notorious for not showing up on X-ray, but if the correct clinical finding of localized bony tenderness is noted over the scaphoid, the wrist should be plastered anyway. Very often the fracture will show on the second X-ray taken a week to 10 days later, even though it did not show on the first. The importance of treating clinical signs is shown by Brown (1995). He looked at a sample of 36 consecutive patients where there were clinical signs of a fractured scaphoid but the radiographs were clear. He demonstrated by radio-isotope bone scanning techniques that there were 18 fractures present in this group, but only three were of the scaphoid, the rest were mostly involving other carpal bones or the distal radius. Recent discussion suggests that an MRI scan should be carried out within a few days of injury to establish whether a fracture has occurred or not. However, this pathway of treatment will be limited to hospitals with this resource.

The scaphoid cast is similar to the Colles cast, except that it immobilizes the base of the thumb (the first metacarpophalangeal joint – mcp) and should leave the interphalangeal joint of the digit free. A fracture through the base of the thumb involving the mcp joint is called a Bennett's fracture and requires the interphalangeal joint to be included in the plaster.

Padding is therefore required around the thumb as well as the rest of the wrist and forearm. The plaster should be started with a 7.5 cm bandage turned twice around the proximal portion of the metacarpals before being taken twice around the base of the thumb, and completed with a 15 cm bandage. The patient should be able to touch finger tips with thumb when the scaphoid cast is complete (Fig. 7.3).

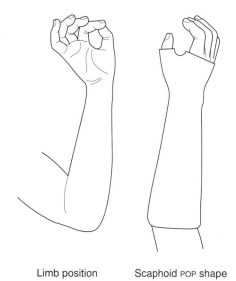

Limb position   Scaphoid POP shape

Fig. 7.3 Application of a scaphoid pop

Full arm plasters

If the elbow is to be immobilized, the plaster will need to extend to the top of the upper arm. Particular attention should be paid to the area of the brachial artery to ensure there is no constriction in this region. Care should also be taken that the plaster is not causing discomfort under the axilla. It is usual to plaster the elbow at 90° with the palm of the hand facing the body. The wrist may be left out of the cast or included, depending on the injury. For example, if a Smith's fracture of the wrist (see page 86) is to be treated conservatively, it is typically done so in a plaster that will immobilize the elbow as well as the wrist. This is due to the risk of the fracture slipping if the forearm is allowed to rotate, a movement that occurs at the elbow. However, a supracondylar fracture of the humerus can be treated by leaving the wrist joint free, outside the plaster (Fig. 7.4).

Plaster casts for leg injuries

Below knee plasters

For a simple below knee plaster, a 15 cm bandage should be used. Most commonly three sides are needed to make a secure cast. One slab for the medial side, one for the lateral and one for the posterior aspect of the leg. This slab should run from the head of the metatarsals up the calf until it is level with the head of the fibula. You should ensure that the patient can bend the knee without rubbing or obstruction. The two side slabs should overlap at the back allowing space at the anterior aspect of the leg, so that swelling cannot occur (Fig. 7.5). One trick is, if you are working on your own, to ask the patient to lie on their front with the leg bent at the knee. The ankle will then fall naturally into a near 90 degree angle. The effects of gravity will also help keep the slabs on for you.

Long leg cylinders

A long leg cylinder is usually applied for fractures of the tibia and fibula or injuries involving the knee. This cast will take a minimum of two people to apply, one to help support the patient, the second to apply the cast. It should extend from just above the

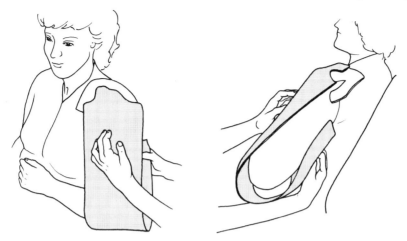

Fig. 7.4 Hanging U slab for humerus fracture

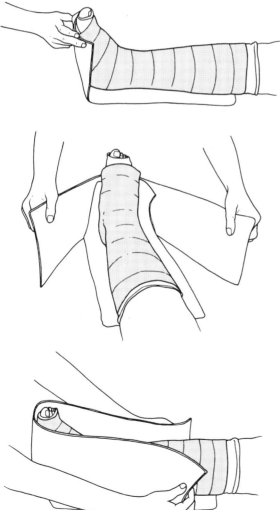

Fig. 7.5 Backslab for ankle/foot injuries

malleoli to the top of the thigh. Flexion of the knee should be allowed of about 5–10°. This will prevent knee stiffness and discomfort. A useful tip is for the nurse holding the limb to encourage the patient to move towards the end of the trolley. The nurse then stands at the end of the trolley with the patient's foot pushed into their chest or abdomen. This pressure will allow the knee to flex to the given degrees needed, you can also support the calf from this position and you are out of the way of the nurse completing the plaster. Within A & E, a backslab may be utilized or, if it is a more chronic problem, then a full cast may be needed. Some operators will use a backslab approach and build on that, others will go ahead and apply the plaster as normal practice. One problem with this cast is that they drop down the patient's leg slightly and rub on the malleolus. This is due to the reduction of swelling that occurs over time. To avoid this problem, place a piece of felt padding over the malleolus and incorporate it into the plaster (Fig. 7.6). This gives extra padding and prevents the cast from dropping. With this cast you also need to ensure adequate plaster is placed around the upper thigh. This is difficult to do but it will otherwise breakdown very quickly once the patient gets home and starts sitting on chairs or toilet seats.

Synthetic casting materials

A variety of synthetic casting materials have become available as alternatives to POP. They are more expensive but have the great advantage of setting very quickly. Thus, an elderly person having a below knee cast for an ankle injury will find it very difficult to be non-weight-bearing on crutches for 48 hours while the POP sets. However, a synthetic cast will set hard for weight-bearing purposes in a fraction of that time, allowing patients to retain their independence and self-care ability. They are, however, rarely used within A & E as most patients are reviewed at a fracture clinic within 24 hours. They are therefore not cost effective in A & E. Backslabs are also more difficult to make using synthetic materials, although more customized 'slabs' are becoming available for this specific use. We may also see a reduction in their cost.

Discharging the patient with a plaster of Paris cast

Two key elements exist when discharging a patient with a cast *in situ*: discharge planning and patient education. It is obvious for a wrist fracture of the dominant hand that a 70-year-old person may encounter different problems to a 16 year old. An individual assessment of the patient's home circumstances is essential. If necessary, community discharge teams that contain physiotherapists and/or occupational therapists as well as social services need to be involved as soon as possible if the patient is being discharged out of 'office hours'. Gone are the days when patients can be admitted overnight to be assessed the following day. If a lower limb is injured, careful consideration should be given to whether the person can manage any stairs that may be at home. This applies to both the young and elderly. The biggest cause of accidental death is falls in the patient's own home. Your cast and discharge planning should help prevent this from happening, not encourage it.

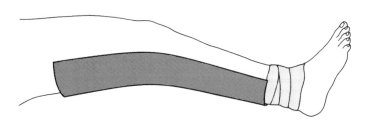

2 × 20 cm backslabs overlapping at the back of the leg. Finish above the ankle which must be well padded. Knee flexed at 10°.

Fig. 7.6 Backslab for knee injuries

Patient teaching and POP casts

It is essential to explain the common complications of living with a cast, not only for the first 48 hours but in the longer term as well. Discussion on pain relief is important so that the person can mobilize within their new restrictions. Exercises should be encouraged to keep all other joints moving. For example, a patient with a Colles fracture should be encouraged to comb their hair in order to keep the shoulder joint mobile. The patient must be taught about the potential problem of constriction as the cast dries. Observation of the limb for discoloration of the extremities, together with being aware of altered sensation and feeling ('pins and needles') need to be highlighted as a potential emergency. Immediate contact with the local NHS Direct number or A & E unit is vital. Elevation to encourage drainage of tissue fluid away from the injured limb under gravity is one of the simplest ways of avoiding this complication The high arm sling for upper limb injuries or elevation of the leg at hip height are effective preventative measures which should be encouraged. Aids to mobilization, such as crutches, need to be properly assessed to make sure they are in working order and clear instructions given to the patient on how to use them safely. Written advice with diagrams is best given to all patients. This will allow the patient to re-examine the information given to them and refer to it if they have problems at home before seeking further help. Diagrams are important as they allow people with reading difficulties, or for whom English is not their first language, to be able to cope with a plaster safely.

Crutches

Two fundamental types of crutches exist; these are axillary crutches and below elbow crutches. Most departments have a selection of both. The below elbow crutches, which are made of metal were originally used for partial weight-bearing patients, whereas the wooden axillary crutches were made for non-weight bearing. Many emergency units now use one type for both situations.

With both sets of crutches it is essential that they are measured correctly for the patient to use. If they are not then the patient may develop associated problems such as back pain,

arm ache or even fall over while using them. Axillary crutches also have the potential to cause axillary nerve problems if fitted incorrectly. This occurs if the patient just rests their weight on the axilla, rather than taking their weight on the hand grip and so through the whole arm.

The crutches are correctly adjusted when a space exists between the armpit and the crutch, which is at least two fingers' width. The wrist should also be slightly bent when holding the crutch. This will allow weight bearing to be concentrated through the wrist. Adjustable nuts and bolts allow the crutch to be altered to the correct length.

Below elbow crutches again require a gap of two fingers' width, but in this case it is from the brachial area down. These crutches are simpler to adjust as they have a metal stud system which, when pressed, resets the crutch height. Some also have the same system for the arm component. Therefore you need to be sure that both are adjusted correctly.

Usually patients are discharged non-weight bearing, most typically with a plaster cast on. Patients with minor sprains may be partial weight bearing. To prevent further falls at home it is essential that the patient is secure and safe on the crutches before being allowed home. The nurse is responsible to ensure this is so and should also document that this is the case.

Most young people will be able to cope with the below elbow crutches for non-weight-bearing casts. Older people may be able to cope with axillary crutches more readily.

When being taught to use crutches for non-weight bearing, the patient should be encouraged always to stand with the crutches in line with their feet. This will prevent stooping, lower back pain, and promote a positive stance, so that they will not fall over. All weight should be on the unaffected or 'good leg'. To move, the crutches are lifted together and placed down approximately 60 cm in front. The patient then pushes their weight onto the crutches and hops forward bringing the feet into alignment with the two crutches. If they hop too far forward or not enough, then the stance will become unstable and they will fall over.

To sit down, the patient should position themselves near the chair then turn around so that they are facing away from the chair. S/he should move backwards until the backs of the legs are against the chair. At this stage the crutch on the injured side is swapped over to join the crutch on the uninjured side. The patient then feels for the arm of the chair and holds it with the free hand to maintain balance. The injured limb is then swung forward as the person sits down slowly.

In order to stand the person simply reverses this procedure with both crutches on the affected side, held by the wrist bar. The patient then lifts himself up pushing down on the wrist bar with one hand and pushing down with the free hand on the chair arm. Once in a stable standing posture, the crutches can be placed in the normal position for walking.

When climbing stairs, the patient will need to keep both crutches in one hand and hold the handrail with the opposite hand. The patient then should push firmly down on the crutches and hold the rail well. The unaffected leg is then put onto the step first. All weight is then pushed onto the crutches and handrail to gain ascent. The injured leg then follows. Putting most weight into the unaffected leg the crutch is then raised to the next step and the sequence repeated.

For the descent, both crutches are held in one hand and the stair rail in the other. Weight is taken on the crutches which should be on the same level as the person, while holding the handrail for balance. The affected leg is then lowered. Weight is taken on the crutches and handrail as the unaffected leg is then lowered. With the weight on the unaffected leg, the crutches are then moved down to the step the person is standing on ready to repeat the manoeuvre.

Zimmer frames are ideal for the elderly or for people who cannot manage with crutches. As they often come as fixed height devices, a large stock is usually needed. They are cumbersome and difficult in small houses or a confined space, however.

Reference

Brown J (1995) The suspected scaphoid fracture and isotope bone imaging. *Injury*, **26**:7, 479–82.

Further reading

Bache J, Armitt C, Gadd C (1998) *Practical Procedures in the Emergency Department*. London: CV Mosby.

Chapter 8

SOFT TISSUE INJURY

Wounds and other injuries to muscles and joints make up a large proportion of an A & E department's workload. Some wounds are old and have become infected by the time the patient presents, while other closed injuries may also be several days old. Many patients with wounds and minor injuries are suitable for treatment by nurses without lengthy delays to see busy medical staff. The nurse practitioner role in A & E clearly has a major part to play in the future treatment of patients with such injuries.

Pathology

Soft tissue injury can either be closed, as in bruising or a ligament sprain, or open, in which case some sort of wound will be present.

Wounds

The wounds seen in A & E are rather different from the surgical incisions that the nurse will have encountered elsewhere: A & E wounds can be in all shapes and sizes, and are all caused by non-sterile agents, with an accompanying risk of infection. Some may be fresh and others several days old.

The normal healing process will produce fresh epithelial cover within 48 hours if the wound has been closed, although the healing process below the surface will take much longer. An impaired blood supply, infection or the presence of foreign material will all delay or prevent healing. The aim in A & E, therefore, is to clean the wound thoroughly, removing foreign material and reducing the risk of infection, and then to close the wound so as to promote rapid healing with the minimum of scar formation and infection risk.

The most feared pathogens are the anaerobic Clostridium family. *Clostridium tetani* gives rise to tetanus, and *Clostridium welchii* and *Clostridium sporagenes* are involved in gas gangrene. The spores of these organisms are found in the soil, and the fact that they are anaerobic means that they can live without free atmospheric oxygen. Therefore, if they are present in a wound that is closed over, they will thrive.

Tetanus is characterized by the toxins released by the *Clostridium tetani* attacking the nervous system. The result is severe muscle spasm that could be fatal once the muscles of respiration become involved. In established

1. *Laceration.* A linear cut in the skin, usually superficial but may involve deep structures.
2. *Crush injury.* Fingers and toes are the most commonly involved. There may be a fracture of the bone underneath which will, therefore, be an open fracture. The force of the impact causes the soft tissue to burst open; a very painful injury with much swelling involved. Crush injuries carry a high risk of infection due to the damaged and devitalized tissue present (Fergusson, 1993).
3. *Penetrating wound.* A narrow but deeply penetrating track is involved. The cause can be anything from treading on a nail to a stabbing or gunshot wound.
4. *Abrasions.* A superficial but very painful injury. Dirt and grit is commonly ingrained or tattooed into the skin and has to be removed by scrubbing.
5. *Bites.* Ragged wounds with crushed tissue are produced by bites and have a high risk of infection. Human bites carry a very high risk of infection as the mouth is heavily contaminated with bacteria, while the risk of hepatitis B or HIV transmission also exists (Kelly *et al.*, 1996). Such wounds should not be sutured due to the risk of infection.
6. *Degloving injury.* If a force is involved that is parallel to the skin, layers of tissue may be torn away, exposing a whole area of deeper structures.
7. *Burns.* (see p. 47).

cases, therefore, the treatment involves long-term ventilatory support.

In gas gangrene, putrefactive changes occur within damaged or dead tissue. Clostridia are responsible for forming various gases which escape into the tissue planes, giving the characteristic foul odour. The gas increases the pressure in the tissues surrounding the wound. This further impairs blood supply. Meanwhile, the toxins released by the bacteria cause a severe toxaemia. The condition is extremely painful and carries a high mortality rate.

A wide variety of other pathogens cause wound sepsis. As the patient in most cases is going home after treatment, it is important that the signs of infection be carefully explained. The patient should be given instructions to return should there be any signs of infection, such as pain, swelling, redness or inflammation tracking up the limb along the line of a vein.

Pre-tibial flap lacerations are usually seen in older people who have fallen at home or in the street. They are often difficult to treat because the elderly have very fragile skin, and suturing is not necessarily the best means of closing wounds in this case as they may simply cut through the skin. They are best treated by the use of steristrips rather than sutures, although complete skin opposition may not be achieved as steristrips cannot always maintain the tension needed to keep the skin edges together. Often there is skin loss from the site or the skin at the edge of the wound has rolled under itself. Careful use of a cotton bud will often allow you to unroll the skin and make for a much better closure. Good patient teaching is essential upon discharge. The limb must be elevated as much as possible to minimize swelling by promoting venous return. The patient must also keep the limb warm, which is one of the few benefits of a wool and crepe bandage over the dressing. Good diet will promote wound healing. If the flap is proximally based (Fig. 8.1), there is a good chance of healing. The distally based flap, however, has a very poor blood supply and often necroses. A skin grafting operation is then needed.

In dealing with gunshot or shrapnel injuries, it is important to consider the velocity and hence energy of the projectile. If the velocity exceeds that of sound, the particle is supersonic and is defined as a high energy missile. It will behave in a very different way from a subsonic particle (a particle travelling below the speed of sound). For example, the muzzle velocity of the average handgun is some 550 feet per second (168 m/s). The velocity of sound is 1100 feet per second (335 m/s). A

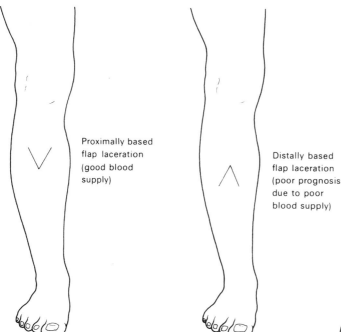

Proximally based flap laceration (good blood supply)

Distally based flap laceration (poor prognosis due to poor blood supply)

Fig. 8.1 Pre-tibia/flap laceration

modern military rifle, on the other hand, has a muzzle velocity of about 2500 feet per second (762 m/s) and the Colt Armalite exceeds 3000 feet per second (914 m/s). At these supersonic speeds, there is a high pressure shock wave preceding the projectile and, in its wake, there is a vacuum. The result on hitting the human body is an instantaneous pressure wave, causing catastrophic damage. This is followed by the vacuum which sucks gross contamination deep into the wound. A volume of tissue roughly equal to that of a football may be destroyed by a single bullet, with only a tiny entrance and exit wound to show for it. Bone is shattered, muscle and soft tissue infarcted and blood vessels destroyed, simply due to the pressure wave and without any physical contact with the projectile.

Fortunately, such wounds are rare in the UK; the knife culture is much more common than the gun culture. Knife wounds may look insignificant but can have devastating consequences. If a patient attends the department with a knife *in situ* then it should not be removed until you have the appropriate facilities available as serious bleeding can ensue and a range of internal structures could be seriously damaged. Many knife wounds are superficial and the result of works accidents (e.g. a Stanley knife), while other superficial wounds may be self-inflicted as a result of deliberate self-harm. Wounds sustained as a result of assault are more likely to be penetrating and often need exploring in theatre where thorough cleaning can take place and surgical repair of damaged structures undertaken. If the wound is superficial (e.g. a slash) this can generally be closed within the A & E department following thorough irrigation and cleaning.

A particular type of accidental knife injury is a pulp laceration which occurs usually as a result of a mishap while preparing food. The pulp of the finger is sliced off which causes the wound to bleed continually. Sometimes elevation in a high arm sling at triage along with direct pressure will stop the bleeding. However, once direct pressure is removed, bleeding may start again. One alternative is to use Kaltostat which, when placed on the wound, will help promote clotting. It can then be included in the dressing. This product is very useful in stopping persistent minor bleeding from wounds.

Patients will sometimes present at A & E with a range of other skin lesions of a non-traumatic origin. These may include various dermatological conditions ranging from eczema to skin cancer and rashes which are associated with infectious diseases such as measles and chickenpox. Such presentations might be more appropriately considered as primary care conditions and the more common ones are summarized in Table 8.1. Walsh *et al.* (1999) discuss nurse-led management of such common skin conditions from a nurse practitioner perspective. More detail can be found in Reifsneider (1997), while a specialist paediatric account is given by Singleton (1997).

Closed soft tissue injuries

Sprains are the most commonly seen closed soft tissue injury. These consist of ligament injury where the ligament is grossly intact, but some individual fibres have been torn. The result is a joint that is painful, swollen but stable. Ankle sprains are probably the most common such presentation and in 90% of cases involve the lateral aspect of the ankle (Greaves *et al.*, 1997). Neck sprains caused by road traffic accidents ('whiplash' injury) are also commonly seen. Bruising is another frequent injury and can have serious consequences because, in areas such as the foot and calf, there may be little room for expansion to accommodate the extra tissue fluid. Pressure levels can rise to such a point that the microcirculation is impaired and serious neurovascular complications can develop. This is known as 'compartment syndrome' and can have many other causes such as a tight POP or circumferential burn (p. 48). The lower leg and foot are most commonly effected but the forearm is also a high risk area (Greaves *et al.*, 1997).

Other commonly seen injuries include trauma to cartilage and bursae. In the knee, a tear of one of the semilunar cartilages is commonly associated with a twisting movement when the knee is flexed, resulting in the patient's knee locking in a flexed position. Repeated wear and tear on the bursae of the elbow or knee can lead to inflammation, swelling and pain, the so-called housemaid's knee or tennis elbow.

Table 8.1 Common rashes seen in A & E

Disease	Chief complaint	History
Herpes simplex Type 1 (cold sore)	Usually around mouth or nose; group of vesicles with yellow crust	Colds, fever, menstruation or overexposure to ruptures leaving painful ulcer. Sunlight may precede outbreak
Herpes simplex Type 2 (genital herpes)	Small grouped vesicles around genitals and mouth	Sexual contact with infected person
Herpes zoster (shingles)	Grouped vesicles or crusted lesions along nerve root	Chicken pox, reactivation of virus may cause attack
Verrucae (warts)	Slightly raised papules	Previous history of warts
Rubeola (measles)	Rash begins with macules on hairline, neck and cheeks, spreads downwards over rest of body. Appears 2–4 days after other symptoms, lasts 4–5 days	Exposure to infected person 10–14 days previously. Cold, cough, fever before rash
Rubella (German measles)	Maculopapular rash begins on face, spreads to trunk	Exposure to infected person 14–21 days previously. Adolescents have malaise, fever, anorexia and headaches before rash
Varicella (chicken pox)	Appears first on trunk, spreads to face and scalp. Small red papules and clear vesicles on red base which break and dry leaving a crust, Itching	Exposure to infected person 13–21 days ago. Malaise and anorexia before rash
Tinea corporis (ringworm)	Intense itching. Round red scaly lesions, central area heals while lesion continues outward	Exposure to infected animals or persons. Most common in children
Tinea capitis (scalp ringworm)	Mild itching, small spreading papules cause hair loss	Exposure to infected persons

Assessment

In order to assign the correct priority to the patient (triage) a good history of the accident and an accurate assessment of the wound or injured part are essential. The findings should be carefully documented and a diagram drawn to illustrate the location of any wound/skin lesion or the exact area which is tender, swollen or painful. The effects of the injury on the whole patient should also be assessed. S/he may be very distressed as the effect of the sight of blood can be very dramatic for some people. You should aim to find out what caused the injury, how and when it happened and how much (if any) blood loss there has been. It is worth remembering, however, that the lay person is prone to exaggerate blood loss.

Taking universal precautions, the nurse should examine the wound itself, carefully removing the patient's own first aid dressing. Assess the patient's pain and give appropriate analgesia. If necessary, the assessment should be stopped until the analgesia has taken effect. If you decide to infiltrate the wound with local anaesthetic prior to suturing, you must have assessed the sensation around the wound first, to ensure that there is no nerve damage. The nurse should examine the depth and extent of the wound, noting if any deep structures such as tendons are visible and if so, whether they are damaged. Any contamination should be recorded and if bleeding occurs it is important to note whether it is pulsatile and therefore arterial in nature.

The assessment should then move on to the area distal to the wound to see if there is any evidence of damage to structures such as tendons and nerves. The nurse should test sensation and movement with this consideration in mind and also note the colour and warmth of the skin.

The possibility of either the patient or a relative fainting as a result of the sight of blood should always be kept in mind. The patient should be laid on a trolley to prevent fainting and it should be made easy for relatives to exit the treatment area should they begin to feel squeamish. It is most embarrassing to have a patient suddenly feel faint and they may suffer significant injury if they collapse onto a hard A & E floor.

The tendons and nerves in any hand injury need also to be assessed. Specialized texts can easily teach how to assess them, although Walsh *et al.* (1999) have described such assessment from a nurse practitioner perspective.

When there has been significant blood loss, or a penetrating injury, it is essential to record vital signs and then monitor them as necessary. If the injury is in a large cavity such as the chest or pelvic region, internal bleeding can be heavy with little apparent external evidence. Hypovolaemia can therefore develop very quickly. Remember that a small entry wound in the case of a penetrating injury can conceal devastating trauma within. The patient must be closely observed with full resuscitation facilities available in case of collapse.

The patient's anti-tetanus status should also be ascertained, together with any other information relevant to wound healing, such as whether the patient is a diabetic or on steroid or current antibiotic therapy.

In assessing closed soft tissue injuries the nurse should examine the whole limb after first obtaining a history. It needs examining for localized bony tenderness, which would raise the possibility of a fracture, and for swelling, pain and degree of function. Assessment of the ankle (the most common site for sprains) has been greatly aided by the introduction of the Ottawa system which substantially reduces the incidence of unnecessary X-rays (Fig. 8.2). Salt and Clancy (1997) showed that these simple rules can be effectively used by nurses in A & E and they are strongly recommended, especially where nurse-led X-ray has been introduced. Patients often complain of hearing a crack when they injured their ankle, thinking this is evidence of a fracture. Reid *et al.* (1996) have shown that there is no association between the person hearing a crack and the likelihood of there being a fracture.

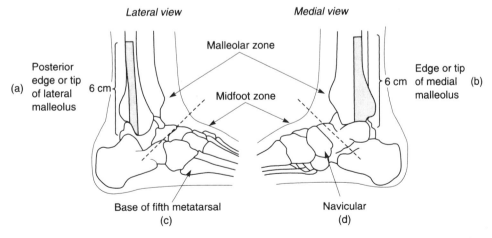

Fig. 8.2 Ottawa ankle rules: Ankle X-ray needed if there is pain in the malleolar zone and any of the following: bone tenderness at (a) or (b); inability to weight bear both immediately and in A & E. Foot X-ray needed if there is pain in the midfoot region and any of the following: bone tenderness at (c) or (d); inability to weight bear both immediately and in A & E.

It is also important to know how rapidly the existing amount of swelling occurred so that a reasonable estimate can be made of future swelling and, therefore, whether there is a significant risk of neurovascular compromise. To reduce swelling it is important to elevate the limb while the patient is in A & E. Many ankle and lower limb injuries will be waiting some hours before diagnosis and treatment, therefore, you should be proactive in reducing further painful swelling. Ice packs should be used in conjunction with elevation if delays are possible

A wound that has become infected because the person did not seek treatment at the time can frequently be seen within the emergency department. In addition, people present with a wide range of abscesses, some of which can be extremely painful. In assessing the patient, the nurse should obtain a history of how long the problem has existed and of any likely precipitating factor. The area should be examined for signs of the infection spreading such as a red prominent track along the line of a vein or the swelling of lymph nodes. Due to the association of infective lesions with diabetes, the patient should have a routine stix test performed for blood glucose levels. Temperature and pulse should also be recorded to assess the degree of systemic involvement.

Bites are very prone to infection and must be assessed very carefully. The animal responsible should be ascertained. Dogs are the most common culprits. Higgins *et al.* (1997) cite a figure of 74% of bite presentations in A & E being due to dogs, however, human bites are the second most common accounting for 18% according to these authors. Human bites are potentially highly infective. A patient with a wound over his knuckle sustained as a result of punching someone in the mouth has effectively sustained a bite wound even though he probably would not describe it in those terms. Such an injury has the potential for serious joint and bone infection and should be surgically explored in theatre according to Kelly *et al.* (1996).

Intervention

Control bleeding

A priority with any wound is to stop bleeding. This may be done by direct pressure over the wound with a firm dressing. Initially this can be held by hand, remembering to use universal precautions, but a firm non-crepe bandage will suffice once the bleeding has been stopped. Elevating the injury will also reduce bleeding, for example, by using a roller towel and a drip stand for a hand or arm injury. There is no indication for the routine use of a tourniquet in A & E other than to provide a temporary bloodless field for a brief examination of the wound.

Cleaning the wound

Whether it is a major wound that will require repair in theatre or a minor wound that can be dealt with in A & E, it will need cleaning out thoroughly. If the wound is major, irrigation with normal saline in large quantities is recommended. This can be followed by a dressing of saline soaks and iodine to keep the tissue in the best condition possible for theatre, where a formal toilet and debridement will take place. The aim is to toilet the wound thoroughly to wash out all contamination and to remove surgically any dead or dubious tissue which may act as a focus for infection (e.g. gas gangrene). The surgeon may leave badly contaminated wounds open for 3 days after surgery, covering them with only a light dressing. Only when absolutely sure that there is no evidence of sepsis, will the surgeon proceed to a delayed primary suture. This procedure is mandatory for all high velocity missile wounds.

In dealing with wounds that can be treated within A & E, cleaning with antiseptics is of little value in preventing infection because the solution is not in contact with microorganisms long enough and resistant strains are increasingly common (Walsh and Ford, 1989). A further major problem is that naturally occurring body fluids can make most antiseptics ineffective (Fergusson, 1993). A thorough cleansing with a sterile saline solution at a pre-warmed temperature is therefore recommended. Drinking water has been recommended for wound irrigation in A & E by Ryatt and Quinton (1997) whose studies indicated that it is free from pathogenic organisms. If the wound is very contaminated, hydrogen peroxide has traditionally been used as a cleansing agent as its effervescent effect may help loosen debris. It should be noted, though, that it has little, if any, antiseptic action, and there have been reports of tissue damage and near fatal air embolism associated with its use (Fergusson, 1993).

Abrasions demand special attention as grit may be tattooed into the wound. If left there, it will cause infection and possibly a permanent disfiguring mark. Traditionally such wounds have been treated by the use of a toothbrush to remove such grit by dermabrasion. This practice is now being questioned and Kenward (1998) offers a range of alternatives, such as high pressure irrigation and the use of dressings to effect debridement less painfully. Needless to say dermabrasion is a very painful procedure and the patient should have the benefit of either topical/local anaesthesia, plus Entonox or IV morphine. In severe cases a general anaesthetic may be needed.

Wound closure

The main techniques used in A & E for wound closure are suturing, steristripping, and tissue glue. Medical staff sometimes ask for wound closure that is quickest for the department rather than in the patient's best interest. The method of wound closure should, however, be determined by what is in the patient's best interest rather than what is most convenient for staff. For example, many departments use steristrip as their main wound closure technique, but certain wounds are better treated with sutures. Apart from obvious clinical factors, such as whether the wound is over a joint, there are also social factors to consider. Once a wound is steristripped the patient is usually recommended to keep it dry for 5 days compared to two or three with a suture. Consider therefore the predicament of single mother with a young child who has suffered a laceration to her hand; suturing would actually be better from a practical point of view. If a wound is closed by gluing or steristrip this causes less scarring than suturing. A laceration to the eyebrow may prove very difficult to stop bleeding sufficiently to steristrip closed, consequently it is very tempting to suture it as a 'quick fix' even though this leaves a worse cosmetic result for the patient.

Whether suture or steristrip is being used, it should always be applied at right angles to the wound, skin edges should never be inverted (turned under) as this delays healing, and the tension in the skin around the wound should be evenly distributed. If there is too much tension in the skin the wound will break down. The nurse should therefore resist the temptation to pull skin edges together tightly. They should only be placed in opposition. Figure 8.3 shows the correct technique for suturing.

The needle should be firmly gripped half-way to one-third along its length by the needle holders. When the needle is introduced into the skin, it is important that the wrist be rotated in alignment with the curvature of the needle, otherwise the needle will be bent. The needle should enter some 4 mm from the wound edge and exit the same distance from the opposite side of the wound. Dissecting forceps may be used to hold the wound edge to facilitate passing the needle through.

The knot is tied as shown in the diagram, some three turns being needed, each in the opposite direction from its predecessor. Each stitch needs to be about 3 mm from its neighbour. In cutting the stitch, the nurse should remember that a colleague will have to remove that stitch in a few days time – 3 days for faces, 5 days for scalps, 7 days for elsewhere. For faces, 5/6–0 size suture material is usually used; 4–0 is used elsewhere, although if considerable force is involved (e.g. over a knee), 3–0 may be used. Scalps are also often sutured with 3–0.

If more than one stitch is required, the area should first be infiltrated with local anaesthetic which should be introduced via a needle inserted parallel to the wound and injected as the needle and syringe are gradually withdrawn. Lignocaine 1% is the agent of choice. However, in a very vascular area, such as the scalp, where bleeding often proves a problem, lignocaine with adrenaline may be used. Such a solution should never be used on a finger or toe as the vasoconstrictor effects of adrenaline are so great that peripheral gangrene may result.

Steristrips are simply thin strips of adhesive paper (Fig. 8.4). They are suitable for many wounds, do not require local anaesthetic and leave less scar than sutures. They cannot, however, be applied to hairy areas such as the scalp, and if the wound is over a joint, they will probably be pulled apart by tension in the skin as movement occurs.

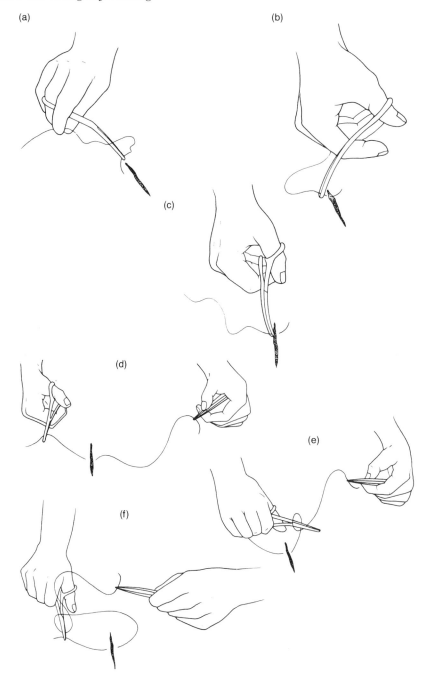

Fig. 8.3 Suturing technique. (a) Note that needle holders grasp the needle approximately one-third along the needle and not at the end. The point of the needle is perpendicular to the skin at point of entry. The point of entry should be 3–4 mm from wound. (b) By rotating the wrist, bring the needle through and out of the wound. (c) Re-enter on the opposite edge of the wound, rotating the wrist to bring the needle out 3–4 mm from the opposite side of the wound. (d) Pull the suture through the wound, ready for tying the knot. (e) Start tying the knot by making a loop with the needle holders. (f) Grasp the end of the suture. (g) Pull the end of the suture through the loop. (h) Pull it firmly but not too tightly, laying the knot to one side of the wound. (i) Then repeat this twice, looping in the opposite direction on each occasion.

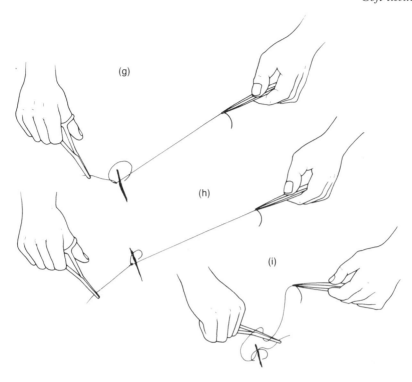

The skin on either side of a wound should be clean and dry. Remember if the wound is still bleeding the steristrip will not stick and an alternative method of wound closure needs to be discussed. For most wounds 3 mm strips will suffice; 6 mm or 12 mm are available for bigger wounds. The strip should be attached first to one side of the wound. The wound is then pulled together and the strip stuck down onto the skin the other side. In large or ragged wounds, it may be necessary to perform a two-stage closure, using some strips initially to approximate the wound edges, and then proceeding to close the wound fully with further strips, removing the first strips in the process.

A gap should be left between strips to allow for drainage of any fluid from the wound. Finally, anchoring strips should be applied parallel to the wound to distribute skin tension evenly.

Tissue adhesive is now well established as a wound closure technique. It is very effective in closing wounds and the recent products are pain free on application. Much discussion is ongoing on whether each vial should only be used once and discarded or if multiple use is permissible. The manufacturer's guidelines should be followed.

The first step in application is to clean the wound thoroughly. The wound edges can then be held together by yourself or a colleague. Ensure that you are wearing gloves and a gauze swab is also useful. Once the wound is held together several drops are applied along the wound edge ('spot welding'). Alternatively, you can run the glue continuously along the wound edge ('layering'). Whichever method is used, you will then need to hold the wound together according to the manufacturer's instructions, usually for around 30 seconds. Ensure you have not glued yourself to the wound, which can be a common mistake for beginners. No other dressing is usually needed, although if the patient is a child, the wound may be covered to stop the child picking at it. The patient must be told not to get it wet for a few days and allow the scabbing to fall off naturally, as less scarring will occur and there is less risk of infection.

As with steristrips, there is the advantage of not requiring infiltration with local anaesthesia. It is therefore very useful in treating children with minor lacerations (Pope, 1993).

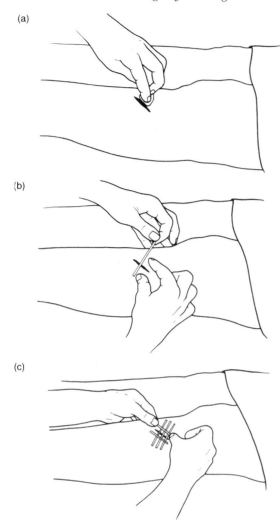

Fig. 8.4 *Steristripping technique. (a) After a thorough cleaning of the wound, wipe the skin on either side of the wound with tinct. benzene. (b) Pinch the skin edges together and lay the strips across it. (c) Leave gaps between the strips and finish by laying two anchor strips parallel to the wound.*

Some minor scalp lacerations can be effectively dealt with by tying together strands of hair from either side of the wound to pull the wound closed.

Dressing the wound

The optimum dressing should produce a moist, sterile environment with minimum trauma to newly forming tissue (Lait and Smith, 1998). Dressings which shed loose fibres into the wound will significantly delay healing. They should therefore be free from toxic or particulate material. Additionally, they should cause the minimum interference to the patient's normal activity, remain in place as long as required and be easily removed.

Plain dry gauze should not be in direct contact with the wound itself because it absorbs blood and exudate to form a hard, adherent mass that can be very difficult and painful to remove. One of the non-adherent proprietary dressings should be used in contact with the wound itself. Eyre (1993) has argued strongly against the use of the traditional paraffin impregnated gauze dressing for abrasions and other wounds, as there are many superior dressings now available which have far less of a problem with regard to adherence and 'strike through', i.e. the dressing soaking through to the outside with wound exudate. Antibiotic impregnated gauze should never be used as it is expensive, ineffective and contributes to the development of resistant strains of bacteria.

The dressing may be secured to the skin with a hypoallergenic tape (e.g. Micropore) applied longitudinally as any swelling may give rise to circulatory impairment if there is a circumferential constriction around the limb or digit. Many modern dressings though are self-adhesive.

The use of an elasticated tube type of bandage (e.g. Tubigrip) is recommended, rather than the traditional crepe bandage, to complete the dressing. It is cheaper, easier to apply, gives a more even pressure over the limb with no risk of the wrinkles that can cause skin problems, and will stay in place far more effectively than a crepe bandage.

Finger dressings can be retained with a tubular bandage (e.g. Tubinette). If swelling is anticipated, the hand should be placed in a high arm sling (Fig. 8.5). The use of Flamazine cream and the finger from a sterile glove is an effective treatment for crushed finger tips (Bache *et al.*, 1998).

Head wounds may need a pressure bandage even after suture. A size F Tubigrip, 10 cm long, worn as a headband provides a very simple and effective solution to the problem, rather than the intricacies of head bandaging so beloved of the first aid manuals. Similarly the elasticated tube bandages (e.g. Netelast)

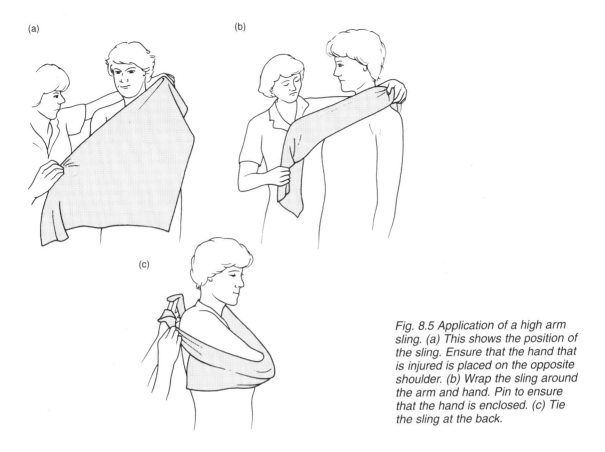

(a)

(b)

(c)

Fig. 8.5 Application of a high arm sling. (a) This shows the position of the sling. Ensure that the hand that is injured is placed on the opposite shoulder. (b) Wrap the sling around the arm and hand. Pin to ensure that the hand is enclosed. (c) Tie the sling at the back.

provide a better means of securing dressings to the trunk than does the traditional body bandage.

Tetanus vaccination

The effectiveness of the anti-tetanus immunization programme in the UK can be judged from the fact that there are no more than one or two dozen cases per year compared to the death toll from tetanus of approximately a million per year in developing countries.

The adsorbed tetanus toxoid that is given to patients in A & E units is a form of active immunization in that it stimulates the patient to manufacture their own antibodies. All children in the UK should have received tetanus immunization as babies followed by booster doses at ages 4 and 14. Further boosters at 10-yearly intervals are needed, but two such boosters should be sufficient for normal adults. Some wounds are said to be more tetanus prone than others. Risk factors include heavy contamination with soil or faeces, puncture wounds, the presence of devitalized tissue or the presence of infection (Wyatt *et al.*, 1999). The DoH recommend that a total of 5 injections in a life time is probably sufficient for life-long immunity (Department of Health, 1990).

If the patient states that they have never received any anti-tetanus immunization, it is possible to give passive immunity in the form of the appropriate human immunoglobulin if the medical staff assess the risk as being significant.

Abscesses and infected wounds

Abscesses are commonly treated by surgical incision and drainage, under general or local anaesthesia. The appropriate preparation of the patient is therefore required in line with hospital procedure, together with a full explanation of what is to happen and how long the procedure will take.

In dressing an old infected wound or a recently drained abscess, the principles of providing a sterile moist environment, which can heal from the bottom up, remain. Wound beds which have a superficial infection should be dressed with Inadine, Iodoflexar or Actisorb. Heavily exuding wounds benefit from the use of the alginate dressings such as Sorbsan or Tegage, although if devitalized tissue is to be removed by autolysis, hydrocolloid dressings such as Granuflex or Comfeel should be used in such cases (Bale, 1997).

The patient will usually be discharged with a course of antibiotics and analgesics. The nurse should ensure that the patient understands the labels on the bottles and knows which are the analgesics and which the antibiotics. The patient also must understand the need to complete the full course of antibiotics, even if

	0–5 min	6–20 min	21–60 min
Documentation	Registration as A & E patient	A & E notes ready	Wound assessment chart started for follow-up A & E notes completed with sketch of wound
Assessment	Triage nurse, check wound for type size bleeding, patient for pain and anxiety	Obtain history from patient. Check wound for FB (?XR) and contamination, also damage to any underlying structures, check Tetanus status	Assess dressing when complete. Patient's understanding of care post discharge?
Medication	–	–	Anti-tetanus Antibiotics Analgesics as needed
Treatment	–	–	Debridement and thorough clean of wound, closure with suture steristrip or glue
Nursing care	Apply pressure dressing, limb elevation, psych support	Maintain as before	Lie patient down, explain procedures, close wound and dress. Give medication and wound care teaching
Referrals	–	–	Follow up in A & E or refer to health centre
Family	Inform if not present, psych support if needed	–	Include in patient teaching
Discharge	–	–	Ensure appropriate referral letter written

NB. FB = Foreign body

Fig. 8.6 Example of critical pathway for wounded patient

the infection appears to clear up before completion. The patient may need follow-up care, which can either be in A & E or at the patient's health centre.

The recent fashion for body piercing has resulted in frequent presentations at A & E with painful or infected pierced body parts, sometimes involving genitalia. The indications for removal of jewellery are localized oedema, infection or bleeding. Khanna *et al.* (1999) cite anecdotal evidence that this can occur in up to 30% of cases. Staff need to be familiar with how such jewellery functions in order to be able to remove an item from a swollen and tender site. In most cases there is a bar and one or two beads at one or both ends, which can be unscrewed. Khanna *et al.* (1999) recommend grasping the bar firmly with artery forceps while unscrewing the bead(s) with another pair of artery forceps. If embedded in oedematous tissue (e.g. the tongue or labia), the jewellery should be pushed through the tissue to expose the bead sufficiently for this manoeuvre to be accomplished. The other common device is a tensioned ring held by a bead. These captive ring beads can be removed by holding the ring either side of the bead and pressing inwards to release the tension on the bead.

Self-care

It is important that the patient be instructed in self-care of the injury before discharge. Key points include the need for elevation, keeping the dressing dry and clean, the length of time until dressing or suture removal, and instructions about how to remove the dressings or where to go to get the sutures removed. The patient should be alerted about the signs of infection and instructed to return immediately if there is any suspicion of infection. If a full course of tetanus is required, the patient should be given a card with the dates of the next two injections and the nurse should emphasize the importance of the follow-up injections. As in all treatment given in the emergency room, treatment should be supported by written information or diagrams. Most patients are in discomfort or pain following a dressing and may be in a hurry to get home. Patients may not therefore absorb the information that you have given them verbally. In order to evaluate the effectiveness

of self-care teaching, it is essential to question the patient to see that they fully understand what has been taught.

Closed soft tissue injury

The usual aim is to treat closed soft tissue injury conservatively by rest and support. Swelling can be reduced by elevation and ice packs if necessary. Gradually the area can be mobilized as pain and swelling ease off. Early mobilization of sprains should be actively encouraged as this produces the best outcome. This is particularly true of ankle sprains (Higgins, 1999) and also 'whiplash' injuries to the neck which should not be immobilized in soft collars (Ritchell-Herren, 1999). A tubular support bandage may be used to lend support to a joint such as the ankle or wrist, but the patient must be encouraged to mobilize and weight bear as soon as possible. If a sprain of the ankle is so severe as to prevent full weight bearing, then non-weight-bearing crutches must be supplied to allow mobilization of the patient, while resting the limb. Crepe bandage or wool and crepe bandages are of little effective use for this type of injury.

Evaluation

In many respects, the only real evaluation of treatment is if the patient returns or not. If the patient does not return, the assumption is that the nursing interventions have been successful. If the patient does return with a problem, however, the nursing staff should try to see how nursing care could have been better carried out. This will benefit other patients in the future. All dressings performed by junior staff should be checked before the patient is discharged, for if they are done incorrectly, they go home wrong and remain wrong.

References

Bache J, Armutt C, Gadd C (1998) *Practical Procedures in the Emergency Dept.* London: CV Mosby.

Bale S (1997) A guide to wound care debridement. *Journal of Wound Care*, **6**:4, 179–82.

Department of Health (1990) *Joint Committee on*

Vaccination and Immunisation: tetanus. *Immunisation against Infectious Disease*. London: HMSO.

Eyre G (1993) Alternative wound dressings in A & E. *Nursing Standard*, 7:25–8.

Fergusson A (1993) Wound infection – the role of antiseptics. *Accident and Emergency Nursing*, 1:79–86.

Greaves I, Porter K, Burke D (1997) *Key Topics in Trauma*. Oxford: Bios Medical Press.

Higgins G (1999) Mobilisation of lateral ankle sprains. *Journal of Accident and Emergency Medicine*, **16**:3, 217.

Higgins M, Evans RC, Evans RJ (1997) Managing animal bite wounds. *Journal of Wound Care*, **6**:8, 377–80.

Kelly I, Cunney R, Smyth E, Colville J (1996) The management of human bite injuries of the hand. *Injury*, 27:7, 481–4.

Kenward G (1998) Dermabrasion: is there a less traumatic alternative? *Emergency Nurse*, 5:9, 12–17.

Khanna R, Kumar S, Raju S, Kumar A (1999) Body piercing in the Accident and Emergency Department. *Journal of Accident and Emergency Medicine*, **16**:6, 418–21.

Lait M, Smith L (1998) Wound management; a literature review. *Journal of Clinical Nursing*, 7:1, 1–17.

Pope S (1993). The use of Histoacryl tissue adhesive in children's A & E. *Paediatric Nursing*, 5:20–1.

Reid P, Aggarwal A, Browning C, Nicolai P (1996) The relevance of hearing a crack in ankle injuries. *Journal of Accident and Emergency Medicine*, **13**:278–9.

Reifsnider E (1997) Common adult infectious skin conditions. *The Nurse Practitioner*, 22:11, 17–33.

Ritchell-Herren K (1999) Mobilisation of neck sprains. *Journal of Accident and Emergency Medicine*, **16**:5, 363.

Ryatt M, Quinton D (1997) Tap water as a wound cleansing agent in A&E. *Journal of Accident and Emergency Medicine*, **14**:165–6.

Salt P, Clancy M (1997) Implementation of the Ottawa ankle rules by nurses working in the A & E department. *Journal of Accident and Emergency Medicine*, **14**: 363–5.

Singleton J (1997) Pediatric dermatoses: Three common skin disruptions in infancy. *The Nurse Practitioner*, 22:6, 32–50.

Walsh M, Ford P (1989) *Nursing Rituals, Research and Rational Action*. Oxford: Butterworth-Heinemann.

Walsh M, Crumbie A, Reveley S (1999) *Nurse Practitioners; Clinical Skills and Professional Issues*. Oxford: Butterworth-Heinemann.

Wyatt J, Illingworth R, Clancy M, Munro P, Robertson C (1999) *Oxford Handbook of Accident and Emergency Medicine*. Oxford: Oxford University Press.

Chapter 9

EYE COMPLAINTS AND EMERGENCIES

Pathology

The human eye has been well-endowed by nature with defences such as the bony orbit and a very fast blink reflex. Despite these defences, however, eye injuries are common. In addition, the A & E nurse will see many patients who bring themselves to the department with a wide variety of eye complaints of a non-traumatic origin, although eye trauma remains the single most likely reason for attendance (Khaw and Elkington, 1994).

Non-penetrating eye injury

Trauma to structures surrounding the eye

The bony orbit that surrounds the eye may be fractured as a result of facial or head injury. The injury may be an isolated fracture, which is called a blow out fracture, or it may be a component of either a faciomaxillary injury or a fractured base of the skull. In a blow out fracture, the cause is a blow to the front of the orbit; the force from the blow is conducted as shock waves by the orbital floor and causes a sudden rise in intra-orbital pressure, the result being that an isolated piece of bone is blown into the adjacent sinus. The problem that this injury causes is that tissue, including muscle, herniates through the hole and becomes trapped; the mobility of the eye is restricted and double vision or diplopia develops.

In the more serious cases, where the orbital fracture is part of other fractures, the eye can be impaired by damage to the optic nerve, or one of the other facial nerves, leading to the development of a nerve palsy.

Soft tissue injury to the eyelids is a common situation; it usually causes bruising which resolves with the passage of time. Most lacerations are easily stitched or closed with tissue glue; however, Greaves *et al.* (1997) recommend that lacerations which go through both surfaces of the lid or involve structures such as the lacrymal duct should be referred to a specialist. Due to the speed with which swelling of the lids can develop, it is essential to examine the damaged eye promptly, as soon afterwards examination may be rendered virtually impossible by the swollen and bruised lids. In burns cases, it may be impossible to close the lids due to the burn damage. As the cornea must not be left exposed, this requires that antibiotic ointment be applied to the cornea and that urgent arrangements be made for a plastic surgery procedure to replace the destroyed tissue.

Foreign body (non-penetrating)

This is probably the most common ophthalmic complaint seen in A & E, the cause being any small particle such as dust, grit, woodsplinters or metal fragments. Low velocity foreign bodies fail to penetrate the eye and will either be found lodged on the surface of the cornea or on the under-surface of the eyelid, the conjuctiva. In this latter case, it is known as a sub-tarsal foreign body (Jones, 1998).

Corneal foreign bodies, such as vegetable material, can produce severe irritation and infection and, in the case of metallic objects, can very quickly stain the cornea with a deposit of rust. Sub-tarsal foreign bodies produce the sensation of 'something in my eye' and, therefore, the eyelids should always be everted to permit careful inspection when a patient presents complaining of a foreign body.

Corneal abrasion

This is an extremely painful condition in which the epithelium of the cornea is removed from the damaged part. It is usually caused by a glancing blow to the eye from any number of objects such as a finger nail, towel or newspaper. Inflammation of the cornea is known as keratitis and can have several causes.

Chemical injury

The extent of the injury is related to the nature and concentration of the agent involved. Alkalis are the most damaging (e.g. substances containing lime, such as wet cement) as they can rapidly penetrate the cornea and produce severe damage to the iris, ciliary body and lens while also causing ischaemia. Acids of equivalent strength are less frequently involved in eye injuries as they are less common in everyday use. They also cause less damage than alkalis as they combine with tissue components to precipitate deposits of protein which form a barrier against further penetration (Marsden, 1999a). Nevertheless, whether the injury is caused by an acid or alkali, the effects can be devastating with a serious injury producing an inflammatory response leading to possible corneal perforation and scar tissue formation. Opacification of the cornea and loss of vision may result. According to Marsden (1998b) the only type of eye injury which is placed in triage category red (most urgent) is a chemical burn.

Radiation injury

Ultraviolet light is the usual culprit, producing damage to the superficial layers of the epithelium of the cornea. Pain, photophobia and watering are the usual symptoms the patient presents with a few hours after exposure. Sun lamps and welding without proper goggles are the usual causes, the latter giving rise to the name of 'arc eye' by which this condition is informally known.

Keratitis or inflammation of the cornea is the usual result of exposure to other forms of radiation. Cataract formation is a long-term complication of ionizing radiation exposure.

Contusion and concussion injury

Contusion refers to injury from the direct impact of the force involved. Damage to the eyelids has already been mentioned; the cornea can also be affected by contusion. The result can vary from corneal oedema through to rupture of the whole globe, depending on the force involved.

Concussion refers to the conduction of shock waves from the point of impact to other parts of the eye. The blow out fracture has already been discussed as an example of this type of injury. Within the globe itself, various very severe injuries are possible, including detachment of the retina or the ciliary body, vitreous or retinal haemorrhages, and/or the development of a hyphaemia. A hyphaemia is bleeding into the anterior chamber and can have devastating effects on sight due to the development of secondary glaucoma and corneal staining. Cataract of the lens or the dislocation of the lens may result from a concussion injury; the iris sphincter may be ruptured in concussion, leading again to the long-term risk of glaucoma.

Penetrating eye injury

Penetrating eye injuries are caused by high velocity particles and may be classified into two groups: those in which the object responsible is withdrawn after penetration and those in which the object is retained in the eye, forming an intraocular foreign body. The prognosis for vision depends upon the size of the laceration in the cornea or sclera, and upon which part of the eye is involved. Penetration to the posterior chamber carries the worst prognosis.

In order that a foreign body may penetrate the eye, it must possess a large amount of energy. Typical objects are glass from a car windscreen (Fig. 9.1), flying debris from industrial processes such as drilling, and material propelled by a blast after an explosion. The most common form of retained foreign body within the eye is metallic; iron and steel account for between 85 and 98% of intraocular foreign bodies caused by industrial accidents.

A much feared complication of penetrating eye injury is sympathetic ophthalmitis, where after injury to one eye, the uninjured eye develops a severe inflammation some time after (from 3 weeks to 4 months has been reported). If untreated, this inflammation may lead to loss of useful vision in the uninjured eye. Prompt post-traumatic surgery and early enucleation of the injured eye, together with the use of steroid therapy, have greatly reduced the incidence of this complication which can lead to complete blindness.

In addition to the obviously disastrous

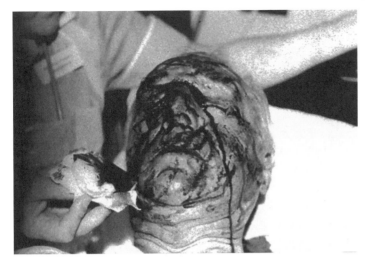

Fig. 9.1 Typical car windscreen injury. Serious damage to both eyes plus multiple lacerations to face

effects that the foreign body may have on the delicate structures of the eye, there is a further risk of siderosis bulbi if the foreign body contains iron. This condition stems from the chemical reactions which occur within the eye due to the iron, its effects being seen some time after the injury. As the iron dissolves, it becomes incorporated into the cells of the eye, leading to chronic damage and eventually blindness. For this reason, it is mandatory that all ferrous intraocular foreign bodies be removed. An electromagnet is commonly used to do this.

Other conditions

There are many varied eye conditions that bring patients to A & E other than trauma. Any sudden disturbance of vision should be treated as an emergency and afforded a high priority for medical attention. Examples include the patient complaining of seeing floating images (floaters) which could indicate a detached retina or vitreous haemorrhage, haloes due to the sudden onset of acute open angled glaucoma or the sudden loss of vision in an eye. This could be caused by arterial occlusion or disciform macular degeneration (Walsh *et al.*, 1999). A range of conditions can cause inflammation of the eye and this is the most common eye problem after trauma seen in A & E. They are summarized in Table 9.1.

Eye symptoms may be associated with a range of systemic diseases such as diabetes, hyperthyroidism, rheumatoid arthritis and systemic lupus erythematosus. AIDS can produce uveitis, retinal haemorrhages and exudates and makes the patient susceptible to opportunistic infections such as herpes simplex or candida (Marsden, 1999a). It is possible, therefore, that the patient may present as an emergency complaining of sudden visual disturbances and loss of visual acuity which turn out to be associated with AIDS. Plona and Schremp (1992) report that, in the USA, 75% of AIDS patients develop ocular conditions and comment that the person may be totally unaware that they are HIV positive when they present. This systemic dimension to acute eye disorders must always be remembered when dealing with patients complaining of eye problems.

Assessment

The first step is to obtain a history of the complaint from the patient. Some of the important symptoms that may be mentioned and which should alert the nurse to give a patient high priority have been mentioned above. These include: haloes around lights, 'floaters' described by the patient as visible wisps or strands, flashing lights and, of course, sudden blindness. The nurse should check whether the patient is experiencing double vision (diplopia) or blurred vision which is due to interference with light transmission caused by cataracts of refractive errors. Other less

Table 9.1 Common causes of inflammation of the eye

Condition	Pathology	Common signs
Stye	Boil on lid margin	
Chalazion	Cyst within tarsal plate (eyelid)	
Allergy	Reaction affecting both eyelid and conjunctiva	Oedema around periorbital area
Conjunctivitis	There is discharge, discomfort but little pain. Bacteria are the usual cause	Redness of conjunctiva
Keratitis	Painful inflammation of cornea. Common causes are an extension of existing conjunctivitis, corneal exposure, the herpes simplex virus which leads to the formation of a dendritic ulcer or corneal abrasion	Damage visible on staining with fluorescein eye drops
Iritis	Acute inflammation of the iris	Small pupil, redness restricted to immediate area of iris
Glaucoma	Raised intraocular pressure. Common cause is blockage of the aqueous circulation from ciliary body via the pupils to the drainage angle in the anterior chamber. It can be acute, chronic or secondary to some other condition such as iritis or hyphaemia. This is a potentially blinding condition.	Painful fixed dilated pupil in acute glaucoma

helpful symptoms (less helpful because they are so non-specific) include photophobia, which may be associated with inflammation of the eye but can be associated with many other illnesses (such as migraine) and pain in the eye. Pain may be of ocular origin (e.g. inflammation of the cornea), but it may also be caused by many other conditions such as sinusitis, where the patient attributes the pain to the eyeball. Furthermore, the pain of acute glaucoma can be described by some patients as being in the forehead and nowhere near the eyes. Relevant past medical history should be noted including whether the person wears spectacles or contact lenses, any previous similar problems or the presence of diabetes.

If the patient is presenting with a foreign body, it is essential to find out if it was a high energy or low energy accident due to the risk of penetration and, if possible, what the foreign body might be composed of. Similarly, if it is a chemical injury to the eye that the patient has sustained, then nurses need to know what chemical, how long ago and what first aid measures have been taken (hopefully copious irrigation with cold water).

After obtaining a history, the next step is to assess the eye in a systematic fashion, starting with visual acuity. This should be done at triage. Irrigation or installation of a local anaesthetic are the only actions to take priority over visual acuity testing and triage (Marsden, 1998). Simple finger counting will assess whether there is any double vision present. The use of the standard Snellen Visual Acuity Test is strongly recommended for all patients with eye complaints. The chart consists of lines of letters of differing sizes which the average eye should be able to read at varying distances, depending on the size of the letters.

The patient is asked to read the chart from a distance of 6 metres, one eye at a time, the other eye being occluded. The results of each eye are carefully recorded, noting the last line to be read correctly. If the patient wears spectacles, this test should be carried out both with and without the spectacles. Each line has a number which refers to the distance at which the average eye should be able to read that line. The result is, therefore, recorded as a fraction, the top number referring to the distance at which the patient stood from the chart, the bottom number being the line number that was correctly read (i.e. the distance at which an average eye would be able to read that line). Thus vision recorded as 6/6 means that at a range of 6 metres the patient can read the same size letters that the average eye can read at 6 metres. If the patient cannot read one or two letters in a line this is recorded as the number of the line minus the number of letters that cannot be read. Reading all but one letter of the 6 line is recorded therefore as 6/6–1 (Marsden, 1998b).

If the patient is illiterate or very young, an E chart is used, consisting of rows of the capital letter E pointing in different directions. The patient is asked to indicate the position of the E using three fingers.

After assessing visual acuity, the nurse should move on to the eye itself, working inwards in a regular sequence which the A & E nurse will find helpful to have as a standard pattern for assessing eyes. Both eyes should always be examined.

The eyelids should first be examined for evidence of disease or damage. This should include eversion to examine the under-surface of the lid (the conjunctiva). This is best done by asking the patient to look downwards, grasping the eyelashes, then gently pulling down, round and up while depressing the upper margin of the tarsal plate with a cotton applicator or similar implement. The under-surface of the eyelid should be readily visualized by this technique. Any swelling around the orbit should be noted as this may indicate an allergic reaction. Obvious abnormalities such as a droopy eyelid, squint or exophthalmos should also be documented.

For assessment of the eye itself, a bright pen torch is essential. First the pupil responses and the shape of the pupil should be tested to check they are brisk to respond and equal and regular in size and shape. Note that some 20% of people have unequal pupils normally, however (Seidal *et al.*, 1995). A pear-shaped pupil indicates significant eye trauma and disruption of internal ocular structures (Hartland, 1993). The cornea should be examined for evidence of a foreign body, a corneal wound or redness

indicative of inflammation. This is best done by shining the pen torch tangentially across the cornea as this will make any abnormality more apparent. Any discharge should be noted. Damage to the corneal epithelium is difficult to visualize under normal conditions, but the addition of a drop of sodium fluorescein will show the damaged area in bright green which is easily visible if a cobalt blue filter is added to either the ophthalmoscope or torch. Ocular position and movement should also be checked; a blow out fracture of the orbit is often associated with an apparently recessed eye, for example (Hartland, 1993).

Finally, the person as a whole must be assessed. Eye injuries produce great fear of blindness in many patients. Patients are, therefore, likely to be very frightened and anxious. Thus an assessment of the psychological state of the patient is needed as nursing intervention is required in this area as much as for the actual eye injury.

Among those patients who do lose their sight, the greatest psychological trauma has been shown to occur at the actual time of sight loss rather than later (Vader, 1992), which underlines the importance of the A & E nurse approaching such patients holistically rather that just focusing on the immediate physical problem.

The medical assessment will include a test of the field of vision, a detailed examination using both an ophthalmoscope and a slit lamp. A slit lamp is a binocular microscope with a strong light source that provides a well-illuminated and highly magnified view of the area in question. X-rays will be required if there is a risk of penetrating injury or fractures. Nurses developing nurse practitioner roles are increasingly using such equipment to examine patients but must ensure that they are competent in these advanced skills. Reference should be made to texts such as Walsh *et al.* (1999) or Seidal *et al.* (1995) for further reading concerning the use of these techniques.

Intervention

The victim of an accident who has suffered serious eye injury will need considerable and immediate psychological support due to the fear of blindness, which will probably be uppermost in his or her mind. It will be the lot of the nurse to deal with difficult questions such as 'Will my sight be alright?' and 'Am I going to be blind?' from a patient whose face will probably be swathed in bloody dressings. The approach described in the chapter on burns is recommended; i.e. sympathetic, honest and realistic.

If chemicals have been spilt into the eye, copious irrigation with water is the correct first aid procedure, and removal of contact lenses if worn. Irrigation will then be continued in A & E. Devices are available which can be plumbed into the main water supply and which will irrigate both eyes at once, this is particularly useful for gross contamination. Bache *et al.* (1998) recommend the use of an ordinary IV giving set, first accustoming the patient to the temperature of the solution (sterile saline or water) by running it onto the cheek. The procedure is best carried out with the patient lying flat and the nurse standing at the patient's head. Sterile gloves should be worn throughout. For effective irrigation to occur, the eyelids must be opened. This will require a great deal of tact and gentleness on the part of the nurse, for most people with an already irritable and possibly painful eye are understandably reluctant to have that eye held open while somebody pours fluid into it. Local anaesthetic such as amethocaine 1% applied in advance may facilitate this procedure. Nurses would do well to try to imagine themselves in the patient's position when deciding how to handle the victim of eye trauma. A kidney dish should be held against the face and the head turned to that side in order to catch the irrigation fluid. A plastic apron should be used to protect the patient's clothes from soaking. The nurse should work from the inner, nasal part of the eye outwards when irrigating and ensure that there is a constant flow of fluid over the eye. The patient should be advised to move the eye around during the procedure. Bache *et al.* (1998) recommend a Snellen visual acuity test after irrigation together with staining with fluorescein eye drops and re-examination of the cornea for evidence of damage. The pH of the eye should also be tested using special ophthalmic indicator paper to ensure it has returned to normal. Sufficient time should be left between irrigation and testing to ensure that it is the pH of tear fluid that is being tested rather than the irrigation fluid which may still

be in the eye. Normally tear fluid is neutral with a pH of 7 (Marsden, 1999b).

A sub-tarsal foreign body can be removed with a cotton applicator after eversion of the eyelid. Gentleness and reassurance are required in carrying out the procedure as the patient may find it frightening. Marsden (1998c) recommends testing with fluorescein after removal to ensure that the cornea has not been damaged by the foreign body. Corneal foreign bodies are removed frequently with nothing more than a sterile hypodermic needle; however, the cornea first needs anaesthetizing with amethocaine 1% eye drops. Local anaesthetic drops should never be used, however, for the management of ocular symptoms such as pain (Khaw and Elkington, 1994).

In the past, chloramphenicol (ointment or drops) has been the mainstay antibacterial agent used in preventing or treating eye infections, frequently coupled with the use of an eye pad. The recent move to evidence based practice has led to serious questioning of such traditional practices. Field *et al.* (1999) carried out an extensive literature review on the safety of chloramphenicol and noted that while there have been occasional reports of adverse reactions (aplastic anaemia), it is still the most cost effective broad spectrum antibiotic for use with eye problems. They therefore encourage A & E nurses to continue to use the agent within properly drawn up group protocols, although fusidic acid is increasingly popular for treatment of staphylococcal infections. A review by Dollery (1998), however, suggests that there is no evidence to support the routine use of chloramphenicol in cases of minor corneal abrasions in order to prevent infection. She recommends that chloramphenicol use should be discontinued in cases of corneal abrasion secondary to corneal foreign body. Mackway-Jones (1999) has reviewed the evidence on the use of eye patches in cases of corneal abrasion and he concluded all the well-carried out trials showed no beneficial effects from the use of a patch. The strongest trial actually showed patients did better without a patch. The traditional treatment of chloramphenicol ointment and patch for a corneal abrasion has no evidence to support it and should be discontinued according to these authors. Jones (1998), however, observed that each patient should be treated on his/her own merits, especially with regard to comfort, rather by adherence to a rigid protocol. Table 9.2 provides information on the main agents used in treating eye conditions, including antibiotics, mydriatics to dilate the pupil and local anaesthetic agents for pain relief.

Patients with damage to the cornea from ultraviolet light (arc eye) often present 6–12 hours after they have been welding. They have a gritty and painful eye(s) and may have photophobia. Topical anaesthetic drops will be necessary before examination is possible as the condition is so painful. Marsden (1998c) recommends mydriatic eye drops, chloramphenicol ointment and oral analgesia for treatment, although the condition usually resolves within 48 hours.

Patients presenting with non-traumatic 'red eye' will usually have either a subconjunctival haemorrhage or conjunctivitis, which could be bacterial, viral or allergic in origin. Subconjunctival haemorrhages do not need any specific treatment, although it is worth checking the patient's blood pressure (hypertension may be a cause) or whether they are on anticoagulant therapy. Reassurance will be needed that the haemorrhage will reabsorb and gradually fade away. A viral cause for conjunctivitis is more likely than bacterial and is associated with a watery rather than a purulent or sticky discharge. Corneal erosions may be seen on fluorescein staining with a viral cause but not when the problem is bacterial in origin (Marsden, 1998a). A bacterial conjunctivitis requires an antibiotic such as chloramphenicol or fusidic acid, while a viral conjunctivitis does not. Artificial tears or a bland ointment may help relieve symptoms if a

Table 9.2 Eye drops and ointments commonly used in A & E

Type	Examples	Reasons for use
Local anaesthetic	Amethocaine	To relieve pain and allow examination. To allow procedures which involve contact with cornea
Miotic drops (pupil constricting)	Pilocarpine	To open the drainage angle thereby restoring the aqueous circulation in glaucoma
Mydriatic drops (pupil dilating)	Tropicamide Homatropine	To obtain a clear view of the posterior segment of the eye. Prevent adhesions between the iris and the lens in chemical burns. Patient should not be allowed to drive after use as the focusing mechanism of the eye will be disturbed
Antibiotics	Chloramphenicol Drops 0.5% Ointment 1%	To treat infection. If both eyes are being treated, two separate tubes should be used and labelled left and right, in order to prevent cross-infection. Drops are rapidly diluted and therefore need frequent application (hourly). Ointment will last longer.
	Fusidic acid drops 1%	Commonly used for staphylococcal infections
Antiviral	Acyclovir	To treat dendritic ulcers caused by the herpes simplex virus. Requires frequent application
Stain	Fluorescein	To obtain visualization of areas of missing corneal epithelium. Green indicates affected areas
Steroids	Betamethasone	To suppress inflammation. Must never be used unless the corneal epithelium is shown to be intact as steroids' suppression of the natural defence mechanisms can have disastrous consequences in the presence of herpes simplex. Never use, therefore, in cases of undiagnosed red eye

Source: BNF 1998.

viral causes is suspected. Good washing techniques are important to prevent spread to other members of the family.

Conditions such as uveitis and acute glaucoma require the urgent attention of an ophthalmologist. This is also true of serious conditions such as a hyphaemia or detached retina. Rest is essential as further sudden movements can exacerbate the situation. It is as well, therefore, to have a general rule in A & E that movement should be minimized for patients suffering from any eye injury. Effective channels of communication must exist between A & E and the nearest ophthalmic unit to ensure prompt specialist treatment for serious eye conditions.

Finally, before discharging a patient home from A & E, nurses must be sure that the patient understands what is required in terms of self-care of their eyes and that they are aware of the correct way to apply the ointment or cream that has been prescribed.

References

Bache J, Armitt C, Gadd C (1998) *Practical Procedures in the Emergency Department.* London: Mosby.

British National Formulary No.35 (1998) British Medical Association, Royal Pharmacological Society of Great Britain.

Dollery W (1998) Antibiotics and corneal abrasion. *Journal of Accident and Emergency Medicine,* **15**:352.

Field D, Martin D, Witchell L (1999) Ophthalmic chloramphenicol: a review of the literature. *Accident and Emergency Nursing,* 7:13–17.

Greaves I, Porter K, Burke D (1997) *Key Topics in Trauma.* Oxford: BIOS Publishers.

Jones G (1998) Foreign bodies in the eye. *Accident and Emergency Nursing,* 6:66–9.

Hartland G (1993). Nurse-aid management of ocular emergencies. *British Journal of Nursing,* 2:823–6.

Khaw P, Elkington A (1994) *ABC of Eyes,* 2nd edn. London: BMJ.

Mackway-Jones K (1999) Eye patches and corneal abrasions. *Journal of Accident and Emergency Medicine,* 16:136.

Marsden J (1998a) Identifying and managing non-traumatic red eye in A&E. *Emergency Nurse,* 5:6, 34–40.

Marsden J (1998b) Systematic eye examination in A&E. *Emergency Nurse,* 6:6, 16–19.

Marsden J (1998c) Care of patients with minor eye trauma. *Emergency Nurse,* 6:7, 10–14.

Marsden J (1999a) The effects of systemic illness on the eye and vision. *Emergency Nurse,* 7:1, 8–11.

Marsden J (1999b) Ocular burns. *Emergency Nurse,* 6:10, 20–4.

Plona R, Schremp P (1992) Care of patients with ocular manifestations of HIV infection. *Nursing Clinics of North America,* 27:793–805.

Seidal H, Ball J, Dains I, Bendict G (1995) *Mosby's Guide to Physical Examination,* 3rd edn. St Louis: CV Mosby.

Vader L (1992) Vision and vision loss. *Nursing Clinics of North America,* 27:705–13.

Walsh M, Crumbie A, Reveley S (1999) *Nurse Practitioners; Clinical Skills and Professional Issues.* Oxford: Butterworth-Heinemann.

Chapter 10

ENT AND DENTAL EMERGENCIES

The ear

Trauma

The external part of the ear, the pinna, is composed of cartilage and is commonly involved in injury. It may be lacerated, in which case it may be sutured and treated as any other wound, or it can suffer blunt trauma leading to the formation of a haematoma. Left untreated this will lead to deformity and the formation of a 'cauliflower ear'. Wardrope and Smith (1992) are pessimistic about the prospects for successful aspiration of such a haematoma and recommend referral to a specialist ENT surgeon for surgical drainage.

In severe injuries the whole of the pinna may be cut or torn off, e.g. in a knife fight. In such cases reattachment may be possible; therefore the wound site should be covered with a saline soak and the missing part retained, preferably dry and in a refrigerator, though not frozen.

Foreign bodies in the external auditory meatus are common problems with small children. They vary from beads to live insects, in which latter case, they should be drowned with olive oil before removal is attempted, as the insects are easier to remove dead than alive. Great skill is required on the part of the nursing staff to gain the cooperation and confidence of the parents and the child. The best approach, after explaining to the parents what is going to happen, is to sit the child on the parent's lap, wrapped tightly in a blanket so as to keep little hands and arms safely out of the way, and then attempt once to remove the object. If the casualty officer cannot remove it immediately, it is best left and the case referred to an ENT specialist. Further attempts with a struggling child may well lead to the object being pushed further into the ear, risking perforation of the eardrum.

The eardrum is most frequently damaged as a result of a sudden pressure change, e.g. after an explosion or on landing or take-off when flying. A blow to the ear with the hand flat or slightly cupped can produce the same effect. Small perforations will usually heal themselves but large tears may require surgical repair. The usual result of a perforated eardrum is deafness on the affected side.

A common reaction is for people to hit themselves on the side of the head affected or to try to poke something down their ear. Both should be discouraged as they may lead to further damage to the delicate structures of the middle ear. In making disaster plans, it should be taken into account that if an explosion has occurred there may be large numbers of people with perforated eardrums and deafness as a result. It is important to attempt to convey the likely temporary nature of such deafness to people in order to allay anxiety.

Diseases of the ear

It is probably true to say that in an ideal world people with diseases of the ear would not often be seen in A & E as they should have seen their GP who would have arranged the appropriate ENT specialist referral if needed.

A & E staff should not, however, be too dismissive of people with earache for two reasons. First, the ear may be very painful and the patient may be in considerable distress, especially if they cannot get an appointment to see their GP for two days, and secondly, ear pain may indicate a disease process which could have serious consequences for the patient if untreated.

The usual cause of a painful ear is infection: otitis externa, otitis media (which can be acute or chronic), or mastoiditis. Chronic disease of the middle ear (chronic suppurative otitis media) can lead to complications such as meningitis, brain abscess, and erosion and destruction of bone.

Otitis externa is common in swimmers and starts as an itchy ear but with gradually increasing pain and a discharge. Topical antibiotics and possibly a topical steroid are the usual treatments together with advice about hygiene, which should be given sensitively. Acute otitis media is most common in young children and presents as earache, pyrexia, lethargy and often with a story of a preceding upper respiratory tract infection. Oral analgesia should be given, although Wyatt *et al.* (1999) consider the prescription of antibiotics such as amoxycillin or erythromycin as of doubtful value.

Infections of the pinna of the ear include herpes (which may be accompanied by involvement of the inner ear leading to deafness, giddiness and vomiting) and the inflamed crusts of a staphylococcal infection seen in children with impetigo. If herpes is suspected it is essential the patient is given a triage category which ensures they see a doctor (Butler and Malem, 1993). A swollen painful earlobe may be associated with a recently pierced ear which has become infected. The earring should be removed and the person advised about hygiene.

One disease involving the ear that can lead patients to attend A & E in a very distressed emergency condition is vertigo. This condition gives rise to an illusion of movement, either that the person is moving, or that the environment is in motion. The cause is a conflict of information from the vestibular sources within the inner ear with information from other sensory systems, or alternatively, when the information supplied by the vestibular system about body movement cannot be coherently assessed by the central nervous system.

Vertigo always produces imbalance, although imbalance is not always caused by vertigo. The person suffering from an attack of vertigo will often fall to the ground and vomiting and nausea are common. The patient will present at A & E collapsed with vomiting. The patient should be laid flat on a trolley with cot sides in place and a vomit bowl available. Acute episodes of vertigo can be very frightening for the patient, therefore, considerable psychological support is necessary. An intramuscular injection of prochlorperazine (Stemetil) 12.5 mg is often prescribed to help relieve the acute symptoms followed by an oral course.

A common cause of vertigo is Meniere's disease, affecting one ear only and most common in onset in people between 30 and 60 years of age. The result is a violent paroxysmal attack, rotary in nature, associated with tinnitus and deafness, which may be one of several attacks clustered together. Migraine is another common cause of vertigo, particularly in adolescent girls.

The nose

Trauma

Fracture of the nasal bones is the most common facial fracture and is usually due to blunt trauma, e.g. a fall on the face or assault. Deformity, which may be obvious at first, will quickly be obscured by soft tissue swelling. Reduction should occur before 3 weeks, as fractured nasal bones will have set within that time span. However, it is necessary to wait for at least one week in order to allow the swelling to go down. If there is obvious nasal deformity or significant swelling, an ENT appointment should be made for 7–10 days time in order that the ENT specialists can manage the problem thereafter.

Nose bleeds

There are many reasons for nose bleeds, ranging from trauma or simply blowing the nose too hard in young people through to hypertension and degenerative arterial disease in the elderly. In young people bleeding is usually venous, while in the elderly an area of multiple arterial anastomosis located on the septum, Little's area, is usually the culprit, giving rise to arterial bleeding.

Nose bleeds are potentially very serious, especially in the elderly, and should be carefully assessed by the nurse in the same way that any other serious bleed would be assessed. Blood loss should be checked by asking the patient how long the bleed has been going on, examining any evidence such as a towel used to try to stop the bleeding, and by asking if the patient has been swallowing any blood as well as spitting it out. Blood pressure and pulse must be measured as hypotension and hypovolaemic shock are possible; an alternative finding is that the patient is hypertensive, and the hypertension has given rise to the nose bleed.

If the patient is hypovolaemic, then the full resuscitation procedure should be activated and should take priority over controlling bleeding in the first stages. Ludman (1993) states that 'An elderly patient who has lost a lot of blood is more likely to die during the next few hours from the effect of loss already sustained than from the results of continued bleeding.'

To try to arrest bleeding, the best procedure is to show the patient how to squeeze the *soft* lower part of the nose tightly. This will control bleeding by compression. Compression should be applied *continuously* for 20–30 minutes. The application of ice packs to the bridge of the nose may also be beneficial due to their vaso-constrictor effect. The patient should be sat upright if possible with their head tilted slightly forward and they should be supplied with a bowl and instructed to expectorate any blood that drips into their mouth. The patient should be instructed not to swallow the blood because it will lead to vomiting and also prevent measurement of the blood loss. If direct pressure is controlling bleeding, however, there should be little or no blood dripping down into the mouth.

If the patient is shocked from the bleed, their position should be modified to promote venous return and perfusion of the vital centres by elevating the legs and lying the patient as flat as possible. Medical staff may attempt to stop the bleeding by cauterization, nasal packing or the insertion of a compressed surgical sponge – nasal tampon (e.g. Merocel).

The sight of blood can have a very distressing effect on some people and, young or old, the patient suffering from a nose bleed may need considerable psychological support and encouragement from the nursing staff who should be aware that this is a potentially fatal condition. This is especially true of the situation where the patient is required to compress their own nose for 30 minutes. The temptation to let go soon becomes very great and all the good work done by 10 minutes of compression can be undone by 10 seconds' curiosity in wanting to see if the bleeding really has stopped.

The throat

Trauma

Reference has already been made to the need to deal urgently with neck injuries due to the twin threats posed by spinal injury and damage to the soft tissues of the throat which may lead to swelling and airway obstruction.

A common problem encountered in A & E is that of adults who feel they have 'something stuck in their throat', usually a fish or chicken bone. Such objects are usually found at the level of the tonsils or in the upper part of the oesophagus and may be visible with the aid of a good light source and a tongue depressor, enabling removal with a pair of forceps.

In assessing the patient, the nurse should be alerted by the patient describing a sensation of sharp pain on swallowing, especially if it radiates to the ear, difficulty in swallowing saliva, and tenderness over the trachea. Any of these symptoms indicate a real risk of an object being lodged in the throat or upper oeso-phagus. Unfortunately, many such objects are radiotranslucent, e.g. fish bones and many dental plates, but radiography is standard procedure still. If a perforation has occurred, even though the causative object may not show on X-ray, air in the soft tissues will allow the medical staff to make a diagnosis.

The picture is complicated by the fact that a sharp object that is swallowed may well scratch soft tissue, leaving behind a sensation of something sticking in the throat, even though the object has long gone on its way down the alimentary canal. Despite reassurance that there is not a problem and that nothing is stuck, the patient can still feel the sensation of something sticking there, and may not be convinced of the diagnosis. Considerable tact and diplomacy are required sometimes in this situation.

Perforation of the oesophagus or the devel-opment of an abscess in the upper respiratory tract due to impaction of a foreign body can have very serious consequences. It is advisable, therefore, to err on the side of caution and most A & E departments refer their patients on to ENT specialists if there is any chance of an impacted foreign body. If the patient is discharged, the nurse should reinforce patient instructions to return if symptoms do not improve or if any feeling of being unwell and feverish or if pain in the upper chest and neck region should develop. Mediastinitis develop-ing from a perforation of the oesophagus will make the patient seriously ill, while if a pharyngeal abscess were to develop, there is a risk of occluding the airway.

The advent of button batteries used in toys, watches, etc., has led to anxious parents presenting at A & E convinced their small child may have swallowed one. They are potentially very damaging as they may become lodged in the oesophagus causing perforation or may corrode and leak toxic substances such as mercury. It is essential to find out exactly what sort of battery has been swallowed and when and confer with the Poisons Information Centre for advice. On no account should any attempt be made to induce emesis. A button battery lodged in the nose can also cause corrosive burns and bleeding after a few weeks (Wyatt *et al.*, 1999).

Hoarseness and stridor in children

Stridor in a child with a previously adequate airway is usually caused by infection, but inhaled foreign bodies, trauma from ingesting corrosive agents and allergic oedema are other possible causes.

Croup is caused by acute laryngitis and can be a very frightening experience for both parent and child, a fact that should be remembered by the nurse. Dyspnoea is usually associated with more serious infections of the respiratory tract from the epiglottis downwards, rarely, but most seriously, epiglottitis. The throat and larynx of such young children in respiratory distress should only be examined by medical staff with considerable experience due to the risk of provoking laryngeal spasm which will lead to a total airway obstruction and cardiac arrest. Tracheotomy in a situation such as this is extremely difficult and the only way of providing an airway may well be by inserting needles into the trachea.

Facial and dental emergencies

Facial trauma

Trauma in the form of a direct blow to the face tends to produce one of several characteristic fracture patterns, which may also involve the base of the skull, leading to CSF leakage (rhinorrhoea from the nose and otorrhoea from the ear).

Blunt trauma to the side of the face is most likely to fracture the cheek or zygoma, characteristically in three places, the zygomatic arch, the posterior half of the infra-orbital rim and the frontal zygomatic suture, giving rise to what is known as a tripod or trimalleolar fracture.

High energy trauma affecting the front of the face can lead to fractures of the maxilla. Maxillary fractures tend to follow one of three characteristic patterns, first described by the French pathologist Le Fort (Fig. 10.1). A Le Fort II fracture produces very heavy nasal and pharyngeal bleeding which endangers the airway. A Le Fort III fracture commonly involves a CSF leak as there is usually an associated fracture of the cribiform plate. The airway is also at risk in a Le Fort III fracture because, as can be seen, the whole of the front of the face is effectively separated from the rest of the skull.

Fractures involving the mandible are associated with injury to the jaw. A midline fracture will usually be associated with a fracture of the condyles as well. Fractures of the nose have been discussed elsewhere (see p. 120).

Assessment of facial injuries

The first priority in assessing the patient who has sustained facial trauma, as in all cases, is to assess the patency of the airway. Noisy, laboured breathing almost certainly indicates obstruction of the airway. The mouth should be examined for the cause of obstruction, e.g. bleeding, vomit, dentures and the tongue. The contours of the face should be assessed, as in a Le Fort III fracture the front of the face is separated from the skull and gives a characteristic 'shoved in' or dish-like appearance. This indicates a serious hazard to the airway due to the abnormal anatomy.

Bleeding should be assessed and its source identified if possible, as clots of blood constitute a major airway threat. CSF should be looked for, indicating a fracture of the base of skull if found.

Facial trauma inevitably means that the brain absorbs a substantial amount of the energy involved, leading to the possibility of brain damage. A thorough neurological assessment, with particular attention being paid to level of consciousness, is therefore required.

If the patient is able to cooperate, the ability to oppose upper and lower sets of teeth correctly should be assessed. Failure to do so indicates a facial bone fracture such as a Le

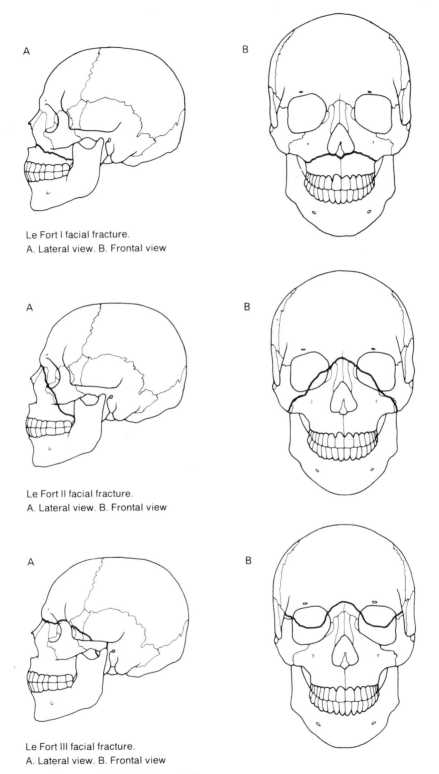

Le Fort I facial fracture.
A. Lateral view. B. Frontal view

Le Fort II facial fracture.
A. Lateral view. B. Frontal view

Le Fort III facial fracture.
A. Lateral view. B. Frontal view

Fig. 10.1 Patterns of fracture, Le Fort Types I–III

Fort or mandibular fracture. Gentle palpation of the face may well allow the nurse to feel the step associated with a fracture. A complaint by the patient of double vision should alert the nurses to the possibility of a blow out fracture causing tethering of the rectus muscle that controls eye movement (see p. 111).

Intervention

The first intervention priority is to clear and maintain the airway which is at hazard from bleeding, clots, dentures, fractured teeth, the tongue, vomit and the abnormal anatomy associated with certain fracture patterns such as a Le Fort III fracture.

The standard measures of mechanically clearing the oropharynx with suction and forceps (or gloved fingers), inserting an oral airway to lift the tongue forward (if tolerated), and positioning the patient on their side with the head down to aid drainage of blood, etc., should be followed immediately. Consideration should also be given to the possibility of cervical injury. In severe cases, intubation or tracheotomy may be required immediately in the A & E resuscitation room. The nurse should therefore know where the necessary equipment is located and be able to give whatever assistance is required by the medical team.

Due to the grave hazard posed to the airway by facial injuries, patients should never be left unattended or lying on their backs. Oxygen may be administered via a high concentration mask. Careful monitoring of the patient's neurological status is required due to the risk of deterioration in consciousness associated with brain trauma. A cervical collar and/or head blocks is a wise precaution due to the risk of spinal injury.

Severe facial injuries can be very distressing to the patient, distress that can be compounded by fear of disfigurement. Psychological support from the nursing staff is therefore very important. Communication with the patient may be impeded as the injuries may interfere with normal speech. Nurses should, therefore, try to phrase questions so that the patient may answer simply yes or no.

Patients with facial fractures will usually have their fractures dealt with by wiring. They therefore need preparing for theatre in the usual way, according to hospital policy.

Dental problems

A & E departments are commonly confronted with patients in severe pain due to toothache for whom there is little we can do apart from offer analgesia and a contact number for any out of hours dental services that may operate in the area.

Bleeding from a tooth socket following an extraction earlier in the day is a familiar complaint seen in the evening at A & E. The presence of blood in the mouth which the patient continually has to expectorate leads to distress and anxiety, while swallowing it will cause nausea and vomiting. The correct procedure is direct pressure to the bleeding socket applied by having the patient bite on a gauze swab for at least 10 minutes. It is helpful to ask the patient if there have been any other bleeding-related problems, as this may indicate a significant blood disorder that requires investigation.

Pain associated with facial swelling and an elevated temperature is indicative of a dental abscess, usually related to non-vital or degenerative pulp, the result of advanced dental caries. The patient will often complain of having been unable to eat, drink or sleep because of the condition.

While the medical staff will probably prescribe analgesics and antibiotics, the nursing staff should ensure that the patient understands the need for complete rest, which tablets are for pain and which are the antibiotics. This last information should be written on the tablet bottle label as patients who have been suffering from a dental abscess are often tired and distressed and may not absorb fully information given verbally. Dehydration may be present; therefore advice should be given about the need to drink plenty of fluids. General dietary information concerning liquid nutrition may be of assistance in some cases. In severe cases, cellulitis may develop involving the soft tissue of the whole jaw. Admission for inpatient management is required in such cases.

References

Butler K, Malem F (1993) Nurse and management of ear, nose and throat emergencies. *British Journal of Nursing*, **2**:875–8.

Ludman H (1993) *Otolaryngology*, 3rd edn. London: BMJ.

Wardrope J, Smith J (1992) *The Management of Wounds and Burns*. Oxford: Oxford University Press.

Wyatt J, Illingworth R, Clancy M, Munro P, Robertson C (1999) *Oxford Handbook of Accident and Emergency Medicine*. Oxford: Oxford University Press.

Chapter 11

CHILDREN IN A & E

Children are a major group of patients in A & E with problems unique to themselves. This raises the question of how well prepared are A & E Departments to meet their needs? Wood (1997), for example, estimated that 30% of A & E attendances are accounted for by children aged 16 and under. Smith (1998) confirms this figure but, based on her national A & E survey (responses received from 204 out of 283 departments), points out that in some departments the figure is as high as 45%. Despite the well-recognized need for special children's areas within A & E, 21% of the departments in Smith's survey reported that they did not have such a facility. Even more worrying was the finding that only 11% reported that they had sufficient children's trained nurses to provide 24-hour cover, despite the fact that it is DoH policy that nursing staff trained and experienced in the care of children should be available at all times in A & E (Department of Health, 1991). This survey also highlighted serious deficiencies in the training available to staff. For example, departments reported that staff did not receive training in the following areas: drugs and equipment used with children (29%); clinical assessment of children (38%); communicating with children (61%); young people's mental health problems (84%). Other areas listed included child protection (12%) and chronic illness in children (77%). As most

A & E nurses are adult trained, education in these key areas is essential.

A fundamental principle is that children should not be treated as small-scale adults. Their needs are very different, whether it is in terms of clinical interventions or psychosocial care. Vital signs for children are very different from adults and normal ranges are summarized in Table 11.1.

Causes of death in children vary with age. Cot death was the leading cause in those aged 4 weeks to 1 year, but the incidence of this has been reduced dramatically in the 1990s as a result of campaigns to alert parents to known risk factors (see p. 133). Trauma remains the leading cause of death in children aged over 1 year. When the time from injury to death is noted, three main groups are apparent; 44% occur within the first hour, 20% within a few hours and a further 36% occur days later (Advanced Life Support Group, 1997). The A & E department is therefore the part of a hospital most likely to witness the death of a child and this has major implications, both for coping with the bereaved parents and for staff supporting each other through this difficult period.

The nature of critical childhood illness is such that children often tend to experience hypoxia, acidosis and respiratory arrest prior to cardiac arrest which has usually followed a

Table 11.1 Normal range of vital signs in children

Age	Respiratory rate	Systolic BP	Pulse rate
<1	30–40	70–90	110–160
2–5	25–30	80–100	95–140
5–12	20–25	90–110	80–120
>12	15–20	100–120	60–100

Source: Castle (1999)

period of profound bradycardia (Castle, 1999). Resuscitation is, therefore, very difficult when compared to an adult who frequently presents in (reversible) ventricular fibrillation as a result of a sudden cardiac episode. Paediatric arrest, therefore, has a low initial survival rate and a high incidence of neurological damage in survivors (Castle, 1999). Circulatory failure leading directly to cardiac arrest can also occur in conditions such as anaphylaxis, septic shock or severe fluid loss as encountered in burns or blood loss due to trauma.

The observation that children are not small-scale adults has particular physiological significance. Drug therapies, for example, are usually weight dependent and therefore an accurate estimate of a child's weight is essential. If it is not possible to weigh the child, various charts based upon average ages, heights and weights may be used. A useful rule of thumb (Advanced Life Support Group, 1997) is that for children aged 1–10, weight in kilograms is approximately given by Wt = 2 × (age + 4). Body surface areas change with age, which is of particular significance in dealing with burns. For example, although the head accounts for 9% of the body surface area in adults, the figure is 19.5% in the new born. The Wallace Rules of 9 are therefore not appropriate for use with small children (see p. 47). Intravenous access is very difficult in small children and intraosseous infusion is used instead. The usual site is the anterior surface of the tibia, 2 cm below the tibial tuberosity. Local anaesthetic must be used if the child is conscious (lignocaine 1%). Strict asepsis is essential and the fluid or drugs being given need gently pushing through the intraosseous needle with a 50 ml syringe as gravity feed will be insufficient to overcome back pressure (Bache *et al.*, 1998).

The assessment of pain in the child is another area where we cannot think merely in terms of a small-scale adult. Devices such as the pain ladder (aged 8 and over) or faces scale (ages 4–8) have to be used (Fig. 11.1). Childrens' perceptions of the world are different at different ages (p. 128–9) and consequently their experience of pain is likely to be different from that of an adult. The greatest single thing that helps a child deal with pain is likely to be the presence of a parent. Talking to and touching the child helps distract attention from an unpleasant procedure and relieve anxiety. Having a child-friendly environment is extremely helpful in reducing fear and distress. Mason (1998) points out that creating a supportive environment for parents to help their child may be the only nursing intervention necessary. However, the nurse should not expect the parent automatically to know what to do, advice and guidance may be needed in how best to help the child through a procedure. Family-centred care has to be reality not rhetoric in A & E.

Given the importance of parents in relieving a child's pain and distress, it is salutary to examine research by Spedding *et al.* (1999). They carried out a 28-day survey of pain relief in children attending A & E. They received 276 completed questionnaires during the study and found that, in 203 cases (74%), no analgesia had been given before taking the child to A & E. When questioned as to why they had not given painkillers to their children, 32% stated they did not have any analgesia suitable for children at home, 28% stated that they thought giving painkillers would be harmful, 21% that they did not give painkillers because the accident did not happen at home and a further 7% thought analgesia was the responsibility of the hospital. These findings, if replicated in your A & E department, indicate the need for a major health education campaign.

The Advanced Support Life Group (1997) recommend the following analgesics as being

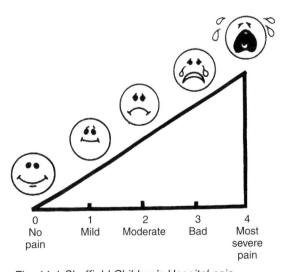

0	1	2	3	4
No pain	Mild	Moderate	Bad	Most severe pain

Fig. 11.1 Sheffield Children's Hospital pain assessment tool (Husband and Trigg, 2000)

suitable for use with children:

- Topical local anaesthetics such as Emla or Ametop gel which can be used under an occlusive dressing. They take at least 45 minutes to work properly but mean that IV cannulation can be carried out painlessly.
- Lignocaine 1% can be used as a rapid acting, sensory nerve block. Bupivacaine 0.25% may be used when a longer lasting effect is required. It takes up to 15 minutes to become fully effective and can last for up to 8 hours.
- Non-steroidal anti-inflammatory drugs are particularly suitable for treating pain due to trauma because of their anti-inflammatory effect. Ibuprofen is probably the drug of choice, although diclofenac can be given by suppository if required. The usual contra-indications for all NSAIDs apply as in adults.
- Paracetamol is widely used in children but has no anti-inflammatory effect. Its taste means it usually has to be camouflaged in a preparation such as Calpol.
- Entonox (nitrous oxide and oxygen) can be used by children as young as 5 years old and is ideal for a short-term effect. It reaches its maximum effect within 2 minutes but wears off just as quickly.
- Opiate analgesics such as morphine are very effective but, as the possible side effects are potentially very serious, drug doses must be carefully calculated and checked and the child should be observed closely at all times for signs of respiratory depression and hypotension. Morphine is best given via the IV or intraosseous route rather than by intramuscular injection. Naloxone (opiate antagonist) should be available at all times.
- Midazolam; this is an amnesic and sedative drug which may be used to perform unpleasant procedures, it is not, however, an analgesic. Davies and Waters (1998) have reported upon a successful trial of the drug used orally at 0.5 mg/kg. At this dose it became effective within 15 minutes and produced amnesia or greatly reduced anxiety levels in 76% of the children upon whom it was used. Ninety per cent of parents stated that they would like the drug used again on their child if similar circumstances arose. Hyperexcitability is a known side effect in

children and this was observed in three of the 50 children in the study.

The assessment tools, medication and techniques are therefore available to treat effectively children's pain in A & E. The important thing, however, is to use them properly and appreciate that the child's perception of things differs substantially from the adult.

When national statistics are examined, the major influence exerted by poverty and other social factors on childhood accidents and mortality rates is apparent. We have already seen in Chapter 1 how social class plays such an important role in determining health. Children in class V are more than twice as likely to die as a result of an accident than in class I, while for some types of accident the differential is even more pronounced. For example, the mortality rate from burns and household fires is six times greater in children from class V families than it is among class I families (Drever and Whitehead, 1995). The Public Health Common Data Set (Department of Health, 1993) shows that gender plays a key role, as the overall mortality rate for boys in England and Wales was 8.96 compared to 6.64 per 100 000 for girls.

Cody and Waine (1992), in their study in North Wales, showed that the two main causes of childhood accidents were environmental hazards and inadequate supervision. The most common presenting condition in children aged under 5 was head injury, accounting for 40% of attendances in the age group 1–4 alone. Findings such as these have major implications for health education and accident prevention programmes as well as for training of A & E staff to ensure they are well prepared to deal with the most common presenting childhood conditions.

The way children think and how it varies with age

A child's way of thinking and of perceiving the world is very different from that of an adult. Psychologists have espoused many theories of child development and while a book such as this cannot explore this area in detail, it is essential that the A & E nurse at least appreciates the key principles involved and their implications for A & E work. Early views saw development of behaviour as a series of predictable, mechanistic reactions to environmental stimuli, which progressed in well-defined stages to adulthood (e.g. behaviourism). A contrasting view saw children develop in response to self-initiated activities that came from within the child, but which also progressed through a series of distinct stages. This model is exemplified by the work of Jean Piaget (1952) and his theory of cognitive development. Piaget's ideas have become widely known and taught within children's nursing courses. His stages may be summarized as follows:

1. *The sensori-motor stage, age 0–2.* Egocentric, needs to learn that the world around is not just an extension of self. For the first 7 months of life, the child is without the concept of object permanence; therefore, if something cannot be seen it does not exist. By 18 months the child can start to work out how to do something before doing it.

2. *Pre-conceptual thought, age 2–7.* Egocentricity is still very pronounced; the child believes that others, including the nurse, think and see the world in the same way that the child does. Reason is dominated by perception and there is no idea of groups or classes. Intuitive rather than logical thought, thus if one medicine tastes nasty, the child decides all medicines taste nasty.

3. *Concrete operational, age 7–11/12.* The child begins to see things from other people's point of view and can now think logically, although in a rather literal way, s/he cannot handle abstract concepts. The child can reverse mental processes and understand quantity. If liquid is poured from one container into another of different shape, a child under 7 will claim that there is more in the container with a higher liquid level and will not be able to see that the volume remains the same. Thus in giving medicine to a reluctant 5 year old, a more successful approach may be to pour the medicine onto a large spoon from the measuring pot as the child may think of this as a smaller volume.

4. *Formal operational thought, age 12–14.* It is only in this age range that the child learns to handle the abstract thought patterns and concepts that are taken for granted by adults.

Piaget's ideas can be summarized by saying that children invent or construct rules which allow them to think logically and make sense of the world around them. Research confirms that children do appear to move through such a series of stages, however, for any one child it is a continuum and their thought evolves gradually rather than jumps forward from one stage to the next. Children in different societies and cultural backgrounds move through these stages at very different rates from those originally proposed by Piaget. This is not surprising as his experimental work was carried out with middle-class Swiss children only. The ages at which children achieve these different stages are therefore likely to be very different from those proposed by Piaget.

Although various criticisms have been levelled at Piaget's work and several alternative theories of child development proposed, Lefrançois (1996) considers his work to be the most important cognitive developmental theory of the last 100 years. Lefrançois, however, points out that psychology has moved on from the mechanistic (behaviourist) and organistic (e.g. Piagetian) views of child development. A third approach involves recognizing the importance of context and the child's complex interaction with the environment as the key to understanding development. The key point is that child will not understand the A & E environment in the same way as an adult and allowances must be made for this. Morcombe (1998) shows the value of this insight in demonstrating how Piaget's ideas can be applied to the problem of reducing fear and anxiety in young children in A & E, while Dolan (1997) has explored the common problem of persuading a 3 year old to take medication, in developmental terms.

Child abuse

Abused children present to A & E every day of the week. There are approximately 35 000 children in England alone on child protection registers and proven cases of child abuse are four to five times more common than they were in the 1980s. Perhaps the most shocking statistic is the fact that this week approximately four children will die as a result of abuse and neglect (Meadow, 1997). It is therefore important for nurses to understand the signs that should arouse suspicions of child abuse and to be aware of the likely forms that abuse may take. The main reasons children are on child protection registers are physical abuse (40%), neglect (30%), sexual abuse (24%) and emotional abuse (6%) with girls accounting for 61% of those on the register (Meadow, 1997). Communication failures are a depressingly common theme that runs throughout all the enquiries that have been held into child deaths from abuse. The A & E department is a vital link in that communication chain that must never fail an abused child.

Child abuse is a symptom of disordered parenting (Speight, 1997) and as such does not depend upon social class. Stereotyping should be avoided at all costs and the fact that a child is from a well-off home background does not mean that it could not have been abused. As Speight observes:

'The most difficult step in diagnosing non-accidental injury is to force yourself to think of it in the first place.' Speight (p. 5, 1997)

Niven (1992) points out there is a strong statistical association between sociodemographic factors such as financial deprivation, single mothers, young parental age, marital disruption and lack of social support with child abuse. However, the vast majority of children from such backgrounds, as Niven reminds us, are not abused, hence the importance of avoiding stereotyping.

In assessing any child in A & E for the risk of abuse the following factors should be noted as warning signs:

1. A delay in seeking treatment.
2. If there is an inadequate explanation of the injury.
3. If the explanation is inappropriate for the extent or type of injury.
4. Signs of previous injury, such as fading bruises.
5. Defensiveness and hostility, or alternatively apathy and disinterest towards the child by the parent.
6. Silence and withdrawal on the part of the child.
7. Evidence of failure to thrive; if the child has not reached appropriate milestones both for physical or mental development.
8. Frequent parental attendances at A & E (often for non-specific reasons) with the child.
9. Signs of physical neglect.

If any of the above factors are present, the child should be completely undressed to allow a thorough examination. As a rough guide bruising less than 24 hours old is usually red/purple but at 12–48 hours is more of a purplish blue colour. At 48–72 hours the colour is more of a brown hue and over 72 hours is yellow. The shape and location of bruises should be checked as they may be finger tip bruises indicating excessive force has been used in gripping or the child has been deliberately pinched. Lash marks may be present where the child has been beaten with an object such as a belt. The behaviour of the child and the parent(s) should be carefully watched as this may reveal clues to abuse that may not be noted if just the physical signs are searched for. Mental cruelty, isolation and neglect of the child's developing mind do not leave physical evidence. Sexual abuse may not either, although the genitalia and rectum should be included in the physical examination. The incidence of sexual abuse of children is difficult to estimate because the better known the person is to the child, the less likely the case is to be reported to the police. It is likely that the abuser will be a member of the family or well known to the child, probably male, and the abuse will be a long-term process spread over years which has devastating long-term psychological implications for the victim.

At some stage in the proceedings, the child should be carefully questioned in private, out of earshot of the parents if this is possible. The stage of cognitive development of the child should be considered in phrasing questions. A doll may be helpful in the case of a young child who can demonstrate which parts of their body were interfered with more readily than they can describe with words where sexual abuse is suspected. The important role of A & E nurses in helping to spot cases of child sex abuse cannot be underestimated (Saines, 1992).

Local authorities maintain a register of suspected and at risk children, a copy of which should be in the A & E department, updated frequently, and accessible to qualified staff. Information that is not accessible is not information. This register should be checked at even the slightest suspicion. Clearly laid down procedures which are followed, teamwork and close links with health visitors are essential. If there is a possibility of child abuse, it is usual procedure to contact the paediatric services who will involve Social Services. Meticulous attention to detail is necessary in recording injuries and marks on the child, together with the child's general appearance as the case may well end up in court.

Dimond (1993) lists the following key sections from the 1989 Children Act which are relevant:

- Section 43: Child Assessment Order; this gives legal authority for a detailed assessment to be carried out.
- Section 44: Emergency Protection Order; this allows a local authority to take a child into care for protection.
- Section 46: Police Powers; this permits a constable to remove a child to a place of safety or prevent anyone removing a child from a hospital or other accommodation.

Cases of child abuse can be very distressing for the staff involved. Feelings of anger and outrage at the sight of a pathetic rag doll of a child covered in bruises and burns are understandable human emotions. The suspicion of sexual abuse may also fill the nurse with revulsion and anger. However, anger is not a constructive force that will help the child. The child is, after all, the victim of anger and may have mixed emotions of guilt and anger as a result of the abuse (Saines, 1992). The nurse must be in control of him or herself if he or she is to be in control of the situation and to act for the child in the child's best interests. Remember we are not employed as judges; it is for others to pass judgement on the parents. It is worth noting the findings of Ward *et al.* (1993) that the mothers of assaulted children are more likely than other women to become the victims of assault themselves.

Some common childhood emergencies

1. *Accidental poisoning.* Burton (1993) found that, in a study of 319 children presenting at a major A & E department, the most common age was 2–3 years old. Tablets were the most common substance taken (31%), followed by liquid medications (15%), household cleaners and paint thinners (10% each). He comments that taste and smell are no deterrent to young children and also that many parents stated they thought substances were safe because they were in high cupboards. This ignores the climbing ability of even young toddlers.

In the assessment of the child, nurses need to discover exactly what was taken, how much, when, and if there has been any vomiting since ingestion. Questioning should be tailored to the child's level of cognitive development and also to the parent's level of anxiety, which can be very high and, as a result, interfere with their ability to think clearly. If there is any doubt about care, one of the national poisons information centres should be contacted by phone. Key information for the poison centre staff, apart from what, when and how much was taken, is the child's age and approximate weight.

The treatment of poisoning in adults is discussed on p. 167. The traditional approach to accidental poisoning in children was to induce emesis by giving 15 ml of syrup of ipecacuanha followed by about 200 ml of water which was flavoured with squash according to the child's taste. However, the BNF (1997) states that this is of limited value as there is no evidence to suggest it prevents clinically significant absorption even if used within 1–2 hours. One of the most common and serious poisonings is that due to iron capsules prescribed for the mother's anaemia; they present a very attractive sight to the young toddler. The result is necrosis of the gastrointestinal wall and poisoning by the iron as it is so rapidly absorbed. Desferrioxamine IV should always be available to deal with this serious emergency.

Poisoning of children may occur intentionally. It most commonly is Munchausen syndrome by proxy carried out by the mother, although other reasons include 'teaching the child a lesson' and homes where the parents are involved in drug abuse (Meadow, 1997). Presentation is usually a child with inexplicable signs and symptoms such as seizures, apnoeic spells, drowsiness, vomiting, hallucinations, hyperventilation or haematemesis. The poisoning is deliberately concealed. A high index of suspicion is necessary together with a willingness to think the unthinkable if the correct diagnosis is to be arrived at.

2. *Febrile convulsion.* Convulsions associated with febrile illness occur in 2–4% of children and represent the most common diagnosis in children who have had a convulsion, followed

by epilepsy. It is during the phase of rising temperature that a convulsion is most likely to occur with children aged 6 months to 5 years (Rogers, 1992). Such a convulsion can be a very alarming experience for the parents, who usually wrap their child up in a blanket, raising the temperature even further, and then rush off to the nearest A & E department in a state of great anxiety.

Great reassurance is necessary, together with an accurate temperature reading. Advanced Paediatric Life Support (1997) guidelines also stipulate that a BM stick reading should be taken as hypoglycaemia can cause convulsions. If the child is indeed pyrexial, then cooling should commence by removal of clothing, blankets etc. The nurse should be explaining to the parents all the time what is being done and why. Medication to reduce the child's temperature, such as paracetamol, should be commenced as soon as the child is able to cooperate. Health education about the risk of pyrexia and convulsions is essential for the parents. The medical staff may choose to admit the child for observation and this should be carefully explained in order to avoid alarming the parents unduly. An audit by Fawcett (1998) showed 8% of children brought to her A & E department with a complaint of fitting were still fitting when they presented. If this is the case the child should be given rectal diazepam 0.4 mg/kg and if this has had no effect in 5 minutes, a further dose of 0.25 mg/kg given IV (APLS, 1997).

3. *Acute respiratory distress.* Pathology: the most common causes of acute respiratory distress in children are:

1. Foreign body: commonly nuts or beans cause an inflammatory response in addition to obstruction; can be anywhere between the nasopharynx and bronchus.
2. Infectious disease causing obstruction of the airway: a common problem is tonsillitis or a tonsillar abscess. Epiglottitis is a serious emergency as the swollen epiglottis can easily occlude the airway; the child is pyrexial, dysphagic, drooling, hypoventilating but not coughing. No attempt must be made to examine the epiglottis as this can cause spasm and respiratory arrest.
3. Croup: a bacterial infection of the larynx, trachea and bronchi leading to inflammation of the lining of the trachea and larynx. The child is very distressed, exhibits respiratory stridor and has great difficulty breathing.
4. Asthma: the bronchioles are in spasm leading to expiratory wheeze.
5. Bronchiolitis/pneumonia: the young child can be acutely ill as a result of infection of the lower respiratory tract. Parents may not always contact their GP and can bring such an ill child to A & E at any time of the day or night.

Nursing interventions

Chapters 4 and 5 have already dealt with the care of adults with serious respiratory problems. The following key points are essential to remember in A & E because children are different in significant ways, not least of which is the obvious fact that a child's airway is smaller than an adult's. Airway blockage is therefore easier in children whether the cause is a foreign body or oedema. Either a head tilt/chin lift or a jaw thrust technique can be used to clear the airway (subject to the usual conditions, p. 30), however, in basic life support the finger sweep manoeuvre employed in adults should not be used. This is because the child's soft palate is easily damaged and bleeding within the mouth will make things even worse. Foreign bodies may easily be forced further down the airway (APLS, 1997). A much narrower endotracheal tube will be used with small children, which means the risk of occlusion is always greater and therefore greater attention should be paid to suctioning the tube. If the child is conscious he or she should be allowed to find the most comfortable position, which may be sitting upright on a parent's lap. Children are much less likely than adults to tolerate an oxygen mask, although the presence of a parent may help, especially if combined with the use of nasal cannula. In a child with serious respiratory distress, pulse oximetry and close observation of respiratory rate and effort, along with pulse, are essential throughout. The nurse should always remember the extreme anxiety of the parents involved, as well as the fear of the child, in such a situation.

Ten per cent of school age children have asthma making this a common presentation in A & E (Caldwell, 1997). Table 11.2

Table 11.2 Signs of severe asthma in children

Under 5 years old	5–15 years old
Too breathless to talk or feed Respirations > 50 breaths/min Pulse > 140 Use of accessory muscles of breathing	Too breathless to talk or feed Respirations > 40 breaths/min Pulse > 120 Peak flow (50% predicted or best value)

NB: the following are life-threatening features for all children; cyanosis, silent chest, poor respiratory effort, fatigue, exhaustion, agitation or reduced level of consciousness (Caldwell, 1997).

summarizes the signs which indicate a severe asthma attack in children.

The child should immediately be given high concentration oxygen and a nebulized bronchodilator via oxygen. Pulse oximetry and vital signs monitoring are essential. Oral steroids will also be given. If the child does not improve or if life-threatening features are present, IV aminophylline and hydrocortisone will be given. Parents should be supported and encouraged to stay with their child at all times. If the child recovers and is well enough to go home from A & E, enquiries should be made about inhaler technique and any health education opportunity taken.

4. *Children with burns.* Although Chapter 4 considered burns in detail, it is worth raising the subject here to remind nurses that children are different to adults. The Rules of 9 cannot be applied to children and if a paediatric burns chart is not available, the fact that the child's hand is 1% of his/her body area will permit an estimate of area to be made. If the burn area is greater than 10%, IV resuscitation is necessary. Analgesia in the form of IV morphine, 0.1mg/kg should be given in all but the most minor burns. Absorption via the intramuscular route is too unreliable (Advanced Life Support Group, 1997).

5. *Cot death or sudden infant death syndrome (SIDS)*

The age most at risk is 2–4 months and, according to some authorities, in this age range SIDS accounts for more deaths than all other diseases put together. The evidence is that most deaths occur in the early hours of the morning when infant and family are all asleep. There has been a welcome reduction in the incidence of SIDS with the implementation of advice to avoid the prone (face down) position. Making parents aware of the association between SIDS and parental smoking may also have helped.

Returning to A & E and the nurse confronted with this situation, it has to be said that usually there is nothing that can be done for the infant, who is usually beyond resuscitation.

The nurse's attention has to focus on the parents. A direct and sympathetic approach is best in breaking the news. Parental feelings of guilt are common, especially if the baby has been left with a baby-sitter. It is imperative to try to dissipate this guilt by pointing out that there is no blame to attach and that there is nothing that could have been done. The grieving process begins in the resuscitation room and the parents should be encouraged to hold the baby. It is the first step in coming to terms with the reality of death, of accepting rather than denying death, of letting go.

It is essential to give immediate support, and arrange continuing assistance for the parents by contacting other members of the family and friends. The numbness and paralysis that accompanies the news of bereavement is utterly devastating to the parents in SIDS. This sense of helplessness and disbelief is movingly described by Stead (1998), an experienced A & E nurse, in her account of what happened when her own son, Dominic, became another SIDS victim. The health visitor, GP and Coroner's Office should be contacted as a postmortem will be required. Support for the parents may be obtained from the Foundation for the Study of Infant Deaths. Their address is given at the end of the chapter. They are a world famous organization offering counselling and support through a network of local self-help groups, among their many other activities.

It remains to say that, in addition to the grief of the family, there is also the grief of the staff.

Such grief is to be expected as a normal human response to any death, particularly a child's death, and staff should therefore be encouraged to verbalize their feelings and emotions. It is the senior nurses' responsibility to see that such discussion takes place and that all the staff involved, nursing, medical and clerical, can help each other through such a distressing event.

There is chilling evidence emerging that a significant number of SIDS cases should be reclassified as murder, however. Meadows (1999) has presented the cases of 81 children who were initially diagnosed as SIDS but in each case were subsequently proved to have been killed by their parents. He goes on to suggest that the term SIDS should be abandoned. While the perpetrator is usually the mother in such cases, the example of Simon Smith, who was convicted recently at Staffordshire Crown Court of killing three of his children and faking each as a SIDS case, points out a major gap in child protection procedures (Bufton, 1999). Records concentrate on the mother, consequently it was only an observant staff nurse in A & E who realized that the same man had fathered three different children with three different surnames and two different mothers, all of whom had apparently become SIDS victims. Bufton points out that there has to be a willingness to think the unthinkable in cases of SIDS, especially when the child lies outside the age range 2–4 months. Careful cooperation between A & E, the Coroner's Office and the police to work out a sensitive policy to handle such cases is needed if forensic evidence is to be preserved and prosecutions brought against other parents who kill their children and escape unpunished.

Summary

Children are a very important group of A & E patients and, like all A&E patients, can present with a wide range of conditions from the life-threatening emergency to the trivial. Most A & E nurses are general/adult trained only and therefore need to appreciate the special needs of children; they are not small adults. Continuing professional education is therefore essential if this very important group of patients is to receive the care it deserves. Above all, there are times when we have to be prepared to think the unthinkable.

References

Advanced Life Support Group (1997) *Advanced Paediatric Life Support*, 2nd edn. London: BMJ.

Bache J, Armitt C, Gadd C (1998) *Practical Procedures in the Emergency Department*. London: Mosby.

British National Formulary (1997) London, BMA/ Royal Pharmaceutical Society of Great Britain.

Bufton S (1999) Infant deaths; investigations, implications and considerations for emergency services. RCN A&E Association Conference, Blackpool, November 4th 1999.

Burton R (1993) Eat, drink and be dead. *Accident and Emergency Nursing*; 1:14–19.

Caldwell C (1997) Management of acute asthma in children. *Emergency Nurse*, 5:7, 33–7.

Castle N (1999) Paediatric resuscitation. *Emergency Nurse*, 7:1, 31–9.

Cody A, Waine N (1992) Preventing childhood accidents: an intervention exercise in Clwyd. *British Journal of Nursing*, 2:1059–64.

Davies F, Waters M (1998) Oral midazolam for conscious sedation of children during minor procedures. *Journal of Accident and Emergency Medicine*, 15:244–8.

Department of Health (1991) *Welfare of Children and Young People in Hospital*. London: HMSO.

Department of Health (1993) *Public Health Common Data Set*, vol. 1. London: HMSO.

Dimond B (1993) Non-accidental injury and the A & E nurse. *Accident and Emergency Nursing*, 1: 225–8.

Dolan K (1997) Children in Accident and Emergency. *Accident and Emergency Nursing*, 5:88–91.

Drever F, Whitehead M (1995) *Health Inequalities Decennial Supplement*. London: Office for National Statistics.

Husband S, Trigg E (2000) *Practices in Children's Nursing*. London: Churchill Livingstone.

Lefrançois G (1996) *The Lifespan*, 5th edn. Belmont Ca: Wadsworth Publishing Co.

Mason M (1998) Setting up a paediatric facility. *Emergency Nurse*, 6:2, 8–9.

Meadow R (1997) *ABC of Child Abuse*. London: BMJ.

Meadow R (1999) Unnatural sudden infant death. *Archives of Disease in Childhood*, 80:7–14.

Morcombe J (1998) Reducing anxiety in children in A&E. *Emergency Nurse*, 6:2, 10–13.

Niven C (1992) *Psychological Care for Families*. Oxford: Butterworth-Heinemann.

Piaget J (1952) *The Origins of Intelligence in Children*. New York: International Universities Press.

Rogers M (1992) Febrile convulsions. *Paediatric Nursing*, **5**:24–7.

Saines J (1992) A considered response to an emotional crisis. *Professional Nurse*, **8**:148–52.

Smith F (1998) Caring for children. *Emergency Nurse*, **6**:2, 10–13.

Spedding R, Harley D, Dunn F, McKinney L (1999) Who gives pain relief to children? *Journal of Accident and Emergency Medicine*, **16**:261–4.

Speight N (1997) Non-accidental Injury. In Meadow R (ed.) *ABC of Child Abuse*. London: BMJ.

Stead C (1998) Sudden Infant Death Syndrome (SIDS) on the 'other side'. *Accident and Emergency Nursing*, **6**: 24–7.

Ward L, Shepherd J, Emond A (1993) Relationship between adult victims of assault and children at risk of abuse. *BMJ*, **306**:1101–2.

Wood I (1997) Communicating with children in A&E: what skills does the nurse need? *Accident and Emergency Nursing*, **5**:137–41.

Young S (1999) Comparing the use of ketamine and midezolam in emergency settings. *Emergency Nurse*, **7(8)**:27–31.

Note: The address of the Foundation for the Study of Infant Deaths is 35 Belgrave Square, London SW1X 8QB.

Chapter 12

THE OLDER PERSON IN A & E

Just as it is inappropriate to think of children as adults only smaller, so it is wrong to think of the elderly as the same as everyone else only older. The profound physiological, psychological and sociological changes associated with ageing mean that nurses must consider older people as having a unique field of problems that is deserving of special consideration. They are an important patient group in A & E as is shown by the fact that Ryan (1996) estimates over 300 000 people aged over 65 attend A & E each year in the UK, while admission rates in the 65+ age group from A & E are four times higher than among younger patients (Strange *et al.*, 1992).

As a person ages, s/he becomes more likely to be affected by various degenerative disease processes which will make that person more likely to attend A & E as an emergency (e.g. after a stroke or myocardial infarction). However, ageing also makes a person much more likely to have accidents and falls and brings with it increasing social problems for many elderly people. The social circumstances of the elderly patient must receive careful consideration by the nurse before discharge from A & E, and there are times when the patient advocate role of the nurse must be strongly to the fore.

Physiological changes with age

There will be a general deterioration of bodily function with age. This is only to be expected, but there are certain key areas which are worth focusing on in some detail, starting with the musculoskeletal system.

There is a loss of muscle bulk and osteoarthritis may affect joints leading to pain and stiffness. In addition, there is also thinning of the bone, osteoporosis, which affects females more than males and substantially increases fracture risk. Other pathological processes affecting bone become more common in the elderly, such as osteomalacia, Paget's disease and bony mestastases from malignancy. Decreases in skin elasticity and subcutaneous tissue increase the risk of bruising and tears in the skin. All these processes make the consequences of a fall far more serious. Unfortunately, other changes associated with ageing, such as diminished vision or coordination, orthostatic hypotension and transient interruptions in cerebral blood flow, make falls more likely (Gray-Vickrey and Colucci, 1999).

Older people experience pain just as much as younger people do, although in a more complex way. It has already been stated that pain is an individual experience and the nurse must assess pain for each individual. Many of today's elders grew up in hard times and were firmly taught that pain was something to bear and stoicism a virtue. An older person is, therefore, more likely to bear pain with less complaint than might be expected.

A major problem area is that of temperature regulation which deteriorates with age in some people. Consequently, older people are prone to hypothermia. A range of social factors, such as poverty and poor housing, act with other physical factors, such as lack of mobility and side effects of drugs, to make hypothermia a significant problem. The signs can mimic other serious conditions such as a stroke (e.g. confusion, drowsiness, bradycardia, dilated pupils), therefore, hypothermia can easily be overlooked.

Older people experience many problems with the special senses. Vision deteriorates with age, due to changes in the cornea and lens shape that affect focusing, leading most commonly to long-sightedness. Problems such as cataracts, chronic glaucoma and retinal detachment all threaten sight. In addition, older people develop problems with the lid margin such as entropion (lid margin turned inwards) leading to eyelashes irritating the conjunctiva, or ectropion (lower lid turned outwards) interfering with normal drainage from the eye (Walsh *et al.*, 1999). If an elderly person is brought to A & E without a pair of spectacles, the nurse should ask the patient if they normally wear glasses. Visual impairment will seriously interfere with the person's ability to understand what is happening to them.

Hearing impairment increases sharply with age. Degenerative changes in the auditory nerve and cochlea cause a preferential loss of hearing for high frequency sounds, i.e. consonants, which are essential for understanding speech. Problems in sound conduction contribute further to deafness and many old people, therefore, rely on lip reading to understand what is being said. However, staff should be wary of the stereotypical assumption that all elderly people are deaf and should certainly refrain from shouting at a person who is hard of hearing. Slower, carefully enunciated speech, ensuring that the patient can see the speaker's lips, and a careful check on any hearing aid (is it switched on?) will be more productive.

The A & E nurse must care for the older person as an individual, not a collection of stereotypes. Respect and dignity must be afforded the patient, not childish sobriquets such as 'deane'.

Psychological problems and ageing

Confusion is often the first symptom to spring to mind in considering the older person. It is however an abnormal and unusual state of affairs as most older people are well oriented in time and space. Confusion can be a sudden and transient phenomenon which is reversible. Such an acute confusional state is known as delirium and can be caused by acute illness, e.g. respiratory disease or heart failure leading to cerebral hypoxia, dehydration/electrolyte disturbance, hypoglycaemia, or infection (Gray-Vickrey and Colucci, 1999). However, confusion in the elderly may not have a simple physical cause, but may be situational in nature, i.e. it may be the environment and situation that the patient is in that is causing the confusion. Sensory deprivation can rapidly cause mood changes, hallucinations and thought disorder. An older person, perhaps without their glasses or hearing aid, lying flat on an A & E trolley, isolated in a cubicle with only the ceiling to look at, can quickly start to experience sensory deprivation. It is important to recognize this possibility as simple environmental manipulation by the nurse may control and diminish the patient's confusion.

Dementia is a loss of intellectual function serious enough to interfere with a person's normal daily life on a progressive basis. It can be reversible when factors such as medication interactions, depression or hypothyroidism are the cause. However, it may be an irreversible condition due to Alzheimer's disease, multiple cerebral infarcts or other disorders. In Alzheimer's disease there is shrinkage of the brain and a tangling of nerve fibres that become affected by plaque formation. Estimates of the incidence of Alzheimer's disease are variable. On one estimate it affects 2% of the population aged over 65 and 5% aged over 75 (Lefrançois, 1996), while the Alzheimer's Disease Society (1997) estimates there are 670 000 cases in the UK. In assessing the patient in A & E, it is essential to know the patient's normal level of mental functioning before making a judgement about any confusional state.

There are many reasons why a person with Alzheimer's disease may be brought to A & E. The following key characteristics of Alzheimer's disease will affect the patient's care in the department (Zimmerman and Ortigara, 1998):

- Presentation is very variable, no two patients are the same and each individual's mental abilities can vary a great deal over time.
- The person is locked into their limited reality therefore they cannot understand new information or change their behaviour in response to requests from the nurse.
- Emotions and feelings remain intact until the very end.
- Behaviour is purposeful, not random, even if the person has lost the ability to explain *why* they are doing something. Increased restlessness, therefore, may well indicate something is wrong even though the person cannot describe what.

Finally nurses ought to consider the ageing patient as a whole and how he or she views the current situation they are in. Physical limitations on activity can produce frustration; for some people retirement brings hours of empty time and a feeling of worthlessness, which results in a fall in self-esteem. Disengagement is a process whereby the older person withdraws gradually from social, physical and emotional interaction with the rest of the world. This may be seen as a positive step as it allows the older person to cope with age related loss (Lefrançois, 1996). The balance between disengagement and activity is important in determining the quality of life enjoyed by the older person. Anxiety and depression are commonly encountered in old age. The presenting symptoms of depression in the elderly can be confused with early dementia; these include memory impairment, poor communication, apathy and muddled thought processes (Donovan, 1991). This only underlines the importance of not stereotyping elderly patients.

Social factors and ageing

A & E departments regularly meet the problem of an older person who is not suffering from an injury or medical condition that alone requires admission, but who cannot cope on their own at home. A fracture, for example, may be correctly aligned and immobilized in a cast, but can the person manage their Zimmer frame with a below knee walking cast? Discharge arrangements from A & E are therefore crucial. Families and neighbours care for and support many older people at home, but sometimes it all becomes just too much and they reluctantly have to call in the GP. This can lead to that well-known diagnosis 'Gone off her legs' used to describe the situation where a complex interplay of multiple pathology and social factors leave an older person struggling to cope at home, but there is no neat medical diagnosis, such as a stroke, that describes their condition. The problems of disengagement referred to above, depression or other mental health problems can all lead to an older person living alone neglecting themselves and becoming cut off from society, living as a recluse. Tragically, they may have been dead for days when their body is finally found.

Elderly patients in A & E are often so determined to get home that they reassure staff they can manage, simply to get out of the department without thinking through how

exactly they will cope (Howe, 1998). They are a very vulnerable group and great care is necessary in arranging discharge. Close working relationships with primary health care providers, social services, voluntary agencies and family are essential. The annual bed crisis that afflicts the NHS every winter hits older persons hardest of all with unacceptable trolley waits in A & E for beds, while early discharges from wards only increases the risks of a speedy return to A & E unable to cope. This is aptly named the 'revolving door syndrome'.

Elderly people who fall over

Many older people attend A & E as a result of a fall. The consequences of falls are very serious for older people, with some 25% sustaining a serious injury as a result. Many others reduce activity for fear of a further fall, leading to further disengagement and a reduced quality of life (Eliopoulos, 1997).

Problems in mobility caused by joint stiffness, muscle wasting and bone disease are compounded by decay in neuromuscular coordination, cardiovascular function, environmental factors and drugs. Elderly people are therefore more likely to lose their balance than younger persons, and once they have done so, are less able to correct their posture, leading to a fall. Falls may be seen, therefore, in terms of intrinsic factors, such as postural hypotension, and extrinsic factors such as loose carpets or poorly fitting slippers. The frequency of falls in the elderly has been found to lie in the 28–35% per annum range in most studies which have looked at the elderly living at home (Downton, 1993). The rate among those in institutions is probably much higher.

Terms used by the elderly tend to be very vague, such as giddiness, blackout, and light-headedness, which makes retrospective medical diagnosis imprecise. The nurse in A & E is more concerned with the effects of the fall, which can vary from the obvious immediate injury to a loss of confidence.

Common injuries suffered by the elderly in falls include fractures to the upper end of the femur, wrist (Colles fracture) and upper humerus, dislocation of the shoulder, and lacerations of the shin, scalp and face. Great care has to be exercised with the case of the confused elderly person with a head injury. Is the confusion due to the head injury? The sudden move to hospital in the middle of the night after falling out of bed? Or was the person already confused?

A fracture of the upper end of the femur is a serious injury that most A & E departments see in an elderly person every day on average. The fracture is usually through the femoral neck or in the intratrochanteric region. The following classification (known as the Garden classification) is applied to fractured neck of femur injuries:

- Grade I incomplete fracture
- Grade II complete fracture without displacement
- Grade III complete fracture with partial displacement
- Grade IV complete fracture with full displacement (posterior component completely free).

The classic clinical sign is shortening and external rotation of the injured leg. However, patients may be still walking on an impacted Grade I fracture ('I thought it was just my arthritis playing up' as one lady said to me), which may not even be obvious on X-ray. The classical picture of shortening and external rotation is often only apparent in Grade III and IV femoral neck and intratrochanteric fractures (Greaves *et al.*, 1997). Sometimes the fracture involves the pubic rami of the pelvis rather than the hip. The fracture is usually due to a fall or, in some cases it appears that the fracture occurred spontaneously as advanced osteoporosis just caused the hip to fail as the person was walking on it. The presentation of an elderly person with pain in the hip region associated with a fall should be treated as a potential fracture until proven otherwise. Two recent large-scale studies both reported mortality rates of 12% for such patients (Fox *et al.*, 1994; Holt *et al.*, 1994) and a female to male ratio of over 6:1. The study by Fox *et al.* showed the mean hospital stay was 31 days, but those patients with dementia averaged 56 days and those with pressure sores 53 days. The Holt study found the best predictor of discharge mobility and postoperative complications were age and mobility pre-injury. The most common complication was chest infection, although the incidence of pressure sores is not referred to.

Every effort should be made to admit such patients as quickly as possible to prevent problems such as pressure sore formation. A fast track policy for admission aimed at having a maximum time in A & E of 1 hour is strongly recommended. Howe (1998) reported that, in his survey of 47 A & E departments, most had either a formal or informal fast track policy concentrating on pressure relief using special mattresses, pain relief, early X-ray and access to the wards. Surgery is performed to fix the fracture internally as soon as possible in order to facilitate early mobility. The complications of immobility are such that the elderly person would be unlikely to survive a lengthy period in bed.

Fractures of the wrist are usually reduced and plastered in A & E under regional anaesthesia and followed up on an outpatient basis. O'Sullivan *et al.* (1996) carried out a national survey on regional anaesthesia (Bier's block) used in manipulation of Colles fractures and found that 65% of departments fasted patients before the procedure despite the fact that there is no rationale for doing so. Complication rates were found to be the same in fasted and unfasted patients which led O'Sullivan *et al.* to recommend that fasting before IV regional anaesthesia was not necessary and should be abandoned. Dislocations of the shoulder are relocated using IV sedation and analgesia. Fractures of the neck of humerus require pain relief and a sling, but can be managed with minimal interference on an outpatient basis. Lacerations in elderly people are better steristripped rather than sutured in many cases due to the fragile nature of the skin. This is especially true of flap lacerations over the shins where careful application of steristrips, a non-adherent dressing and an elasticated tubular bandage (never crepe as it always falls down) will produce the best results. On occasions, however, skin grafting is necessary.

The possibility remains that the injuries may not be the product of an accident but have been caused by abuse of the older person. Howe (1998) notes that while there is a high level of awareness concerning child abuse in A & E, the same cannot be said of elder abuse. His survey reported that few units showed any recognition of the need for policies or procedures in this field. Risk assessment schedules have been developed in the USA for elder abuse and are available (Staab and Hodges,

1996). Several of the factors which should make the nurse suspicious of child abuse are equally valid in elder abuse. These include prolonged intervals between accident and presentation, inconsistency between history and physical findings and multiple injuries of differing ages. Abuse in institutions caring for older people is related to depersonalization of the patient by staff, older people being seen in a negative light as helpless and burdensome (Lefrançois, 1996). Risk factors in private homes include caregivers who are inexperienced, socially isolated or who may have been the victim of abuse at the hands of the older person when children themselves (Staab and Hodges, 1996).

Assessing the elderly patient in A & E

Assessment should include the psychological and social setting of the patient. Vital information about the state of the person's home can be obtained from the ambulance crew who bring the person to hospital: is it clean, warm and looked after or dirty, cold and neglected? What is the situation with regard to neighbours and family? This and much more key social information is to be gained from the ambulance crew. In undressing the patient, further information may be gleaned about social background by looking at the state of the clothes, skin and general hygiene. Bennett and Ebrahim (1992) rightly stress that the assessment of the patient's social networks in A & E is just as important as the physical state.

Talking to the patient will enable further information to be gleaned. A first assessment should be made of how oriented the patient is, and of any disabilities due to visual or hearing impairment. Short-term memory should be checked by asking the patient to remember some item and then repeating the question five minutes later. Some elderly people suffer from pathological short-term memory loss yet are able to keep a remarkably good facade of normality in conversation, so short-term memory should always be checked. Check whether the patient does know where they are and why they are there.

History taking is made more difficult in the older person as their perception of pain may alter. A condition such as an MI or acute pancreatitis, which usually produces severe pain in the middle-aged person, may not be perceived in the same way by the older person. Multiple pathology may mean that the older person has severe pain from more than one cause. This makes it difficult to link pain, the key symptom, to the acute pathology which has brought the person to A & E (Seidal *et al.*, 1995). Pain assessment will be assisted by use of the PQRST approach recommended by Walsh *et al.* (1999) and described more fully on page 53.

In assessing the patient for physical injuries, the nurse should look beyond the obvious and examine the whole patient. Bruising and skin marks should be carefully observed, particularly if there are bruises of different ages suggesting repeated injury. Grip marks around the arms and wrists, accompanied by bruising of different ages is suggestive of elder abuse. In all cases of trauma, a full set of vital sign observations is needed as there may be significant underlying pathology. Careful temperature recording is essential to eliminate the possibility of hypothermia. An ECG is fairly standard procedure to eliminate cardiac arrhythmias or a silent MI. Blood sugar should be estimated by a 'stix' test and a sample of urine also tested.

Intervention – care for the older person in A & E

The dangers of sensory deprivation have already been discussed. Provision must be made for the poor memory, if present, by repeating vital information. Spectacles and hearing aids should be obtained if at all possible and great care exercised to secure effective communication.

If the patient has Alzheimer's disease, Zimmerman and Ortigara (1998) recommend the following approaches:

- Limit environmental stimuli, keep noise and activity around the person to a minimum.
- Keep communication short and simple, one idea at a time in simple sentences is more likely to be understood.
- The sense of touch remains intact long after other mental functions have gone, it can therefore be used to reassure and establish contact.

- Family members may feel very angry at watching the deterioration of their loved one and be inclined to vent their feelings on health professionals as safe targets so do not become defensive and anticipate anger and frustration in family members.
- Sometimes you have to use a 'therapeutic fib' to deal with repeated requests such as 'I want to go home as my baby needs feeding'. To the patient, this is reality despite the fact that their children are grown adults. Reassurance that the baby is fed and safe with relatives is not an immoral lie according to Zimmerman and Ortigara, it is actually doing right by dealing with the reality of the moment for the patient.

A & E trolleys are notoriously hard, and pressure sores can have their origins in a long wait in A & E. Pressure area care is therefore essential if patients are to be in A & E for over 2 hours. Turning is difficult but not impossible on narrow trolleys. If the patient has a fracture of the femur, turning will be impossible since the fracture will not be stabilized. Special trolley pressure relieving mattresses are now available and should be reserved for older people.

Old people are more likely to accept their lot uncomplainingly; they should not be forgotten, therefore, in the hustle of a busy A & E department. The offer of a cup of tea while waiting and a few kind words can mean a great deal, and can also obtain for the nurse information that might not have been otherwise volunteered. Elderly people often see real problems as 'something that you just have to put up with', rather than an important symptom.

The problems associated with discharging patients have already been discussed, however, the importance of good discharge arrangements cannot be overemphasized. Given the communication difficulties that arise from declining vision, hearing and short-term memory, it is obviously important to be sure that what has been taught has been learnt with regard to points such as plaster instructions, medication, and follow-up appointments. Simple instruction cards in bold type and medicine bottles that can be opened by older people, whose manual dexterity may have declined, are simple examples of planning for the special needs of the older person.

Empathy, the importance of seeing things from the patient's point of view, is a key part of nursing. When making arrangements for sending an older person home, you would do well to reflect upon how you might cope under these circumstances, not as you are, but as the patient is. At the end of the day the nurse should not forget her or his role as patient advocate, and if you are unhappy about a medical decision that, since the old lady did not break anything when she fell over she must go home, then you must say so. Busy but junior and inexperienced medical staff often overlook the social element of how the patient will cope at home. At the very least, you should ask the doctor to see if the patient can walk unaided, the basic requirement for going home. Many intended discharge decisions have been reversed by such a simple step. Most casualty officers are willing to listen to advice from nursing staff about the care of elderly people and their suitability for discharge or about how to get the community services involved, provided that the nursing staff go about it in a constructive way.

Summary

It is in the nature of A & E work that you will only see an older person when something has gone wrong. This can lead to a stereotyped and atypical view of older people. The vast majority are independent and getting on with their lives. As Lefrançois points out, some 86% of the elderly may suffer from one or more major conditions but the majority do not consider their health to be a serious problem and remarkably few are dependent or hospitalized. It is regrettable therefore that the survey carried out by Howe (1998) paints a picture of services for the elderly in A & E that is sporadic and fragmented with audit frequently revealing poor performance. There are few survivors left from the generation that went through World War I, we can and must do better for the generation that fought World War II.

References

Alzheimer's Disease Society (1997) *What is Alzheimer's Disease?* 3rd edn. St Louis: Mosby.

Bennett C, Ebrahim S (1992). *Health Care for the Elderly.* London: Edward Arnold.

Donovan L (1991) Mental health problems in old age. In Garrett G (ed.) *Healthy Ageing: Some Nursing Perspectives.* London: Professional Nurse.

Downton J (1993) *Falls in the Elderly.* London: Edward Arnold.

Eliopoulos C (1997) *Gerontological Nursing,* 4th edn. Philadelphia: Lippincott.

Fox H, Pooler I, Prothero D, Bannister G (1994) Factors affecting the outcome after proximal femoral fractures. *Injury,* **25**:297–300.

Gray-Vickrey P, Colucci R (1999) Taking charge in a geriatric emergency. *Nursing,* **99**: January, 41–6.

Greaves I, Porter K, Burke D (1997) *Key Topics in Trauma.* Oxford: Bios Medical Publishers.

Holt E, Evans R, Hindley C, Metcalfe J (1994) 1000 femoral neck fractures: the effect of pre-injury mobility and surgical experience on outcome. *Injury,* **25**:91–5.

Howe C (1998) Current provision of care for older persons in A&E units in the UK. *Accident and Emergency Nursing,* **6**:211–18.

Lefrançois G (1996) *The Lifespan,* 5th edn. Belmont Ca: Wadsworth Publishing Co.

O'Sullivan I, Brooks S, Maryosh J (1996) Is fasting necessary before prilocaine Bier's block? *Journal of Accident and Emergency Medicine,* **13**:105–7.

Ryan N (1996) A study of the contribution of effective pressure care on elderly female patients attending A&E who have a suspected fractured neck of femur. *Accident and Emergency Nursing,* **4**:21–4.

Seidal H, Ball J, Dains J, Benedict W (1995) *Mosby's Guide to Physical Examination,* 3rd edn. St Louis: Mosby.

Staab A, Hodges L (1996) *Essentials of Gerontological Nursing.* Philadelphia: Lippincott.

Strange G, Chen E, Sanders A (1992) Use of Emergency departments by elderly patients: Projections from a multi-center data base. *Annals of Emergency Medicine,* **21**: 819–24.

Walsh M, Crumbie A, Reveley S (1999) *Nurse Practitioners; Clinical Skills and Professional Issues.* Oxford: Butterworth-Heinemann.

Zimmerman P, Ortigara A (1998) Caring for the patient with Alzheimer's disease. *Emergency Nurse,* **6**:5, 11–14.

Chapter 13

MAJOR DISASTER PLANNING AND RADIATION CASUALTIES

Major disaster planning

Disasters are characterized by their suddenness and unexpectedness, with the result that hospital plans need to be simple, flexible and integrated with the plans of all the other emergency services (Walsh, 1989). The NHSE's definition of a major incident is as follows: 'A major incident can have a huge impact on one part of the health service, while leaving others relatively unaffected. In a similar way, an NHS major incident is not necessarily a major incident for other emergency services such as police, or local authority services and vice versa' (National Health Service Executive, 1998). A major incident is, therefore, a situation in which normal NHS provision is overwhelmed by the numbers of casualties involved. However, a major incident may relate to a major outbreak of illness such as the Lanarkshire food poisoning epidemic of 1998 or a major failure of hospital systems such as the evacuation of University College Hospital in 1996 caused by a flood in the boiler room (Dethick, 1999b). Major incident plans should always be subject to improvement and should be continually reviewed in the light of lessons learnt the hard way as incidents occur.

In 1990 the HSE issued guidelines for major incident planning and stipulated that all health authorities were to ensure that comprehensive plans were in place for all health services to respond to a major incident. However, a study by Carley (1996) showed that out of 224 British hospitals that have an A & E unit seeing over 30 000 patients a year, only 65 had plans that were deemed comprehensive enough to include all staff likely to be involved in a response to a major incident. He also found that only six hospitals out of the 224 complied fully with the HSE guidelines of 1990.

Planning for a major incident should be based upon a risk assessment strategy. A fundamental question is who is at risk? Within your department the answer is obviously staff and patients. Points to plan for therefore are staff information, contamination, personal protective clothing, training, equipment and occupational health surveillance. With regard to patients this approach raises issues such as injuries, decontamination, treatment and transport (Dethick, 1999a).

The basic principle that should run through a good plan is that people perform best, especially under stressful conditions, when they are doing the things with which they are most familiar. Thus plans should avoid major changes in work practices and departmental layout, aiming to have the department functioning like an ordinary, although very busy, day as far as possible.

A second key principle is that of flexibility and simplicity. A rigid plan that will cope with all eventualities is not possible, as it is not possible to foresee all such eventualities. After all, if disasters could be predicted they could be largely avoided. Simplicity has the virtue of allowing flexibility while the simpler a plan is, the easier it is for staff to follow. The more there is in a plan that can go wrong, the more will go wrong.

Within the department, the person who should be in charge is the senior sister/charge nurse on duty, in other words, the person who would normally be in charge. The place for senior management is doing what they normally do – organizing the rest of the hospital, providing extra staff where needed and supplying the A & E unit with back-up facilities such as extra equipment, trolleys and pairs of hands.

Once the alert has been received, there is a need to evacuate A & E immediately of all patients, either by sending them to wards or moving them to a holding area (e.g. outpatients clinic), in order to free staff and facilities for casualty reception. A designated disaster ward that will receive all admitted casualties is essential, not only for immediate logistic reasons, but also for long-term psychological reasons in the days and weeks after the disaster when its victims can give each other vital mutual support.

Provision should be made for relatives of those involved to be accommodated away from the department as the large numbers that may be involved will be disruptive. Similarly the media should be catered for elsewhere, and ideally the department should be closed by the police to all but staff and disaster casualties. Routine casualties should be informed of the situation and told that they will have to wait a long time before being seen due to the disaster (assuming their clinical condition will permit such a delay) and advised to go to another hospital or their GP. The notion of attempting to operate a non-disaster A & E unit in tandem with a department on major disaster plan is clearly a non-starter and will only result in substandard care for everybody. Liaison with the ambulance service is essential so that, as far as possible, 999 calls may be routed to another department.

Action cards for staff which describe their various functions are an excellent idea, for it is likely to be quite chaotic preparing to receive casualties if different groups of staff are all trying to read through the same lengthy copy of the plan in an attempt to find 'their bit'.

Staff should realize that they may get no official notification of an incident occurring; the fires at Manchester Airport and Bradford City FC in 1985 were examples of this, while communication may remain non-existent with the field for hours on end as happened in the Hungerford Massacre in 1987. Casualties may just start pouring through the doors, under-lining the need for a speedy response and immediate triage. This happened after the Canary Wharf bombing in 1996 and at the three other cases cited above. Notification may also come through informal routes before official notification as happened in the Paddington Rail Disaster in 1999. Horsfall and Slowie (1999) have described how a surgical nurse rang the hospital at 08:20 to say she would be late as she was on a train held up 'because the one in front has crashed'. A ward sister at the same time was looking out of her eighth floor window and saw the smoke rising

from the scene, realized something dreadful had happened and began identifying patients who could be quickly moved if the disaster plan was put into action. Staff were using these snippets of information to begin setting the wheels in motion when the formal notification of the disaster from the police finally arrived.

The feeling of apprehension and chaos at the beginning of a major incident is vividly described by Horsfall and Slowie (1999) but so, too is the sense after the first 30 minutes or so of things clicking into place as a well-rehearsed plan really gets into gear. In those crucial first few chaotic minutes, casualties must be sorted into categories as they arrive so that those who need the care first get it first, and are not delayed by either less urgent cases, or more problematically, those who will die whatever care they are given. This needs considerable expertise and the senior nursing and medical staff on duty will need to be involved in this function.

The A & E unit also has a responsibility to send a team to the site of the incident. This has been carefully discussed by Salt (1989) and he has stressed that the team should be equipped with weatherproof clothing that, for safety reasons, is brightly coloured, including fluores-cent tabards marked 'Nurse' and 'Doctor'. There should also be helmets with lights and Wellington boots in a full range of sizes. Equipment should be carried in backpacks rather than in one big trunk that may be impossible to carry near to the site of the disaster, although a back-up trunk containing reserve equipment is worthwhile.

The functions of the mobile team are variable. Most commonly the team provide skills complementary to the services already there for patients trapped within the wreckage. Other functions include staffing the on-site casualty clearing station, treating patients in the field and assisting with transportation to appropriate receiving hospitals. Triage on site is usually carried out by senior ambulance personnel or the medical Incident Officer who may be part of your team or belong to an organization such as BASICS (British Association of Immediate Care). The A & E team need to take equipment which the ambulance service does not carry, e.g. chest drains or equipment for rapid sequence induction or multiple intravenous fluids.

On-site triage is performed in two ways. First, triage sieve and then a more detailed examination at the casualty clearing station, called triage sort. The sieve identifies walking patients and those unable to walk are categorized according to simple physical parameters such as the ABCs. The sort is based on the more complicated Revised Trauma Scoring System (Dethick, 1999a). Whichever triage method is used, it is vital that all services use the same one and that the process is repeatable. By utilizing this form of triage the team can ensure that the right patient gets treated at the right time.

The value of stabilizing patients at the scene of the incident is stressed by Dethick (1999b), who cites the example of the Clapham rail crash in 1988. Thirty-five people were killed in that disaster, but of all the people who were alive when the emergency services arrived on scene, not one lost their life subsequently.

During the sort phase of triage the team can be splitting up the caseload so that the ambulances distribute the casualties among the various departments in the area. This may not be possible in a rural area where there may be only one department within 30 miles but, in urban areas, this is possible and greatly to be desired. In the Harrods bombing, St Stephen's Hospital received 39 casualties and the Westminster Hospital 37 – a good example of sharing the workload.

Psychological first aid is important as well as the obvious physical care needed by survivors. It is crucial they start the process of coming to terms with the horrific events they have survived by being able to talk about their experiences. A & E staff should recognize this need in the survivors and they should not try to switch the subject. Haslum (1989) has stressed that much needs to be learnt about the psychological needs of survivors and the Bradford Fire of 1985 seems to have marked the beginning of serious attempts to explore this area. Nobody could have remained unmoved at the spontaneous way the people of Liverpool transformed the Kop at Anfield into a memorial to the dead of Hillsborough. Just as the much smaller community of Aberfan still bears the scar of the terrible disaster that destroyed a school full of children, so, too, the much larger city of Liverpool will remember Hillsborough for many decades to come.

Chemical injuries

With the widespread use of chemicals in the UK every department needs to be aware of the potential for patients arriving following a chemical incident. If this occurs during a major incident then many expert agencies are already likely to be involved from the very beginning. A more worrying scenario is exposure to toxic chemicals that may have been dumped illegally; a problem that is on the increase. People may not even realize they have been contaminated for some time and the spread of chemical contamination to other family members can be unnoticed at first. The patient can easily walk into A & E suffering from local irritation and further spread the contamination throughout the department within 30 minutes. Triage nurses need to be alert to the potential problems of contamination with any patient complaining of exposure to chemicals (solid, liquid or gas).

Decontamination is often left to the fire or ambulance service before the patient's arrival in A & E. Given the breakdown in communications that may occur in any major incident, a clear system needs to be used so that A & E staff are aware of who has been decontaminated.

Decontamination of the patient needs to occur following advice from the national Chemical Incident Response Service (CIRS). They can be contacted via the National Poison Centre in London. In 1997 they had recorded 931 chemical incidents.

A contaminated patient needs to be isolated and staff afforded the maximum protection that is compatible with their work. Complete protection for A & E staff is not possible, however, as this requires the extensive specialist equipment used by the fire service including respirators. Eye protection, aprons and appropriate hand protection are easy to provide, however, and must be considered as the bare minimum standard. Full protective suits with an air filter mask, as used by the chemical industry, are more appropriate. Staff need to be aware that there is still a risk, even when wearing this personal protective equipment. Most fire services use water in copious amounts to decontaminate patients at the scene. This method is effective either from a hose reel or a more sophisticated shower device so long as the casualty is not critically injured or ill. Hypothermia is a possible complication, however.

Contaminated patients who arrive at the department unannounced should be taken outside again or treated in a decontamination room if available. The patient's clothes must be removed, preferably by the patient and placed into sealed bags and clearly marked. If a number of patients arrive, then 'dirty' and 'clean' areas of the department should be established. Ideally, the dirty area should be outside the department and staff should not be able to move from the dirty to the clean area without undergoing decontamination (Wheeler, 1998). Removing clothing and washing hands, face and hair will usually remove all but traces of the contaminant, after which the patients are allowed in for treatment. If the patient is critically ill then the focus will need to be on the essential resuscitation elements, such as securing the airway, before decontamination can occur. This must be done with the minimum number of personnel to reduce exposure. Some ambulance trusts have set up, in conjunction with the fire service, specialist teams who can wear protective breathing apparatus and go into contaminated areas to triage and give basic medical care. Some BASICS teams have also developed this capacity while a few hospitals are looking into providing a mobile medical team who could operate in a contaminated environment. Their training, accountability and function are still open to debate.

Every department should have an awareness of the needs of patients involved in chemical incidents. The Accident and Emergency department needs to be ready for any eventuality and that includes the contaminated patient. Planning is therefore essential.

Radiation casualties

After Chernobyl, no A & E unit can afford to pretend that it may never have to deal with radiation casualties. If nurses are to understand the principles of care, they first need to know a little about ionizing radiation.

Atoms consist of a central nucleus composed of a cluster of positively charged particles (protons) and particles with no charge (neutrons), all held together by very strong forces. Surrounding the nucleus is a cloud of negatively charged particles called electrons that are almost one two-thousandth the mass of a proton and whose number equals that of the number of protons. The atom is, therefore, electrically neutral. Neutrons and protons are similar in mass, and the number of neutrons in the nucleus of a given element can vary, giving rise to the different isotopes of that element. The chemistry of an element is defined by the number of electrons orbiting the nucleus – from one in the case of hydrogen, two for helium, through to 92 in the case of uranium – and the number of protons in the nucleus, which should be the same.

This account of atomic structure is a great

Table 13.1 Summary of common forms of ionizing radiation

Radiation type	Nature of radiation	Penetrating power	
		Air	Body tissue
α ray	Particle stream, each particle consists of two protons and two neutrons.	6 cm	<1 mm
β ray	Stream of electrons.	5 m	<2 cm
X rays	Energy released by electrons changing position in atom.	10–100 m	Whole body
γ rays	Energy released by nuclear particles reorganizing position.	100 + m	Whole body
Neutrons	Stream of neutrons.	100 + m	Whole body

NB. The penetrating power of γ rays and neutrons is such as to make wearing lead aprons as used for radiology of little use.

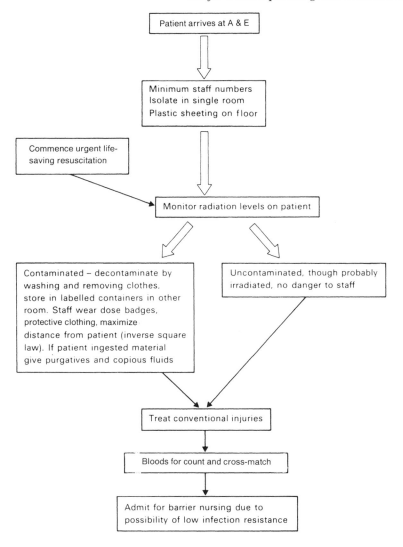

Patient arrives at A & E

Minimum staff numbers
Isolate in single room
Plastic sheeting on floor

Commence urgent life-saving resuscitation

Monitor radiation levels on patient

Contaminated – decontaminate by washing and removing clothes, store in labelled containers in other room. Staff wear dose badges, protective clothing, maximize distance from patient (inverse square law). If patient ingested material give purgatives and copious fluids

Uncontaminated, though probably irradiated, no danger to staff

Treat conventional injuries

Bloods for count and cross-match

Admit for barrier nursing due to possibility of low infection resistance

NB. Inverse square law means that the intensity of radiation decreases inversely with the square of the distance. Therefore by doubling your distance from the patient, you reduce the radiation intensity to one-quarter of previous level.

Fig. 13.1 Flowchart for radiation casualties in A & E

simplification, but it will suffice for our purposes. The effect of ionizing radiation is to knock out an electron from an atom or molecule, leaving it with a surplus positive charge; in this state it is known as an ion. Radiation damages cells in the human body most commonly by forming water radicals – hydrogen atoms or hydrogen–oxygen atom combinations, with an electron missing. They are written as H^+ and OH^- and are more correctly called ions. This occurs by the radiation knocking electrons out of water molecules in the cells. These radicals can chemically oxidize and destroy parts of the DNA molecule, disrupting normal functioning of the cells.

The effect of radiation on the human body will depend upon the energy of the ionizing radiation, the frequency with which it will ionize atoms and molecules (knock out electrons), and its penetrating power. Table 13.1 summarizes the penetration potential of the different forms of radiation that we may encounter.

In practical terms the penetrating power of α rays is such that they are unlikely to go beyond clothing or the outer layers of skin, while β rays penetrate only a few millimetres of tissue. Other forms of radiation, while causing fewer ionizing events for a given length of track, do, however, fully penetrate the body and therefore are able to damage rapidly dividing cells such as the cells in the bone marrow (blood-forming tissue) and in the lining of the gut.

The amount of energy in radiation is measured in Grays (old units were rads and 100 rad = 1 Gy), while the amount of absorbed energy dose in human tissue is measured in Sieverts (old units were rems and 100 rem = 1 Sv). For practical purposes 1 Gy equals 1 Sv in most cases.

The likely A & E scenarios that we would encounter are that there is a patient who has been exposed to ionizing radiation, or has ingested and/or inhaled radioactive material or has radioactive material on their body, with or without conventional trauma in each case.

A person who has been exposed to ionizing radiation, but not contaminated with radioactive material, is *not* radioactive and therefore not a danger to anybody else. The damage has been done, just as somebody who has been shot is no longer a danger to anybody else: the bullet has done its damage and gone, the ionizing radiation has gone. They may be treated in the normal way in A & E, but will need special inpatient care depending on which aspect of the radiation sickness syndrome develops according to the absorbed dose. Regular blood counts are required together with antibiotics and blood transfusions, consideration being given to the need to barrier nurse the patient in view of their lowered resistance to infection.

If a person is contaminated, urgent life-saving measures must take priority over decontamination, otherwise the result may be death.

The basic principles of reception and treatment in A & E are to decontaminate the patient; to prevent the spread of contaminated material around the unit by isolation and by reducing the number of staff involved to the minimum; to protect staff looking after the patient. Monitoring equipment must be obtained and personnel from the hospital physics department immediately involved. Protective clothing such as plastic gloves and aprons should be worn but they will not prevent radiation affecting staff; they will simply prevent skin and clothes becoming contaminated with radioactive material. Conventional injuries should be treated as far as possible in the normal way, with great importance attached to psychological support for the patient.

Local authority emergency planning officers make an important contribution to planning for major disasters (Walsh, 1989). Given the clear need for a coordinated national disaster plan, it would be logical to develop their role, and that of their NHS colleagues, in line with a peacetime function.

The possibility of a single nuclear explosion, however, has to be borne in mind, either as a result of a tragic accident or a rogue state acting in pursuit of some megalomaniac dictator's fantasies (Iraq and North Korea are examples from the 1990s), or even state-sponsored terrorism. A national disaster plan could usefully explore the response to a single nuclear detonation.

References

Carley S (1996) Are British hospitals ready for the next major incident? Analysis of hospital major incident plans. *BMJ*, **13**:1242–3.

Dethick L (1999a) Co-ordinating major incident trauma care: international responses. *Emergency Nurse*, 7:4, 8–12.

Dethick L (1999b) Declaring a major incident. *Emergency Nurse*, 7:3, 21–5.

Haslum M (1989) The psychology of disaster. In Walsh M (ed.) *Disasters: Current Planning and Recent Experience*. London: Edward Arnold.

Horsfall K, Slowie A (1999) The Paddington rail disaster. *Emergency Nurse*, 7:8, 14–16.

National Heath Service Executive (1998) *Planning for Major Incidents: The NHS Guidance*. London: NHSE.

RCN (1983) *The Consequences of Nuclear War Civil Defence Planning for Nurses*. London: RCN.

Salt P (1989) The mobile team. In Walsh M (ed.) *Disasters: Current Planning and Recent Experience.* London: Edward Arnold.

Walsh M (1989) *Disasters: Current Planning and Recent Experience.* London: Edward Arnold.

Wheeler H (1998) Major incident planning: particularly those involving chemicals. *Emergency Nurse,* **6**:1, 12–17.

Chapter 14

WOMEN'S HEALTH PROBLEMS IN A & E

The ratio of male to female patients in most A & E departments is around 2:1. However, a significant number of women who attend A & E do so with complaints that are unique to women and therefore deserving of special attention. The presence of a female nurse can be a source of great comfort to a woman in A & E, especially if the cause of her hospitalization has been a man.

Stress and women

Stress among women results from a diversity of internal and external factors. Society, encouraged by the media, expects certain stereotypical behaviours from 'normal' women, e.g. the housewife, mother or working woman. Rarely in these images are women seen in combined roles. Guilt and disharmony occur as women perceive that they are unable to perform all these roles simultaneously. Other factors which induce stress include any significant life change, e.g. divorce, separation and single parenting. Statistics provide us with the occurrence of each of these events; however, the sociopsychological impact cannot be measured, although 'risk scores' of stress provide some indicators to susceptibility.

There is a strong feeling of guilt when a single mother looks at her children and sees them totally as her responsibility. There is no one to share decisions or control of the children, no one to help to decide which bills should be paid now and which can wait. It is a great burden to fall on one pair of shoulders, but is the daily reality which many women have to struggle with after they leave the A & E department. You should reflect on how realistic your health education advice really is in such circumstances.

Stress may manifest itself differently, but among women self-poisoning (parasuicide),

alcohol abuse, and smoking are well-recognized signs of stress.

WHO (1993) figures indicate that the incidence of parasuicide among women is three times greater than men. The reasons for this discrepancy may not always be clear, although it may be the culmination of a period of stress which may have been treated with antidepressants. There is strong evidence that some female survivors of childhood sexual abuse regularly inflict self-injury upon themselves, usually by cutting, when they reach adulthood. The reverse is not true, however, self-injury does not automatically mean the person was abused as a child (Reece, 1998). In trying to help such women it is important to treat the person, not the injury, and avoid being judgemental as this only leads to labelling. Conversation and dialogue are essential rather than a cold detached approach (Arnold, 1994).

The victims of domestic violence

Historically, violence against women in the home was endorsed by society as acceptable; the principle of zero tolerance is a new concept. Violence can occur within any social group and the perpetrator is usually known to the woman. The abuse is often cyclical in nature with a gradual build-up of tension and verbal aggression leading to the actual assault. This is then followed by what is known as the 'honeymoon' phase when the man is full of remorse and pleads for another chance as 'nothing like this will ever happen again' (Davies and Edwards, 1999). Of course it usually does as another cycle of abuse and violence unfolds. The abusive behaviour usually involves physical violence, rape and emotional abuse, such as systematic humiliation and deliberate isolation of the woman from her family or friends. It may also include the threat or reality of harm to any children involved. Women typically live in fear and have low self-esteem; the abuser has power and control (Hadley, 1992).

Women attending A & E departments are often reluctant to state that their injuries are as a result of domestic violence because of the stigma attached to such problems, fear of what might happen if the police are involved and a view that A & E staff are unsympathetic. The A & E nurse therefore has to combine taking a good history with careful assessment and a knowledge of factors which indicate the probability of abuse. Table 14.1 summarizes such indicators for female victims.

No two women are the same and no two cases of domestic violence are the same. Each woman will present differently with various combinations of some of the indicators listed in the table.

It is easy for A & E staff to wonder why the woman does not leave her abusive partner. It is not so simple, however, for as Davies and Edwards (1999) observe, the woman must first overcome the fears that are keeping her there in the first place. These include the fear of reprisals and further violence as it is usually easy for the man to track her down to friends or family members. There is the fear that she might lose her children, false optimism that things will improve, financial dependence on the man and the fact that she may have been so psychologically and physically traumatized that she is just too frightened to do anything. We should not indulge in victim blaming but rather offer the woman help in a non-judgemental way. She must feel able to come to A & E for assistance without feeling judged as the author of her own ills or without fearing lectures on why she should leave her partner. A secure and sensitive environment should be coupled with confidentiality and careful record keeping. The nurse has to remain neutral, however difficult it may be and respect the woman's decision about what to do next (Davies and Edwards, 1999).

It is helpful to be able to pass on information concerning the local women's refuge or

---

Table 14.1 Indicators of domestic violence in A & E

Attendance
- Delays in attendance
- Attitude of male partner, woman reluctant to speak in front of him
- Tendency to minimize injuries
- Injuries do not tally with history
- Pattern of frequent attendance

Presentation
- Anxious, tense non-verbal behaviour, appears distressed
- Apathy, fatigue
- Complaints of sleep disturbance, ill-defined pains, palpitations and dizziness

Psychological
- Feels powerless, unable to cope, guilty, fearful or angry
- Low self-esteem, lacking self-confidence
- Anxiety, depression, panic attacks
- Alcohol /drug use
- Self-harm, parasuicide, suicide attempts

Physical signs
- Bruises of various ages, especially around the face, arms, breasts
- Fractured facial bones, spiral fracture of radius/ulna (indicating severe twisting forces), old healed fractures
- Subconjunctival haemorrhage
- Violence may actually increase during pregnancy

Source: Lane and Beal (1998)

telephone help line and, where children are involved in domestic violence, child protection guidelines must be followed. Lane and Beale (1998) stress the need for a fast track emergency access system from A & E to refuge accommodation. They also urge departments to have a private, less clinical, room to interview victims and to have a camera to preserve an accurate photographic record of injuries as possible evidence. Posters and leaflets carrying information on domestic violence should be displayed in the waiting room and there should be a policy of making *all* staff aware of the problems of domestic violence, which of course requires good in-service training.

Rape and sexual assault

'What I felt most strongly was the look in his eyes which completely negated my existence as a human being. I was no longer a person, I was only an object, *his* object.' This description by a rape victim illustrates the psychological impact of rape upon an individual. Sexual assault is any attempt by one individual to coerce another into any form of undesired sexual contact with or without penetration, either of which may lead a woman to the door of an A & E department.

In many cases, the assailant is known to the victim. Sexual assault and rape in particular are emotive issues widely reported by the media, particularly where unusual circumstances prevail, i.e. age or gang rape. Why rape occurs is not clearly understood, although Roberts (1989) suggests the act requires a victimizer and victim. She goes on to propose a correlation between men's contempt of women and women's passivity, at least in relation to the role portrayed by the media. Roberts also indicates that there may be an association between male aggression against women who fail to conform to the aggressor's notion of femininity. It is questionable whether there is sexual satisfaction for the male, the aim being humiliation of the victim. Social class is not a discriminatory factor; however, class and education may be associated with those prepared to disclose the crime. For this reason statistical data about occurrence is of little benefit. Women who attend the A & E department may well have been the victim of additional physical violence, therefore the immediate physical care is of paramount importance.

Where staff suspect rape they should offer peace and privacy, avoiding assumptions that 'she asked for it' because of the woman's appearance or location of the incident, for these are judgements which are inappropriate for anybody to make. Only the victim can make an allegation of rape to the police. If she chooses to do so the police will attend with a police surgeon to organize and participate in the collection of forensic material, for example semen and swabs for analysis. Ideally the optimum place for this intimate examination is in a location away from the busy areas of the A & E department. Units now offer suites where intimate consultation and examination can occur.

After rape many women feel dirty and contaminated and have a great desire to wash themselves. This should be discouraged until after the forensic examination as vital evidence may be destroyed in this way. This includes advising the woman not to bathe, shower, clean her teeth, throw away clothing or defecate in cases of alleged anal penetration. While the woman is in the department a female member of staff should be continually available for psychological support. The nurse should be prepared to listen, in addition to being able to provide contact names and telephone numbers for future counselling needs.

The victim may demonstrate a range of emotions and fears reflecting the impact of the trauma upon her, including self-blame and guilt. The fear of pregnancy and sexually transmitted disease are more tangible anxieties than the anticipated reactions of partners, family and friends. Apprehension about being believed by hospital staff, loved ones, the police and possibly a jury will enhance feelings of isolation and desperation. Whatever the circumstances, there is no justification for sexual crimes against any individual. Rape is no longer recognized as a purely female phenomenon – the victim may be male.

Emergency contraception

A recent nationwide survey (Gbolade *et al.*, 1999) revealed that requests for emergency contraception or post-coital contraception (PCC) had been received by 96% of the 355 units that responded. Women therefore see A & E as a legitimate source of help when emergency contraception is required. Unfortunately, only 57% of the A & E units surveyed actually provided treatment, indicating that women are entering something of a lottery when going to A & E in need of PCC. Such inequalities of provision are not acceptable in what is supposed to be a *national* health service.

The most likely reason for presentation is after isolated unprotected sexual intercourse, although a 'lost' or burst condom may also cause a woman to seek help. The usual approach is to prescribe a high dose combined oestrogen/progesterone pill which must be taken within 72 hours of intercourse. Wyatt *et al.* (1999) recommend 2 tablets each of levenorgestrel 250 µg and ethinyloestradil 50 µg to be followed by two more 12 hours later. The woman must be advised to return immediately should she vomit soon afterwards. There is still a 1–2% chance of pregnancy occurring and the woman should be advised to use alternative contraceptive methods in the meantime (e.g. condoms) and visit her GP in 3 weeks time to confirm that menstruation has occurred and that she is not pregnant. It is anticipated that a progestogen only method will be licensed in the UK soon involving two 750 µg doses of progestogen given 12 hours apart, the first being within 72 hours of unprotected sex (Quinn, 1999). An alternative approach is the insertion of an IUCD which must be performed within 5 days of unprotected sex. This method is even more effective than the combined pill method and should be used when there is a history of thromboembolism (Quinn, 1999). Whichever method is used, Wyatt *et al.* (1999) point out that both methods work by making the endometrium hostile to egg implantation. The treatment does not therefore constitute abortion and it is helpful to reassure the woman of this fact.

The circumstances surrounding a request for PCC may be very embarrassing for some women. McDonald (1998) has described a way to reduce this problem which grew out of Emergency Nurse Practitioners in his department developing protocols to allow them to administer PCC. They drew up a form which the woman could complete in private, recording all the key information without the need for a detailed question and answer session with a nurse (who may have been male). The protocol includes the under 16s providing they are judged to show an adequate level of understanding, which is the test of so-called 'Gillick Competency' that applies to the under 16s (McHale *et al.*, 1998). McDonald's experience suggests that not only can ENPs successfully administer PCC under protocol but that it is 'morally, ethically and professionally right they should' (McDonald, 1998).

Women clearly feel this service should be available from A & E departments. Reducing the rate of teenage pregnancy is a major health target for the government and PCC can play a significant role in achieving that target. It is regrettable therefore that only 56% of the departments who responded to the Gbolade *et al.* survey felt that PCC should be provided by A & E departments.

Trauma and the pregnant woman

Pregnancy is a state of normal health. Despite this fact, however, many A & E nurses feel very anxious when confronted by a pregnant woman who has suffered trauma because of the specific ways that trauma can affect the pregnant woman. On admission always ask for the woman's clinic card, as this will provide a wealth of information.

Blunt trauma

1. *Placental abruption (abruptio placenta)*. The placenta is sheared from the uterus. This is the second most common cause of fetal death; maternal death is the most common. The uterus will be very painful and tense in this situation and maternal blood loss may be heavy.

2. *Uterine rupture*. This is rare but unfortunately fetal death and hysterectomy are the usual outcome.

3. *Rupture of liver and spleen*. The gravid uterus acts as a shock absorber and protects many of the abdominal organs from trauma. However, in pregnancy, the liver and spleen become distended and displaced making them more vulnerable to injury.

4. *Placenta praevia*. While not associated with specific trauma, any separation of a low-lying placenta may cause torrential blood loss and is potentially fatal for the mother.

Penetrating trauma

This is usually the result of gunshot or knife wounds and therefore relatively rare in the UK. Nevertheless, it is possible given that pregnancy does not exempt a woman from the risk of assault. The gravid uterus protects the woman's abdominal organs very effectively, though at the expense of the fetus. Fetal injury is possible in both blunt and penetrating trauma, however, the fetus is more likely to suffer from maternal hypoxia/hypovolaemia or placental abruption (see above). This emphasizes the need for high concentration oxygen therapy and aggressive IV resuscitation to reduce the risk of hypoxia or hypovolaemia (see below).

Maternal shock

A woman's plasma blood volume increases by as much as 50% during pregnancy with associated haemodilution. Serious bleeding with pooling in the abdominal cavity can occur, hidden by the gravid uterus. The increased blood volume of the woman means that she can lose up to a third of that volume before any signs of hypovolaemic shock appear. The normal response of compensating by shutting down the blood supply to non-vital organs means that the fetus is at great risk in maternal shock, for even in pregnancy, the uterus is non-vital. The increased oxygen requirement of the pregnant woman means that hypoxia then develops more quickly while, as an additional complication, she is at greater risk of regurgitating gastric contents.

Assessment of the pregnant woman after trauma

The usual signs indicating abdominal trauma may be masked or complicated by pregnancy. Stretching of the abdominal wall means that guarding and rigidity are often absent. They are, therefore, unreliable indicators. The increased blood volume associated with pregnancy leads to a situation whereby hypotension and tachycardia may only become apparent when the woman has lost a third of her blood volume.

Any complaint of pain should be taken seriously by the nurse who should ask the patient to describe the pain. Vaginal bleeding is obviously a very significant sign. Monitoring of the fetal heart rate will indicate fetal distress and the potential need for emergency delivery by Caesarean.

The psychological state of the woman, together with that of her partner or other friends and relatives, should be monitored closely throughout what may be an extremely distressing experience.

Intervention

Resuscitation should proceed along the standard lines described earlier, except with the addition of the basic principle that the life of the mother takes precedence over the fetus.

The woman should never be kept in a supine position as the pressure from the uterus causes compression of the vena cava resulting in hypotension and fetal hypoxia. By placing the woman in the lateral position blood flow will increase to vital organs and the uterus. The fetal heart should be monitored using a portable sonic aid. If the fetal heart is not audible then an ultrasound scan will confirm viability. Any signs of fetal distress will indicate that delivery should be precipitated immediately. The nurse should be aware of non-verbal actions as these may increase the anxiety of the woman and her partner. The woman and partner's psychological state is likely to be eased by being provided with up-to-date accurate information in an empathetic manner. The midwife on call or the maternity unit should be contacted immediately.

If spontaneous delivery does occur in A & E remember that childbirth is a perfectly normal event that women have been managing to perform successfully throughout the history of humankind. The woman should be allowed to give birth in whatever position she finds most natural, wherever she feels comfortable, i.e. chair, floor with mattress. She may or may not have made plans for delivery and anxiety will be increased with the realization that she may not attain her personal goal in the environment she had envisaged.

Vaginal bleeding

Most women between the menarche and the menopause experience vaginal bleeding at approximately monthly intervals. What actually happens to individuals varies enormously. For some women a normal period occurs every 3 weeks and lasts 8 days. For others it occurs every 8 weeks and lasts 3 days.

In assessing the patient who attends A & E complaining of vaginal bleeding, the nurse needs to discover the following:

1. Date of last menstrual period.
2. Normal frequency and heaviness of periods.
3. Why is this bleeding different?
4. Is there any pain, and if so, its location, type and duration.
5. Is there a possibility of pregnancy?
6. Psychological state of patient.
7. Baseline vital signs.

There are many reasons for abnormal vaginal bleeding. In the first trimester of pregnancy, spontaneous abortion or a ruptured ectopic pregnancy are the most likely. A spontaneous abortion can still occur in the second trimester but now so can abruptio placentae or placenta praevia. These latter conditions can also occur in the third trimester as can trophoblastic disease. Vaginal bleeding may also occur for reasons unconnected with pregnancy such as vaginal trauma, infection, inflammation or cervical erosion/polyps.

The patient should be interviewed in strict privacy, especially if the nurse is dealing with an adolescent/teenager accompanied by her parents. Pregnancy testing equipment should be available in the department.

If the pregnancy test is positive, it is usual to admit the patient to the care of the obstetric or gynaecological medical teams, depending upon the stage of the pregnancy. Keep the woman comfortable and dry. Any material passed vaginally should be kept for inspection and blood loss estimated from the number of pads used. If the patient is hypovolaemic then urgent resuscitation is required as, for example, a ruptured ectopic pregnancy can cause catastrophic bleeding.

If the pregnancy aborts in the A & E department or en route, the nurse needs to provide pain relief and psychological support. The grieving process may have already started. Placatory comments such as 'Think of your other children' or 'There is always another chance' are inappropriate. The term 'miscarriage' should always be used within earshot of the patient as this carries less distressing connotations than the medical term 'spontaneous abortion'.

Finally, the possibility of a criminal abortion should be borne in mind if there are any suspicious circumstances.

Concealed pregnancy

Despite general information and open discussions about pregnancy, occasionally some women are admitted to A & E complaining of acute abdominal pains only to be told they are in labour. One may assume that this occurs to teenagers who have denied the pregnancy through fear and/or ignorance. It can potentially happen to any woman who does not expect to be pregnant, particularly if menstruation is expected to be irregular, i.e. when becoming menopausal. The woman not only has to deal with the labour but has to begin the adaptation towards motherhood that would normally occur during acknowledged pregnancy. Ideally the woman should be transferred to the local maternity unit. While this is not always feasible, the midwife on call will usually attend. If delivery is imminent the best policy is one of hands off. Provided the fetal heart is established the woman in labour requires attendants who are friendly and calm during contractions, analgesia such as Entonox and usually the person, if any, who came with her.

Lost tampons

This is a highly embarrassing but frequent cause of attendance at A & E, caused usually by either a faulty tampon, sexual intercourse during menstruation with the tampon in place, or an attempt to cope with a heavy period by inserting a second tampon. The result of either of these latter two events is to push the tampon high into the vagina where it cannot be retrieved.

Tact and sympathy, a Cusco's speculum, a good light source, and a pair of long-handled forceps will usually permit a female member of the nursing staff to remove the offending article promptly. In order to try to prevent a recurrence of the problem, advice should be offered about the wisdom of sexual intercourse with a tampon in place or of attempting to cope with heavy bleeding by using two tampons.

Toxic shock syndrome

Toxic shock syndrome (TSS) occurs in women, generally under 25, during menstruation, who are using high absorbency tampons. It is believed that the high absorbency of the tampon dries the normal protective secretions of the vagina, allowing a sudden multiplication of *Staphylococcus aureus*. Women present with flu-like symptoms followed by hyperpyrexia and hypotension, swollen mucous membranes, abdominal tenderness which may lead to delirium, renal failure and death.

Vital signs need to be recorded and maintained. Removal of the tampon as soon as possible is essential, then admission may be required for monitoring and antibiotic treatment. A & E nurses have a health role in endorsing the advice on tampon packaging to use the lowest absorbency tampon wherever possible.

References

Arnold L (1994) *Women and Self-Injury; Information Booklet No. 1.* Understanding Self-Injury, Bristol Crisis Service for Women, Mental Health Foundation, Bristol.

Davies K, Edwards L (1999) Domestic violence: a challenge to accident and emergency nurses. *Accident and Emergency Nursing*, 7:26–30.

Gbolade A, Elstein M, Yates D (1999) UK accident and emergency departments and emergency contraception: what do they think and do? *Journal of Accident and Emergency Medicine*, 16:35–8.

Hadley SM (1992) Working with battered women in the emergency department: a model program. *Journal of Emergency Nursing*, 18:1, 18–23.

Lane M, Beale J (1998) Health promotion in relation to domestic violence. *Emergency Nurse*, 6:1, 26–30.

McHale J, Tingle J, Peysner J (1998) *Law and Nursing*. Oxford: Butterworth-Heinemann.

McDonald H (1998) Moral, ethical and professional issues in prescribing emergency contraception. *Emergency Nurse*, 6:8, 28–32.

Quinn S (1999) Emergency contraception: implications for nursing practice. *Nursing Standard*, 14:7, 38–43.

Reece J (1998) Female survivors of abuse attending A&E with self injury. *Accident and Emergency Nursing*, 6:133–8.

Roberts C (1989) *Women and Rape*. Hemel Hempstead: Harvester Wheatsheaf.

World Health Organisation (1993) *Psychology Report*, 72:3, part 2, 1202.

Wyatt J, Illingworth R, Clancy M, Munro P, Robertson C (1999) *Oxford Handbook of Accident and Emergency Medicine*. Oxford: Oxford University Press.

The patient with behavioural problems

Chapter 15

SUBSTANCE MISUSE

The nurse will not be long in A & E before realizing that alcohol is a major causative factor in attendances, especially at night. In addition, there is now a marked increase in the use of various other drugs ranging from solvents to heroin. Effective care planning in A & E requires some background knowledge of who uses drugs and why and of the social setting within which drug use occurs.

From the outset it is important that the A & E nurse avoids the twin traps of stereotyping and making judgements about patients who attend A & E as a result of substance misuse. The use of terms such as 'alcoholic' or 'drug addict' should be avoided as they are value laden and judgemental. It is better to talk of a dependence upon various substances which may have physiological, psychological and sociological dimensions.

Some of the key aspects of physiological dependence, according to Johns (1990), are tolerance, neuroadaptation and withdrawal states. Tolerance refers to the need for ever bigger doses of a drug to produce similar effects which, in turn, means that regular users can tolerate doses that would be lethal to others. This is caused by the ability of the brain to adapt to larger doses, which leads to the term neuroadaptation. Withdrawal of the drug leads to decompensation and rebound symptoms which tend to be the opposite of the drug's main effects.

The psychological aspect of substance misuse may be understood by considering operant conditioning in which reinforcement of behaviour occurs if there are pleasurable or beneficial effects for the individual concerned. There is, however, no evidence for any personality type who might be particularly prone to substance misuse. How the individual perceives their situation might influence the ability to withdraw successfully from substance use, for example a 'learned hopelessness' view that things are beyond the person's control will make action to give up drug use unlikely to succeed.

Users may associate certain stimuli with the pleasures of use; the chance offer of a drink or the sight of a needle and syringe may suffice to restart the person's habit.

Finally, the sociological dimensions of substance misuse must be considered. Wright (1995) looked at the knowledge and experience of young people regarding drug misuse. He found that over a 5-year period the proportion of 14–15 year olds who had been offered drugs had increased ninefold from 5% to 45% and the amount who knew someone who was taking some form of drug had quadrupled from 15% to 65%. Interestingly, he also showed that the main reasons to try drugs for the first time was to 'feel big, to show off, look grown up'. The study also showed that the knowledge of drugs and their effects was poorly known to the group studied. In different societies there may be widely varying views about the same drug. Islamic and western societies, for example, have very different views about cannabis and alcohol. The presence of a multi-million pound advertising industry actively encouraging people to smoke and drink in the UK cannot be ignored in any discussion of substance misuse. On a smaller scale, the role of peer group pressure and the social norms of the individual's environment all play a part in substance use behaviour.

These factors come together to produce a wide range of substance use behaviours which have been summarized as lying on a continuum which has three phases. There is an initial experimental stage which, if seen as having beneficial effects, may lead to the recreational stage in which the user still has control over drug use, but which may have by now become a regular feature of life. The final phase in this career is reached as control is lost and drug use becomes compulsive, taking over the person's whole life regardless of consequences. This model is supported by Preston (1992) who is critical of the traditional medical model approach which sees substance misuse in disease terms. As Johns (1990) points out there is little support for a disease model either from research findings or clinical evidence, yet it remains a popular model for explaining substance misuse.

It is against this background that the A & E nurse should try to understand the patient presenting with alcohol or other drug-related problems, rather than media hype and the prejudiced views of stereotypes such as 'Skid Row alcoholics' and 'drug addicts'. The growing impact of drug use (excluding alcohol which is also a drug, but it happens to be legal) can be gauged from the fact that drug-related deaths that were accidental in nature grew from just over 700 in 1993 to over 1200 in England and Wales alone. A further 400 drug-related deaths were classified as suicide and another 350 drug deaths were recorded as 'undetermined', meaning that death was either accidentally or purposively inflicted. These figures relate only to England and Wales (Social Trends, 1999).

Alcohol abuse

Paton (1994) suggests there are 4 million heavy drinkers in the UK of whom 800 000 are problem drinkers and 400 000 are alcohol dependent. Statistics published in New Scientist (1999) suggest that 18% of young men in their early 20s are alcohol dependent compared to 4% of females in that age group. By middle age (40–60 years old) this has dropped to 2–4% for men and 1% for women. Alcohol's role in violence is borne out by the work of Yates *et al.* (1987) who studied patients presenting late at night to two A & E units in Manchester. They found 78% of patients after midnight were inebriated, while 60% of assault victims had positive blood alcohol readings even over the whole 24-hour period.

In low doses alcohol acts as a stimulant and increasing brain activity leads to a decrease in inhibitions (Motluk, 1999). However, large quantities of alcohol act as a central nervous system depressant leading progressively to complete loss of control, sedation and

eventually coma (Smith *et al.*, 1996). Apart from increasing the risk of violence and accidents this also increases the risk of unprotected sex occurring, with the problems of unwanted pregnancy and sexually transmitted diseases.

In the A & E department, there are two types of alcohol-related problems. First, there is the patient who has some significant other pathology (e.g. a lacerated wrist or a drug overdose) but who is also under the influence of alcohol, and second, there is the person whose problems are solely related to alcohol. This person may be either inebriated or alcohol dependent and demanding admission to a psychiatric unit.

In assessing a patient, whichever of these two categories they fall into, there is a need to ascertain how much they have drunk and how this compares to their normal drinking pattern, how much control they have over their physical and emotional behaviour, and how much insight they have into their present situation. Finally, there is a need to know how long it is since their last drink.

A frequent injury seen in drunk people is severe laceration of the arm from falling on glass. Unfortunately, the patient is rarely cooperative enough to permit a thorough examination of the wound, and certainly cannot receive an anaesthetic. In such cases it is best to concentrate on first aid measures to stop the bleeding and, if possible, loosely to close the wound and wait for morning when the patient will have sobered up enough to be able to go to theatre for proper examination and exploration of the wound, with repair of damaged structures as appropriate. If the patient insists on walking out of the department, this should be allowed; they invariably return in the morning with a hangover, but prepared to cooperate in most cases.

Alcohol makes the assessment of head injuries very difficult as one of the key signs is altered consciousness, which could be produced by the alcohol as much as by trauma.

Patients are frequently brought to A & E in a collapsed state due to alcohol intake. In such a situation, their airway must be the first consideration, not only because they may become unable to protect it for themselves, but also because they are highly likely to vomit if they have been drinking heavily. They should be thoroughly examined for other injury, specially head injury. If they are to be kept in the department for some time for observation, it is recommended that they be kept on a mattress on the floor rather than on a trolley. There is less risk of them falling off a mattress and injuring themselves than there is of falling off a trolley.

The effect of moderate to heavy alcohol intake can be to produce aggression. It is important first of all to recognize that it is alcohol that is responsible for aggressive behaviour in an individual rather than other causes such as a psychotic state or a stress reaction, as this will influence the handling of the situation.

Sometimes more sober friends or relatives can be prevailed upon to calm the situation. Whatever happens, the nurse should not respond to shouting or abuse and must keep in control of the situation at all times. Usually the best approach is to inquire politely what the problem is and how the person can be helped; this will often defuse a potentially explosive situation. It is futile to become drawn into an argument with a drunk person as the powers of logic are one of the first casualties of alcohol, and an argument can quickly escalate into violence.

Patients with alcohol problems will occasionally present in A & E asking to see a psychiatrist for 'drying out'. The usual approach of the psychiatric services is that they will only consider a patient for admission if the person is sober and therefore able to exercise clear judgement. If the patient in A & E is under the influence of alcohol, it is unlikely that the psychiatric service will admit them. They are best advised to present to a GP in a sober condition with their request, although if sober in A & E there is no reason why an admission should not be arranged there and then for detoxification and treatment. Conversely, many alcohol dependent patients go through a stage of not wanting any help. The person has to recognize there is a problem first, for themselves, before help will be sought, therefore attempts at persuasion are futile in themselves, however well intentioned the nurse may be (Shepherd, 1991).

A valuable quick screening tool which the nurse can use in A & E is known as 'CAGE' (Goodwin, 1994). If a person answers yes to any of the following questions they have an alcohol problem:

Have you ever felt:

- You ought to **C**ut down your drinking?
- **A**nnoyed when others criticize your drinking?
- **G**uilty about your drinking?
- You need to use alcohol as an **E**ye-opener, i.e. need a drink to get started in the morning?

At the end of the day, however, despite a 'low profile' approach, it may not prove possible to help a patient under the influence of alcohol, and if they refuse to leave the department when asked, then the solution is to call the police and have the person removed. Nursing staff should not have to act as 'bouncers' in situations such as these.

The opioids

In the last decade there has been a dramatic increase in the supply of these drugs, especially heroin, to the illegal market in the UK and consequently in the number of dependent individuals. The problems associated with their use can be divided into three groups: the direct effects of heroin itself, side effects associated with illegal injection practices, and the abstinence syndrome.

Direct effects of opioid injection

Heroin produces a euphoric feeling. However, like most drugs, it requires a progressively larger dose to produce the same effect as tolerance develops. There is therefore a risk of accidental overdose leading to coma and respiratory arrest. The greater part of a heroin injection will be excreted within 24 hours and is detectable in the urine as morphine glucuronide (Madden, 1990).

Furthermore, the heroin bought on the street is impure, having been diluted with additives as the pushers try to increase their share of the profits by making each quantity go further. Police seizures of 'heroin' throughout the 1990s have consistently shown that, on average, the substances seized have been only 40% pure (Social Trends, 1999). The result is that if the user were accidentally to obtain some pure heroin, there would be an overdose by a factor of more than two. Accidental overdose is therefore a common hazard of narcotics abuse.

The overdosed patient will usually be in an unresponsive state, comatose with pin-point pupils and severely depressed respirations, if not respiratory arrest. A further tell-tale sign that should be looked for is the presence of injection sites, although these need not be present if the patient had inhaled heroin, which is an alternative to injection. This involves heating heroin in a metal spoon and inhaling the fumes. This is known as 'chasing the dragon'.

Any patient brought to A & E, aged 15 to 40 years, in a collapsed or comatose state with no apparent cause, should alert the nurse to the possibility of heroin or other drug overdose, and the first steps in assessment should be to check the respiratory effort of the patient and the pupil size before looking for evidence of injection sites. Overdoses outside this range of ages can occur, but they are much less likely. Great care should be taken in undressing the patient as he or she may have used needles and syringes about their person, posing a hazard of accidental needle stick injury.

The immediate aim of intervention is to clear and maintain the airway and, if necessary, institute positive pressure ventilation. The patient will need an IV injection of the specific antagonist for the opiate group of drugs, naloxone. Wyatt *et al.* (1999) recommend starting with 0.8 mg IV and giving repeat doses at 2–3 minute intervals until a response is observed. This will produce a dramatic change in the patient's condition in a matter of minutes, bringing them to a state of consciousness, although they may be a little confused for a few minutes. However, as the half-life of naloxone is only an hour, and its peak effect much shorter than that, it is common also to give an intramuscular dose as well as the IV dose. If the patient then leaves the department quickly the naloxone will last longer for the patient. The respiratory depressant effect of many narcotics is in practice much longer, and the immediate improvement that is observed from naloxone administration may only be transient. It is essential, therefore, that a very close watch be kept on the patient for some time, and several further injections of naloxone may be required depending upon the clinical condition of the patient.

The situation may arise where the patient does not wish to stay for observation. In this case, whoever is with the patient should be informed that the drugs given to counter the effect of the heroin will wear off after a while and the patient may again become comatose. They should be told to keep a close watch and if necessary ring for an ambulance should this occur.

Other effects of opioid injection

Most people are now aware of the risk of HIV or hepatitis B transmission from the use of shared injecting equipment, whatever the drug that is being used. Nurses working in A & E should observe universal precautions against blood-borne infection at all times. Any patient could be an IV drug user and any patient could be HIV positive. The importance of avoiding stereotyping patients cannot be underestimated in this regard. It would be helpful if the A & E nurse is aware of local needle exchange schemes and other sources of advice and help for IV drug users, such as methadone maintenance schemes. These schemes are controversial. Their aim is harm reduction by prescribing the person an oral opioid substitute, methadone, in the hope of helping the person move away from the chaotic drug culture and into regular contact with helping agencies. The controversy is fuelled by the fact that while there were 187 deaths from heroin use in England and Wales in 1996 (and 32 in Scotland) there were 357 deaths from methadone overdose (Social Trends, 1999). Avoiding IV injection, however, greatly reduces the risk of HIV and hepatitis B infection. Intravenous drug users may also present with abscesses around injection sites and septicaemia among other side effects of injection.

Withdrawal syndrome

The withdrawal syndrome is caused by the withdrawal of the drug after the body has become physiologically dependent upon it. The typical picture in the case of heroin is one of sweating, stomach cramps, vomiting, headaches and tachycardia.

In this situation, the dependent user is desperate for heroin and may well present in A & E. Extreme caution is required in handling the person as the desperation can easily lead to violence against members of staff.

Under current legislation and guidelines, however, the prescription of drugs to users is strictly limited to certain doctors specializing in the field. It is not, therefore, the place of A & E departments to be prescribing drugs for dependent users no matter how desperate they may appear. Advice should be given about registering with a GP in order to obtain a referral to either a drug treatment centre or to a psychiatrist with an interest in the field. If a person refuses to leave when refused drugs, the police should be called to deal with the situation. In practice, a user will usually be able to obtain drugs if turned away from A & E.

Cocaine

Cocaine is a highly dangerous drug capable of producing profound dependence and its illicit use is expanding dramatically as a stimulant and euphoric agent. It used to be thought of as the Rolls Royce of the drug scene but the market is now being flooded with large quantities at much lower prices. The development of 'crack', a highly addictive, concentrated and purified form of the drug which is smoked, is now regularly seen within A and E departments. Data on police seizures of crack show it is typically 80–85% pure. Cocaine and crack accounted for 15 deaths in England and Wales during 1996 (Social Trends, 1999).

Hallucinogenics

The effect of these drugs is to produce hallucinations as well as bizarre sensations and feelings, such as being able to hear colours and feel sounds. The best known drug is LSD (lysergic acid diethylamide), although there are other substances, such as the so-called magic mushrooms that grow wild in the UK and contain psilocybin as the active ingredient, but whose effects are less potent than LSD. A very powerful agent not found much in the UK is phencyclidine (PCP) or 'Angel Dust'.

The use of LSD declined considerably after the 'Swinging Sixties' and their associated psychedelia but has increased again in recent years. LSD is usually taken in the form of a tablet and usually in a group situation in order that anyone who is on a 'bad trip' may be talked down. However, the effects of the drug may be so alarming and disturbing that the users' behaviour constitutes a danger to themselves and possibly others. It is then that the patient ends up in A & E.

The patient's behaviour will often be totally unreasonable and unpredictable as the sensory input will be bizarre and deranged. The need is for a secure environment where the patient may be safely detained without injury; for example, a bare cubicle with a mattress on the floor. If behaviour is disturbed, sedation is required; experience has shown that what is needed is a quick-acting IV injection (e.g. diazepam 10 mg) and a long-acting IM injection such as chlorpromazine (100–200 mg). Considerable physical restraint may be needed in the first instance to give the IV sedation, and this should only be attempted when there are enough pairs of hands available to do the job safely.

After sedation the patient should be left to sleep off the effects of the drug, under observation, with particular attention being paid to airway and breathing. The patient should also be assessed for injuries that may have been sustained while under the influence of the LSD, as these can be most readily treated at this stage.

Cannabis

Cannabis is commonly seen and used. McMiller (1996) showed that 43% of boys and 38% of girls between the ages of 15 and 16 had used cannabis. The drug may be smoked or incorporated into food and eaten. If smoked, its effects appear within minutes. If eaten, it takes approximately one hour to produce its effect. After use, the general feeling is one of mild euphoria and well-being, although this is heavily influenced by factors such as the group situation and the users' expectations.

There is little evidence to suggest that smoking cannabis is harmful in the short term, although the occasional patient may present in A & E after their first use of the drug complaining of feeling unwell. It is likely that this feeling is more associated with the anxiety of the individual about the drug experience, than the drug itself. After a short period of observation, such persons can usually be discharged with reassurance. In the long term it is worth noting that cannabis smoke is more carcinogenic than tobacco smoke (Smith *et al.*, 1996).

The drug may be injected, sniffed or smoked and acts as a central nervous system stimulant. Effects include euphoria, agitation, exaggerated reflexes, tachycardia, ventricular arrhythmias, hypertension and hallucinations.

Ecstasy

This drug has appeared since 1990 and is very popular with young people engaged in late night parties, 'raves' and club scenes. Its correct pharmacological name is methylene-dioxymethamphetamine (MDMA) and it is a hallucinogenic amphetamine. Preston (1992) summarizes the effects of the drug as producing initially a mild euphoria followed by sensations of serenity. Stamina is enhanced along with the sensual experiences associated with sex, while visual distortions and heightening of perception are also present.

It appears that while the majority of users experience few long-term ill effects, a minority has severe and potentially fatal reactions. During 1996, 12 deaths were recorded in England and Wales from Ecstacy (Social Trends, 1999). Preston (1992) and Jones and Dickinson (1992) describe the presenting signs of a severe reaction as convulsions and collapse, dilated pupils, hypotension, tachycardia, hyperpyrexia and death from respiratory failure associated with disseminated intravascular coagulation (DIC). Such reactions have been recorded among established users, which suggests this is not some sort of allergic reaction and that the effects of the extreme heat and activity associated with dancing and the 'rave scene' combine with the toxic effects of the drug to lead to this fatal outcome.

The signs that should alert the A & E nurse to an Ecstasy-induced collapse include admission from a late night party/disco of a previously fit young person who has collapsed for no apparent reason. Tachycardia, hypotension and signs of hyperpyrexia (e.g. sweat-soaked clothing, elevated temperature) are all important indicators as would be any evidence of clotting disorder such as abnormal bruising. Early recognition of hyperthermia in A & E is crucial and prompt nursing action to cool the patient or at least reduce the rate at which

temperature is rising is needed. Urgent intervention is needed including giving activated charcoal to prevent further absorption of the drug and treating as for heatstroke (dantrolene 1mg/kg IV) with admission to ITU indicated for ventilatory support (Wyatt *et al.*, 1999). The prognosis is not good, however, if DIC becomes established.

Amphetamines

These stimulant drugs are popular on the drug scene, used either alone or in conjunction with other drugs. Klee (1992) has reported an increase in their use, particularly by injection, which is a worrying trend given the HIV and other risks associated with IV drug use. The risk of HIV transmission is potentially greater with this group as Klee's research indicated that they were significantly more sexually active than a matched group of heroin users and 71% of her sample reported that they had not used condoms during casual sexual encounters.

The user may go for several days without sleep while injecting amphetamines and be brought to A & E eventually in a collapsed state. Regular use leads to serious behavioural disorders such as aggression, hallucinations, profound mood swings and paranoid delusions, making such individuals very difficult to handle in A & E. Other drugs such as barbiturates and cannabis may be used to deal with the symptoms that occur after a period of usage. Barbiturates have a respiratory depressant effect, making monitoring of respiratory rate particularly important in any patient who is suspected of attending in a collapsed state after amphetamine usage.

Solvent abuse

The inhalation of substances for mind-altering reasons has a long history that extends back from the adolescents of today through to the likes of Sir Joseph Priestley, who discovered nitrous oxide in 1776 (N_2O inhalers included Coleridge, Southey and Wedgwood), and back to the Ancient Greeks.

The first solvents to be widely abused were different forms of glue in the USA in the 1960s, the habit spreading to the UK in the

1970s. The substances used are now many and varied, but are mostly based on organic solvents (e.g. toluene, benzene and butane) ranging from glue to nail polish remover, from polystyrene cements to hair spray, and from oven cleaners to petrol. Aerosols are also abused for the effects of the propellants (freons).

The substances are inhaled from a plastic bag (crisp packets are commonly used) held to the face. However, more dangerous practices include placing the bag completely over the head to get a stronger effect (and increasing the risk of death from asphyxiation) and spraying aerosols directly into the mouth, which can cause laryngospasm and death. During 1995 there were 57 recorded deaths from solvent abuse in England and Wales (Social Trends, 1999).

Mild intoxication is achieved within the first few minutes and can last up to 30 minutes. With careful usage, a user may achieve a 'high' lasting as long as 12 hours. Intoxication is an appropriate word to use in describing the experience felt by many abusers and their behaviour is similar to that of an adult who is drunk. However, there may also be hallucinatory experiences, which can lead to extremely dangerous behaviour.

Any adolescent brought to A & E found collapsed or behaving strangely should be suspected of being under the influence of inhaled solvents. In assessing the patient, the clues to look for are redness around the mouth and nose, a smell of solvent, the presence of plastic bags/crisp packets in the pockets or the actual substance itself, and changes in behaviour such as an unsteady gait, aggressiveness, slurred speech and inappropriate emotional responses.

The possibility of adolescents in the department sniffing while actually waiting with a friend should also be borne in mind as their behaviour can cause considerable problems. The changes in behaviour described already should be watched for, and frequent visits to the toilet are highly suspicious indeed. The substance involved can usually be smelt on the person concerned.

The aim is to prevent harm to the individual; therefore, airway care is the first priority, coupled with detention in a place of safety, if there are hallucinations. Sedation may be necessary. It is important to involve the GP and the boy's family as soon as possible. The family's social worker, if it has one, needs to know as well. Finally, some parents may be unaware that their son is indulging in solvent abuse, so the knowledge should be broken to them tactfully to prevent a hostile rejection of offers of help. Solvent abuse has been found to affect children of all social classes, so the nurse should beware of the trap of falling into stereotyping and overlooking the likely cause of an adolescent's behaviour simply because he appears to be from, for example, an upper-class background.

The difficult area of children using drugs has been discussed by Harding-Price (1993), who points out that the Children Act gives children the right to refuse treatment even though under 16 years of age. The nurse may also find that the young person or child may refuse to consent to parents being told of the problem. The Northern Drug Services Child Care Group has drawn up a set of criteria to cover this difficult dilemma which would allow nurses and others to work with the child without parental consent. Harding-Price stresses the importance of the child's best interests, his or her ability to understand fully the situation and the probability of harm coming to the child without intervention, as the key principles upon which these criteria are founded.

Summary

Whatever substances have been abused, the patient will probably have a distorted picture of reality and their mood and thinking patterns will have been substantially altered. Ward (1995) suggests the following key points should be considered when working with a person under the influence of drugs:

- Speak plainly in simple language that is easy to understand
- Speak slowly
- Stay out of arm's length and avoid touching the person
- Keep your hands in front of you, this is for your own protection and reduces suspicion on the part of the client.
- Try to work in pairs
- Avoid arguing with the patient or being patronizing/judgemental.

Remember that a cocktail of drugs may have been taken including sedatives such as temazepam and also alcohol leading to a complex mix of mind altering substances. It is as well, therefore, always to expect the unexpected in dealing with individuals under the influence of alcohol and other drugs. Above all a zero tolerance policy applies towards aggressive behaviour whether the patient is sober, drunk or under the influence of other substances.

References

Fleming J (1991) Alcohol-induced head injury. *Nursing Times*, **87**:29–31.

Goodwin D (1994) *Alcoholism; the facts*. Oxford: Oxford University Press.

Harding-Price D (1993) A sensitive response without discrimination: drug misuse in children and adolescents. *Professional Nurse*, April, 419–22.

Johns A (1990) What is dependence? In Ghodse H, Maxwell D (eds) *Substance Abuse and Dependence*. London: Macmillan Press.

Jones C (1993) MDMA: The doubts surrounding Ecstasy and the response of the emergency nurse. *Accident & Emergency Nursing*, **1**:193–8.

Jones C, Dickinson P (1992) From Ecstasy to agony. *Nursing Times*, **88**:28–30.

Klee H (1992) A deadly combination. *Nursing Times*, **88**:36–8.

Madden S (1990) Effects of drug dependence. In Ghodse H, Maxwell D (eds) *Substance Abuse and Dependence*. London: Macmillan Press.

McMiller P (1996) Drinking, smoking and illicit drug use among 15 and 16 year olds in the United Kingdom. *BMJ*, **13**:394–7.

Motluk A (1999) Jane behaving badly. *New Scientist*, November 27, 28–33.

New Scientist (1999) Boozing by numbers. *New Scientist*, November 27, 82–3.

Paton A (1994) *ABC of Alcohol*. London: BMJ.

Preston A (1992) Pointing out the risk. *Nursing Times*, **88**:24–6.

Shepherd A (1991) Dealing with dependency. *Nursing Times*, **87**:26–9.

Smith C, Sell L, Sudbury P (1996) *Key Topics in Psychiatry*. Oxford: Bios Scientific Press.

Social Trends No.29 (1999) London: Government Statistical Service.

Ward M (1995) *Nursing the Psychiatric Emergency*. Oxford: Butterworth-Heinemann.

Wright J (1995) Knowledge and experience of young peoples regarding drug misuse 1969–94. *BMJ*, **10**:20–4.

Wyatt J, Illingworth R, Clancy M, Munro P, Robertson C (1999) *Oxford Handbook of A&E Medicine*. Oxford: Oxford University Press.

Yates D *et al.* (1987) Alcohol consumption of patients attending two A & E departments in the north west of England. *Journal of the Royal Society of Medicine*, **80**: 486–9.

Chapter 16

DELIBERATE SELF-HARM AND PARASUICIDE

Patients attending A & E having committed acts of deliberate self-harm (DSH) or parasuicide can be among the most difficult to handle. These terms are used in different ways by different people but, in this chapter, deliberate self-harm refers to self-inflicted injury such as cutting, while parasuicide refers to self-poisoning, another type of DSH. These acts represent, in many cases, outbursts of aggression which have been turned inwards or acts calculated to manipulate others. Either way the A & E nurse may find the aggression or manipulation that the patient is displaying focused on him or her.

The ultimate act of DSH is suicide. Over the current century the number of suicides has risen from 3121 in 1901 to average around 4600 through the 1980s and remaining around the 4000 mark ever since (Chew, 1993). In 1997 the UK total was 4143 (Office for National Statistics, 1999). There are marked variations in suicide rates in the UK with men having three times the rate of women (16 per 100 000 compared to 5 for women), while in Scotland suicide rates among men and women are 66% higher than they are in England (Regional Trends, 1998). Of particular concern is the high rate of suicide among young men. Males aged 15–44 accounted for 44% of all suicides in England and Wales in 1997 (Office for National Statistics, 1997). Although there is an association between suicide and previous attendance at A & E with episodes of self-harm, patients who indulge in self-harm are a separate group from potentially suicidal patients (Warncken and Dolan, 1999). The vast majority of self-harming patients are not suicidal in intent. The difficulty lies in deciding between DSH and a failed suicide attempt (see p. 169).

If a person has committed suicide then, as in all cases of death in A & E, attention should focus on the living. In addition to the devastating effects of a sudden death, the knowledge that it is suicide puts an intolerable strain on the family. The nurse must be aware of this in dealing with relatives of suicide victims as an extra dimension to the grief they experience.

Parasuicide and self-poisoning

Self-poisoning is frequently seen in A & E and accounts for 20% of admissions to acute medical beds (Wyatt *et al.*, 1999). The numbers seen and treated overall by GPs and A & E units has been estimated at around 200 000 per year (Dunleavey, 1992; Davenport, 1993; Palmer, 1993). Parasuicide seems to be most frequent among the younger age groups and is more common in women than men.

It remains, therefore, to ask why do people poison themselves? In talking to the majority of overdose patients, it quickly becomes apparent that they were not trying to kill themselves. However, within this large number of patients there is a significant number who *are* suicidal, and a trivial overdose may be a 'trial run' before a serious attempt is made. An important task in the nursing assessment is, therefore, to try to identify those individuals for whom there is a significant risk of suicidal intent (p. 169).

A frequently found cause of overdose is manipulation of some other person or persons or simply to attract attention. Domestic disputes and relationship problems figure high in the list of reasons, the aim being to bring back a boyfriend or wife, for example, who has left or is in the process of leaving the overdose patient. Many a reluctant reunion occurs in A & E. It is frequently the case that the patient themselves will raise the alarm, which is consistent with an 'attention seeking' behaviour pattern.

Palmer (1993), however, argues that it is wrong to see parasuicide automatically as attention seeking behaviour, citing Strengel (1970) who argued that it is a mistake to focus on the outcome rather than the act. This underlines the importance of not stereotyping patients and adopting a holistic approach to care. Some patients may be attention seeking, but many are not and their behaviour is underpinned by major psychological disturbance. Bent-Kelly (1992) has written critically of those A & E staff who pass judgement on patients who have committed acts of parasuicide without attempting to understand why the person acted the way they did. Stereotypes are no substitute for a thorough patient assessment.

Evidence supporting the view that relationship crises cause many acts of parasuicide comes from Evans *et al.* (1992) in describing the work of a parasuicide team working in a large London hospital. They are of the view that the behaviour is triggered usually by a crisis that is connected to the patient's dependency needs and which the patient sees as producing an unbearable situation to which the only solution is an overdose. Painful feelings of rejection and loss are frequently involved and a desire to hurt the other person who is seen as responsible.

Self-poisoning can, therefore, be seen largely as a coping mechanism, aimed at seeking attention or manipulating other persons or situations, though in a number of cases, real suicidal intent may be involved.

Self-inflicted injury

Self-mutilation frequently takes a chronic form of repeated episodes of self-laceration, usually involving the forearms and varying from the superficial to the occasionally deep. Occasionally other areas of the body may be attacked, such as the abdomen or legs, while in some very disturbed individuals, the face or genitals may be mutilated. Other forms of self-harm include self-inflicted stab wounds and swallowing objects such as safety pins.

Common reasons given for self-harm include managing feelings, as a response to beliefs or habitual thoughts and as a means of communicating with other people or managing interactions with them (Allen, 1995). It is rare for there to be any significant arterial damage because the areas attacked are often not adjacent to major arteries in their superficial portions. In the case of the wrist, the radial and ulnar arteries are well protected by tough tendon sheaths that require considerable force to cut through. Consequently many self-inflicted wounds are easily closed by sutures or steristrips in A & E and blood loss is minimal. Deep structures are rarely damaged and, if so, it is more likely to be a tendon or nerve than an artery. Greenwood and Bradley (1997) draw attention to the fact that while overdose patients are usually admitted and given the benefit of a psychiatric assessment, most self-injury patients are discharged from A & E with little or no follow up. A 5-month audit of their department revealed that 70% of the 351 overdoses who presented were admitted and assessed by a psychiatrist and a further 10% seen in A & E by a psychiatrist without admission. Of the 50 self-injury patients only 25% were referred to a psychiatrist and hardly any were admitted. There was little evidence in the notes of any attempt by medical or nursing staff to assess the mental health needs of these 50 patients. Greenwood and Bradley acknowledge these can be very difficult and frustrating individuals to treat, but rightly point out that A & E staff cannot ignore them. A multiprofessional approach to meeting the needs of this group of individuals is required.

In trying to understand why people behave in this way it has to be recognized that, as in cases of overdose, there is usually no suicidal intent but there is certainly a strong streak of low self-esteem in persons who have inflicted self-injury. They have frequently been the victim of child sexual abuse which is consistent with low self-esteem. The aggression is often very near the surface, and while it is turned in on themselves in committing the act, the nurse should remember that that aggression could easily be turned outwards if the patient is mishandled.

Carbon monoxide poisoning

Carbon monoxide (CO) poisoning is the commonest form of fatal poisoning in the UK and frequently self-inflicted via the exhaust pipe of a car. In 1996 there were 877 deaths in England and Wales from CO poisoning, the majority of which were car exhaust suicides (Office for National Statistics, 1996). Henry (1998) dismisses the traditional view that CO toxicity is caused by its high affinity for haemoglobin which, in turn, reduces the oxygen carrying capacity of blood and causes organ hypoxia. Turner *et al.* (1999a) cite extensive evidence supporting Henry's views. It seems that a whole series of complex metabolic mechanisms involving CO are actually responsible for its high toxicity. Clinical manifestations of CO poisoning include loss of consciousness, disturbed gait and a range of other neurological signs, hypotension, arrhythmias and cardiac ischaemia.

Assessment of DSH

The approach to the patient is broadly similar for acts of DSH whether they be by overdose or self-injury. A key question is one of suicidal intent and the individual's mental state.

In approaching the patient, the nurse must remember that the emotional cues given out by the nurse (reflecting his or her attitude) will affect the emotional state of the patient. To minimize the risk of aggressive behaviour and obtain maximum cooperation from the patient, there is a need for a very definite effort on the nurse's part to be friendly and helpful, even though the patient may be hostile, abusive or sullen and withdrawn. An attitude of 'not another overdose' may well rebound back onto the nurse and have an undesirable effect on the patient's emotions and behaviour.

The initial interview should be conducted in privacy and aim to explore the immediate physical aspects of the self-harm and also the equally important psychosocial aspects of the incident. If a self-inflicted wound is present, obviously the nurse should first examine its depth, type of bleeding (arterial or venous) and assess blood loss and whether any nerves or tendons have been damaged, applying a dressing as appropriate.

Questioning should be sympathetic and carried out in such a way as to allow the patient the maximum opportunity to talk and explain the feelings and emotions behind the act in order that the suicide risk may be assessed. High-risk factors include being male, the presence of alcohol, the absence of close family/friends, the middle to elderly age group, and an existing psychiatric problem which is under treatment. The severity of the overdose is not a reliable guide to suicidal intent but the use of a more violent method of self-harm such as attempted hanging or shooting indicates a high level of suicidal intent. Chronic disease and recent bereavement/divorce are further high-risk factors.

A useful quick assessment scale for suicide risk is known as the 'sad persons scale' and is given in Table 16.1. Points are awarded as shown and the score may be interpreted to give a suicide risk and suggested course of action.

The use of this scale coupled with extra training in the management of deliberate self-harm can produce real benefits to an A & E department. Cook (1998) describes how setting up a DSH Team in his department based on these principles has improved patient care, avoided unnecessarily directing some people into the psychiatric system and changed the attitude of all A & E staff towards patients who have harmed themselves. Further evidence in support of this approach comes from Crawford *et al.* (1998). They showed that a simple one-hour teaching session about

Table 16.1 The 'sad persons' scale

Item	Score
Sex Male	1
Age <19 or >45	1
Depression or hopelessness	2
Previous suicide attempts or psychiatric care	1
Excessive alcohol or drug use	1
Rational thinking loss (psychotic or organic illness)	2
Separated, widowed or divorced	1
Organized or serious attempt	2
No social support	1
Stated future intent (determined to repeat or ambivalent)	2

Interpretation:
<6	May be safe to discharge (depending upon the circumstances)
6–8	Probably requires psychiatric consultation
>8	Probably requires hospital admission

Source: Wyatt *et al.* (1999)

deliberate self-harm coupled with the use of the 'sad persons' scale made a substantial and statistically significant improvement to the quality of patient assessment, documentation, knowledge about and attitude towards DSH. These improvements applied equally to both medical and nursing staff.

If the patient is found to be very drowsy or unresponsive, then a first priority in assessment must be airway patency and other vital signs, in addition to attempting to work out what was taken and when. Hypothermia cannot be ruled out if the patient has been lying unconscious for many hours. The vasodilator effect of alcohol would increase this risk and alcohol is found commonly in association with overdose. Temperature measurement is essential. There is a high risk of vomit being inhaled in such cases so that, in addition to assessing the patency of the airway, respiratory rate is an important parameter.

Tricyclic antidepressants (e.g. amitriptyline and Anafranil) in overdose have an antiparasympathetic effect which, among other effects, can cause life-threatening cardiac arrhythmias. A patient who has taken an overdose of tricyclic antidepressants should, therefore, have a 12-lead ECG performed as part of their assessment, and be monitored subsequently. Antihypertensive medication, not surprisingly, usually produces hypotension in overdose and ECG abnormalities may also occur after a beta-blocker overdose, such as prolonged PR interval, disappearance of P waves, first degree or total AV block (Bara, 1999).

Throughout the assessment, particular attention should be paid to the level of consciousness as a deterioration can endanger the airway. Benzodiazepines are frequently taken in overdose and produce drowsiness, confusion, slurred speech, dizziness and ataxia. Coma, hypotension and respiratory depression can subsequently occur (Kamanyire *et al.*, 1997). Alcohol greatly increases the effect of drugs such as the benzodiazepines in decreasing consciousness and is frequently taken by individuals who overdose.

Paracetamol is responsible alone or in part for many deaths as a result of self-poisoning. This is due to its toxic effects on the liver and the fact that only 12 g (24 tablets) is capable of producing severe liver damage. Biochemical evidence of such damage may not be apparent until 3–4 days after the overdose, however, a specific antidote is available (N-acetylcysteine or NAC) which, if given soon enough after the overdose, can reduce liver damage. Such is the efficacy of the treatment, if NAC is given within 8 hours, patients may subsequently be declared fit for discharge without needing medical follow up. However, after 8 hours the efficacy of NAC treatment rapidly declines (Bialas *et al.*, 1998). It is, therefore, essential to find out exactly when the patient took the tablets, especially as bloods taken *less than* 4 hours after ingestion do not produce results that can be interpreted with reliability. Blood results for substances taken in overdose can only be interpreted if the time from ingestion is known as there may be further quantities of the drug in the process of metabolism or absorption yet to make their presence felt in the serum levels. Peak levels of serum iron, for example, only occur at 4–6 hours post-ingestion in overdose patients (McRea and Bates, 1999).

Although textbooks state that victims of CO poisoning appear cherry red, Turner *et al.* (1998a) point out that this is rare. The decreased level of consciousness that characterizes CO poisoning may be confused with other possible causes and, therefore, simple tests such as blood glucose should be performed to exclude hypoglycaemia. Turner *et al.* (1998a) stress the need for either venous or arterial blood to be taken and tested for COHb levels in all cases of patients with undiagnosed unconsciousness as well as in cases of known attempted suicide. There is no significant difference in the COHb values obtained whether the sample is arterial or venous. Pulse oximetry will, however, give misleading readings as haemoglobin combined with CO absorbs light at an almost identical frequency to normal oxyhaemoglobin. Metabolic acidosis will be revealed when arterial blood gases are taken. The ECG may show changes indicating ischaemia, such as ST depression or even the classic ST elevation of myocardial infarction (p. 57) even though no infarction has occurred due to the ischaemic effects of CO poisoning.

Nursing intervention

Close and frequent observation is required to monitor vital signs and consciousness, and also to detect any further attempts at self-harm. A discreet check for potentially harmful items or other tablets should be carried out and any such objects quietly removed.

In cases of overdose, administration of activated charcoal solution may be considered. It binds to the drug in the stomach, preventing absorption, however, it should be given within 2 hours of ingestion to be effective. Some drugs delay gastric emptying (e.g. tricyclic antidepressants) and in these cases activated charcoal may still be effective after the 2-hour deadline. Activated charcoal is usually in powder (Carbomix) or granule form (Medicoal) or comes ready prepared (Actidose-Aqua). Either way the patient has to drink up to 500 ml of very unappealing black sludgy liquid. This takes considerable persuasion and repeated swilling around of the drink container to prevent sedimentation. Vomiting is possible but Boyd and Hanson (1998) reported that only 6–8% of patients actually vomited in their study of activated charcoal administration. When Boyd and Hanson looked at how much charcoal had actually been ingested after nurses had done their best to persuade and cajole patients to drink the preparations, they found that Carbomix was superior to Actidose-Aqua (26.5 g compared to 19.5 g). In each case the dose prescribed was 50 g. This indicates that the difficulty experienced by patients in swallowing activated charcoal preparations means that they are only taking half or less of the prescribed dose. The difference between the two preparations was statistically significant so that while neither performed very well, Carbomix was the better of the two. Nurses need to be both persistent and persuasive to ensure the patient takes the maximum possible amount of whatever preparation is used.

There are few specific antidotes to overdoses, although NAC has already been mentioned in the context of paracetamol poisoning. There are national guidelines on treatment based upon a graph showing plasma paracetamol levels and time since ingestion. This should be prominently displayed in all departments. The guidelines recommend that if the person presents 8–15 hours after ingestion and it is thought that 12 g or more has been taken or a dose of more than 150 mg/kg body weight, NAC should be given immediately without waiting for the results of plasma levels (Bialas *et al.*, 1998). A & E departments therefore need to be aware of these guidelines as it is going to be their responsibility rather than the medical wards to commence immediate treatment with NAC.

If the person presents unconscious after CO poisoning, hyperbaric oxygen treatment at a specialist unit is indicated. Turner *et al.* (1998b) report that in their experience of treating CO poisoning in this way, initial COHb levels do not correlate well with the severity of poisoning. The extent of metabolic acidosis is a more reliable guide indicating the complex metabolic processes at work in this condition.

An interesting discussion of the ethical and legal issues has been provided by Davis (1993) who points out that the suicidal but competent patient could legally be left to die. In practice, doctors and nurses feel professionally obliged to intervene even though detaining a patient against their will in A & E entitles the person to sue for damages as a result of the battery committed upon the person. The key to the problem is the competency of the patient to make rational decisions when all the facts have been explained. Young (1994) offers the pragmatic view that either the patient will ultimately be grateful that staff prevented them from taking their own lives or will make a further successful attempt at a later date. Either way they will not sue for damages under the legal tort of battery.

Patients who have practised self-injury may attempt further acts while in the department. Physical intervention is not recommended; talking quietly to try to defuse a potentially violent situation is the best way to proceed. The nurse should explain that there is no benefit from such acts and point out that the wounds will be treated appropriately if the patient is willing to allow the staff to help. However, it is very dangerous for the staff and for the patient to engage in a physical struggle as the result may be to produce accidentally a far worse wound than the one that the patient would have inflicted on their own. In addition, the nurse would be rewarding any attention-seeking motivation that may lie behind such behaviour, thereby increasing the likelihood of further episodes of the behaviour.

If the patient is threatening self-harm with a more serious implement than a piece of glass for example, the best way forward is to talk to the patient and to try to let him or her express their feelings in words rather than in deeds, paying particular attention to what has been said about emotions. Physical intervention is the last resort in such a situation and, if necessary, it should be planned so as to have the maximum degree of surprise and sufficient concentration of force so that the patient is overwhelmed and separated from the implement before they realize what has happened.

The value of developing a DSH team approach and using assessment tools such as 'sad persons' has already been stressed. Improving liaison with local mental health services is essential. Perego (1999) stresses the advantages of having a psychiatric liaison nurse in the A & E department to help this most vulnerable group of patients. Such a nurse can act as a resource for other staff and facilitate improvements in staff attitudes, knowledge and ultimately the care offered.

The nursing interventions around those patients who have practised DSH can therefore be seen to be of a conservative, supportive nature – safeguarding the airway, observing closely, and offering psychological support where needed. The high risk of aggression that is present should the person turn their self-directed anger outwards should always be remembered. This is increased in cases of significant alcohol intake.

Evaluation

Data relating to how DSH patients evaluate their care is scarce but an interesting study by Dunleavey (1992) of 17 such patients is available. She found the patients talked of the nursing staff being cold and distant leaving the patient feeling isolated, so much so that Dunleavey felt their interaction lacked any therapeutic quality; it merely extended the misery of the patient. Staff who respond in a stereotypical way, relying on negative first impressions, will contribute to this type of patient evaluation. It is to be hoped A & E staff will seek a more desirable outcome and aim for care that is holistic and reflects the social and emotional trauma that frequently lies behind DSH or parasuicide.

If the patient talks to the nurse about the events that led up to the DSH episode, we may recognize our intervention as being successful, and further self-harm or outbursts of anger are much less likely to occur. The psychological support offered has been effective. One final check on the nursing care of patients who have practised DSH is the attitude of the staff towards the next patient who has taken an overdose. If the attitude is one of 'Not another overdose, what a nuisance they are', then the care given is likely to fall short of what is required.

References

Allen C (1995) Helping with deliberate self harm: some practical guidelines. *Journal of Mental Health*, 4: 243–50.

Bara V (1999) Antihypertensive drug overdose. *Emergency Nurse*, 7:4, 13–18.

Bent-Kelly E (1992) Too busy for trivia. *Nursing*, 5:32–3.

Bialas M, Evans R, Hutchings A, Alldridge G, Routledge P (1998) The impact of nationally distributed guidelines on the management of paracetamol poisoning in A&E departments. *Journal of Accident and Emergency Medicine*, 15:13–17.

Boyd R, Hanson J (1998) Prospective single blinded randomised controlled trial of two orally administered activated charcoal preparations. *Journal of Accident and Emergency Medicine*, 16:24–5.

Chew R (1993) *Compendium of Health Statistics 1992.* London: Office of Health Economics.

Cook A (1998) Assessing deliberate self harm: a team approach. *Emergency Nurse*, 6:1, 21–4.

Crawford M, Turnbull G, Wessley S (1998) Deliberate self harm assessment by A&E staff – an intervention study. *Journal of Accident and Emergency Medicine*, 15:18–22.

Davis J (1993) Ethical and legal issues in suicide. *British Journal of Nursing*, 2: 777–80.

Davenport D (1993) Structured support at a time of crisis. *Professional Nurse*, June, 558–62.

Dunleavey R (1992) An adequate response to a cry for help? *Professional Nurse*, Jan., 213–15.

Evans M, Cox C, Turnbull G (1992) Parasuicide response. *Nursing Times*, 88:34–6.

Greenwood S, Bradley P (1997) Managing deliberate self harm: the A&E perspective. *Accident and Emergency Nursing*, 5:134–6.

Henry J (1998) Carbon monoxide: not gone, not to be forgotten. *Journal of Accident and Emergency Medicine*, 16:91–2.

Kamanyire R (1997) Acute poisoning; benzodiazepines, phenothiazines and antihistamines. *Emergency Nurse*, 5:7, 14–18.

McCrea S, Bates N (1999) Acute iron overdose:

clinical features and management. *Emergency Nurse*, 7:5, 18–23.

Office for National Statistics (1996) *Mortality Statistics Cause: England and Wales*. London: HMSO.

Office for National Statistics (1997) *Mortality Statistics Cause: England and Wales*. London: HMSO.

Office for National Statistics (1999) *Annual Abstract of Statistics*. London: HMSO.

Quinn S (1999) Emergency contraception: implications for nursing practice. *Nursing Standard*, **14**:7, 38–43.

Palmer S (1993) Parasuicide: a cause for concern. *Nursing Standard*, 7: 37–9.

Perego M (1999) Why A & E nurses feel inadequate in managing patients who deliberately self harm. *Emergency Nurse*, **6(9)**:24–7.

Regional Trends No.38 (1998) Office for National Statistics, HMSO.

Strengel E (1970) *Suicide and Attempted Suicide*. Harmondsworth: Penguin.

Turner M, Hamilton-Farrell R, Clark J (1998a) Carbon monoxide poisoning: an update. *Journal of Accident and Emergency Medicine*, **16**:92–6.

Turner M, Esaw M, Clark J (1998b) Carbon monoxide poisoning treated with hyperbaric oxygen: metabolic acidosis as a predictor of treatment requirements. *Journal of Accident and Emergency Medicine*, **16**:96–8.

Warncken B, Dolan B (1999) Psychiatric Emergencies. In Dolan B, Holt L (eds) *Accident and Emergency; Theory into Practice*. London: Bailliere Tindall.

Wyatt J, Illingworth R, Clancy M, Munro P, Robertson C (1999) *Oxford Handbook of Accident and Emergency Medicine*. Oxford: Oxford University Press.

Young A (1994) *Law and Professional Conduct in Nursing*, 2nd edn. London: Scutari.

Chapter 17

THE MENTALLY ILL PATIENT IN A & E

The A & E unit frequently sees mentally ill patients, some of whom may be very disturbed and who have lost touch with reality. It is this loss of contact with the real world that characterizes psychosis, a term which should be used with care. Sometimes the person is brought to A & E by friends or family; often they are brought by the police or ambulance service after acting in a bizarre way in public. The possibility of drug usage and the effects of cultural differences should also be borne in mind in interpreting the person's behaviour. The closure of large mental hospitals with inadequate community support services has led to significant numbers of mentally ill people presenting at A & E in a very dishevelled and often disturbed condition.

There are many other patients with less obvious psychiatric difficulties who frequently present in A & E. They may be identified and helped by the development of a community psychiatric nursing service within the A & E unit. Patients engaging in deliberate self-harm may be helped by the setting up of a special 'parasuicide team' which works closely with the A & E department (see Chapter 16). It is important that A & E staff fully appreciate their involvement in caring for people with mental health problems.

It will be useful, therefore, to look at some of the common types of behaviour that the mentally ill patient may exhibit, along with the conventional psychiatric diagnosis. The nurse, however, is not trying to make a psychiatric diagnosis in A & E, but rather assess the behavioural problems displayed by the patient in order to plan care which will help the patient and prevent disruption of the department. It is also essential to assign a triage category for such patients, although the more formal algorithms are not really appropriate. Professional judgement and common sense are likely to be more useful.

Schizophrenia

Schizophrenia is conventionally described as a profound disorder of thought associated with disturbance of mood, perception and behaviour. There is a growing body of evidence that schizophrenia is a brain disorder with a physical basis and a strong genetic component. The risk of developing schizophrenia is approximately 1%, although in 25–30% of these cases there is only one major episode of illness, for the rest it is a life-long disorder with a pattern of acute episodes in between lengthy remissions which may be characterized by some degree of impairment. The age of onset is usually 15–25 (Smith *et al.*, 1996).

Although the signs and symptoms of mental illness are much more subjective than in physical illness, it is possible to arrive at a consensus about common presentations of schizophrenia. The person's mood is characterized by a poverty of feeling, conversation typically being in a flat monotone with the mood colourless, bland and emotionally dull. There is also said to be an inappropriate effect, i.e. disharmony, between what a person says and how they say it.

Perceptual disturbance is associated with hallucinations, usually auditory as the person hears voices telling them what to do next or giving a running commentary on events that are happening to the patient. There may be more than one voice audible to the patient. The patient becomes concerned with self, withdrawing from the outside world to live in their own world.

The thought processes become disorganized, illogical and disjointed, leading to the classical thought block where a person stops in mid-sentence, their thoughts having seemingly run into a brick wall. Woolly thinking sometimes characterizes schizophrenia; the patient will go 'all the way round the houses' in giving a simple explanation or answering a simple question.

Delusions creep into the patient's thoughts which may be paranoid or result in the person thinking that he is Christ or God. Another commonly seen phenomenon is that of ideas of reference, where the person thinks there are hidden messages contained in newspapers or TV programmes, for example.

As a result of such profound disorganization of the mental processes, there is often very bizarre and inappropriate behaviour on the person's part, or they may become withdrawn and inert leading to confusion with depression. Violence may occur in response to what the voices that they hear are telling them.

Depression

Everybody at some time or another has a 'low' in life; for some people, though, their lows are much deeper than others, so low that all is black and despair and there is no point to life. It is a short step from there to the decision to end life – suicide.

Depression is a state characterized by a mood of despair, worthlessness, guilt and a decrease in self-esteem coupled with an inability to concentrate. Associated with this mood are physical changes such as loss of appetite and weight, constipation, poor sleeping and early morning wakening. Some patients will talk of their despair, others will not. Signs of self-neglect may be apparent as the patient complains of having no energy or enthusiasm, everything is just too much for them. Impotence or amenorrhoea are also possible. Depression has a life time incidence in women of 1 in 5 and in men of 1 in 10, it is therefore a common and very distressing illness (Smith *et al.*, 1996).

Mania and manic depression (bipolar disorder)

The manic individual suffers from excessive elation of mood, irritability, flight of ideas, talkativeness and hyperactivity, all of which combine to produce extreme and bizarre behaviour. There may also be grandiose or persecutory delusions and auditory hallucinations.

They are frequently very irritable and potentially aggressive or violent in response to even minor frustrations. This latter point is worth remembering when carrying out triage on a patient displaying bizarre, manic behaviour.

It is unusual for a person to display signs of mania (or more commonly a less extreme form known as hypomania) without also having a history of mood swings to the other extreme and becoming depressed, hence the term bipolar disorder or manic depression. It is possible to see these extremes in the same person on different occasions. In between they may function normally for long periods with full insight into their illness.

Anxiety states and phobias

Anxiety is a natural feature of life that we all experience, acting often in a beneficial way in motivating us to work hard for an exam because we are anxious that we may fail or in making us careful in crossing the road.

However, anxiety can build up for some people to pathological levels, with no apparent cause or focus. Such anxiety is called free floating and may lead to acute panic attacks where the person is convinced that they are seriously ill or about to die. Patients may be brought to A & E in the grip of an acute anxiety attack, exhibiting signs associated with sympathetic nervous system stimulation such as tachycardia, palpitations, sweaty palms and a rapid respiratory rate (hyperventilation).

Hyperventilation lowers blood CO_2 levels, upsetting the pH balance making the blood more alkaline which, in turn, lowers serum calcium levels causing muscle spasm (tetany) and tingling in the fingers. There is a characteristic carpopedal spasm of the fingers and abdominal cramps that are associated with hysterical hyperventilation. Their effect is to make the patient even more anxious and therefore more likely to hyperventilate. The solution is to try to calm the patient with reassurance and to encourage them to use a rebreathing bag to increase the CO_2 levels to normal as they rebreathe their own exhaled CO_2. After about 15 minutes, their respiratory rate will be back to normal and the muscle cramps will have abated.

If a person's anxiety is not free floating and instead is attached to some specific object (usually by classical conditioning), then a phobia is said to exist. The most likely phobic state that the A & E nurse may see is agoraphobia – fear of being outdoors – when a phobic patient has a panic attack and is brought to A & E as a result.

Assessment

The nurse will usually be the first point of contact for the patient with the department. Remembering the importance of first impressions, greet the patient in a friendly and sympathetic manner. The patient is an unfamiliar environment, possibly very distressed and seeing things from a very different perspective to you. Try to use empathy and imagine yourself in the patient's shoes. This approach will make triage easier as you assign a priority to the patient and decide which is the best environment in which the patient may be cared for.

The first step is to sit the patient down in a quiet room. Although most patients with mental health problems are not violent, you should consider your own safety. The room door should open outwards if possible and you should be sitting nearer to the door than the patient. A quiet cubicle may be preferable to a relatively inaccessible relatives' room. The offer of a cup of tea may help relax the patient and if he or she insists on smoking then they should be allowed to do so. Introduce yourself so that the patient knows who you are and that you are trying to help. Try and sit slightly to one side rather than square on to the patient – this is less threatening – and make sure your distance is not so close as to intrude on the personal space of the patient (this is potentially threatening) or too far away (suggesting disinterest). You should be out of arm's length for your own safety, a metre is usually an appropriate distance.

The amount of stimuli in the environment should be kept to a minimum as this may exacerbate the patient's misperception problems or overwhelm somebody who is already feeling overwhelmed by life in general.

Seeking eye contact is an important first step in commencing a therapeutic relationship (see Chapter 18 for an exception). Try to get the patient to talk about their problems, if possible

gently keeping them on the subject if they try to wander. It is futile to argue with delusions and hallucinations. This will only provoke anger and aggression in the patient, so the approach should be a non-committal one, no matter how far-fetched the story told by the patient. It is best simply to say you cannot hear the voice the patient hears rather than deny its existence.

Body movements are useful indicators for the observant nurse. Hyperactivity and agitation characterize a manic state while fidgeting, restlessness, facial grimacing and parkinsonian movements are among the side effects of the powerful phenothiazine drugs still used in the treatment of schizophrenia and, if observed in a person, might give a useful clue to their previous medical history. A dishevelled appearance suggests the person has been living rough and underlines the need for the assessment to include a social history. Has he or she recently been discharged from a mental hospital?

Once the nurse has engaged the patient in speech, useful information may be gained from the manner in which the patient talks. A straight refusal to speak suggests withdrawal from the outside world. A reluctance on the part of the person to initiate speech, which is then slow and hesitant, is associated with depression. Not surprisingly, the opposite situation, an uninterruptable flood of speech, is associated with manic states.

The content of the person's speech will tell us much about their thought processes. Pressure of speech and leaping from idea to idea suggest a manic thought process while despair, worthlessness and guilt indicate the person is probably depressive. Psychotic illness, such as schizophrenia, is characterized by disordered thought and this is reflected in the speech of the person, it being vague, woolly and halting and incorporating looseness of association, e.g. if the patient is a virgin, so is the Virgin Mary, therefore the patient is the Virgin Mary. Thought block manifests itself by the patient stopping suddenly in the middle of a sentence, their mind a blank – in the midst of thought, there is no thought. The chaotic state of their thoughts leads the person to move randomly between unconnected statements. In addition, the person may describe delusions and hallucinations, and may be seen conversing with the voices that they can hear inside their head.

Orientation in time and space should be assessed together with how much insight the person has into their illness. If the person does not think they are ill they are likely to become very upset if you suggest they are.

It remains to try to find out something of the person's life history, where they are from, whether they have been ill before, what their family background is, marital status, employment, any medication they take, use of recreational drugs including alcohol. Some persons may be known to the local psychiatric service already, others may be presenting with illness for the first time, while others may have come from afar, which should make the nurse alert to the possibility of psychiatric Munchausen's syndrome (see p. 183).

After the initial assessment, the person's family should be interviewed also if they are present, and they should be involved in the person's care throughout their stay in the department, provided that meets with the approval of the patient.

During the assessment, the nurse should also consider the possibility that the patient's behaviour may be due to drugs. This possibility must be raised with the patient and evidence of drug taking should be looked for. Solvent abuse, LSD, psilocybin and alcohol withdrawal (delirium tremens) can all lead to hallucinations. Stimulants such as amphetamines and cocaine can produce acute psychotic states, while Ecstasy can produce psychological effects ranging from mild anxiety to outright psychosis (Jones, 1993).

In summary, after asking the person to describe their problems as they see them, assessing any physical problems and obtaining a social history, the following key factors should be assessed to determine the patient's mental state:

- Appearance and behaviour (unkempt, agitated, unpredictable etc)
- Speech (rapid, slow, logical, contains neologisms, i.e. made up words)
- Mood (how does the patient see the future? Suicidal thoughts)
- Thought abnormalities
- Hallucinations (auditory, visual)
- Cognitive function (orientation, level of consciousness, long- and short-term memory)
- Insight (does the patient accept they are ill?) (Wyatt *et al.*, 1999).

Intervention

The safety of the patient and the staff are the paramount concerns. There should be a quiet, separate room, with minimal stimulation where the patient may be kept. This room should be carefully furnished to avoid providing ready-made ammunition to a very disturbed patient and should have windows that cannot be opened fully so that the patient cannot leave or attempt to leave via that route. Continual observation of the room from outside should be possible, and the patient should not be left alone at any period. If the family is not able to stay with the patient, a nurse should be assigned to this task.

The same nurse should stay with the patient throughout their stay in the department, in order to give a feeling of security and to try to build up some sort of relationship. Duxbury (1999) recommends that a quiet, consistent approach is most useful, speaking directly to the patient but in simple and easy to understand language. Give the patient time and space to express themselves. Try to use empathy to see things from the patient's perspective. Be approachable and accessible but do not make promises that you cannot keep. Be prepared to negotiate care and explain what is happening as events unfold. As Duxbury observes, while you are not a mental health expert or a counsellor, the use of basic counselling skills can still greatly help patient care.

After the patient has been seen by the medical staff, admission may be arranged to a psychiatric bed. The A & E department is, therefore, assessing the patient and carrying out a holding action until admission can be arranged and therapy commenced. Should violence look likely, the nurse should act in accordance with the principles laid down on p. 186.

Many people arrive at A & E departments in an acutely disturbed state, noisy and behaving in a very bizarre fashion, but leave quietly an hour or so later for a psychiatric hospital and treatment, simply because the nursing staff sat and talked with the patient, in between medical assessments. Force or drugs are not used, the secret being simply to let the patient talk and say what they want to say. The nurse need neither agree (and thereby collude with the patient's delusions) nor disagree (and provoke aggression), but simply allow the patient the opportunity of self-expression. It is worth considering that patients today who are labelled as schizophrenics would in another time and place have been hailed as great prophets and holy people due to their visions and ability to hear God talking to them.

While A & E staff are inevitably going to be the first point of contact for patients with mental health problems, providing a specialist service for these patients in A & E should be the goal. Putnam (1998) has described how an Extended Hours Community Mental Health Nursing Team is able to provide rapid backup to the local A & E department between 1700 and 0100 h. The significance of mental health support can be gauged by the fact that during one year, between these times, the department saw 842 cases of chest pain and 555 patients with mental health problems. Mental health is therefore of the same order of importance as chest pain as a cause for presentation. The team was responsible for discharging 394 patients home (71%) but a key group of 50 (9%) required admission to the mental health unit. The remainder were either admitted elsewhere, took their own discharge or discharged into the care of the police/prison system. This is a model that other A & E units could find very useful to follow in providing services for patients with mental health problems.

In concluding the chapter we need to look at the situation in which the patient will not cooperate, and treatment/detention in hospital against the patient's will is called for. This requires invoking a section of the Mental Health Act 1983, and Table 17.1 summarizes the sections of the Act most likely to be used in A & E.

As can be seen from a study of Table 17.1, the A & E department may receive patients brought by a member of the police force, under section 136, due to their behaviour in a public place. Alternatively, departments may receive a patient whose physical health requires treatment before their mental health, under section 135. Such patients are usually elderly and living alone, suffering from malnutrition, hypothermia and gross neglect.

The other section of the Act most likely to be applied is section 4, where the patient is in A & E and the decision is taken that for their own protection and well-being they must be taken into psychiatric care against their will. However, patients from a psychiatric hospital, who are detained under section 2 or 3 already, may also attend A & E due to injuries or illness.

Part IV of the Act establishes several categories of treatment, each with specific legal safeguards, which can be administered to certain patients without their consent, e.g. ECT or drug therapy. Part IV does not apply to various types of patients, including all involuntary patients and those detained for 72 hours or less. Before treating a patient, therefore, the A & E department needs consent which, if withheld by the patient, means that the department should check carefully with psychiatric colleagues that it is permitted to administer treatment under Part IV, before proceeding against the patient's wishes.

The A & E nurse should be familiar with the various provisions of the Mental Health Act 1983 as it affects A & E, and should always have a readily available supply of section papers, particularly section 4. Nurses in Scotland will be aware of the Mental Health (Scotland) Act 1984 which regulates treatment in that country (Killen, 1993) but nurses moving to Scotland from elsewhere in the UK need to familiarize themselves with Scottish law.

Many patients presenting in A & E will not however be suffering from a major psychotic disturbance, but will be anxious, lonely and unhappy – this is particularly true in the night. Listening and the use of counselling skills may make a valuable therapeutic contribution to the individual's well-being and should be just as much a part of the A & E nurse's repertoire as resuscitation and other technical skills.

Evaluation

If a mentally disturbed patient has gone through the department with the minimum of fuss and into the appropriate treatment facility, the care given may be evaluated as successful. However, if there has been violence, it is important to look at what happened but to do so within a blame-free culture so that staff do not feel defensive or scape-goated. Debriefing is beneficial to help staff work through a violent incident and learn whatever lessons there are to be learnt. If the patient has absconded from A & E, this also needs critical examination in order that the reasons for such a failure may be

Table 17.1 Summary of Mental Health Act, 1983

Legislation	Criteria	Application	Medical Recommendations	Effect
Section 4. Admission for assessment in an emergency. [NB Section 24 of the Mental Health (Scotland) Act 1984 is similar in effect.]	Admission for assessment required as a matter of urgent necessity.	Nearest relative or Approved Social Worker (ASW) of Pt. must be seen by applicant during the 24 hours before application is made.	One written recommendation by any doctor, but if possible, one with previous knowledge of the patient.	Pt. detained for a max. of 72 hours unless 2nd medical opinion given and received by hospital management in that period. Provisions of Part IV on consent to treatment do not apply.
Section 136. Mentally disordered persons in public places.	If a ~c finds a person in a public place who appears to be suffering from a mental disorder and is in immediate need of care or control.	A Police Officer	Nil	Person can be taken to place of safety to be interviewed by ASW or doctor, e.g. A & E or Police Station. Maximum 72 hours.
Section 135. Warrant to search for and remove patient.	There is reasonable cause to suspect that a person believed to be suffering from a mental disorder has been ill-treated or neglected, or is unable to care for him or herself and lives alone.	ASW to a JP (on oath)	Nil	pc, ASW and doctor can enter patient's premises and remove him or her to a place of safety. Maximum 72 hours.
Section 2. Admission for assessment.	Mental disorder warranting detention in hospital for assessment and treatment. The patient ought to be detained in interests of own health and safety or for the protection of others.	Nearest relative and ASW who must interview Pt.	Two doctors, one of whom must be approved under Section 12. Doctors not to be from same hospital.	Patient detained for maximum of 28 days. Part IV applies for treatment without consent.
Section 3. Admission for treatment.	Mental illness or severe impairment. Psychopathic disorder or mental impairment of a nature or degree which makes medical treatment in hospital appropriate.	As for Section 2. but ASW cannot make an application if the nearest relative objects.	As for Section 2.	Patient detained for maximum of 6 months. Renewable for a further 6, then for 1 year at a time.

Adapted from *A Practical Guide to Mental Health Law*, MIND (1983).

identified. If it was because there were not enough nurses on duty to keep adequate watch on the patient, then questions have to be asked of management whose responsibility it is to staff the unit.

References

Duxbury J (1999) Therapeutic communication. In Walsh M, Crumbie A, Reveley S (eds) *Nurse Practitioners; Clinical Skills and Professional Issues.* Oxford: Butterworth-Heinemann.

Jones C (1993) MDMA: the doubts surrounding Ecstasy and the response of the emergency nurse. *Accident & Emergency Nursing,* 193–8.

Killen J (1993) The Mental Health Acts: the UK and Eire. In Wright H, Giddey M (eds) *Mental Health Nursing.* London: Chapman & Hall.

Putnam S (1998) Extended hours community mental health nursing service. *Accident and Emergency Nursing,* **6**:192–6.

Smith C, Sell L, Sudbury P (1996) *Key Topics in Psychiatry.* Oxford: Bios Scientific Publishers.

Wyatt J, Illingworth R, Clancy M, Munro P, Robertson C (1999) *Oxford Handbook of Accident and Emergency Medicine.* Oxford: Oxford University Press.

Chapter 18

THE DIFFICULT PROBLEMS THAT NOBODY ELSE WANTS

Most A & E departments have their share of 'regulars', the frequent attenders who are constantly turning up, often because nobody else can think of what to do with them. They include the footloose, those who are alcohol/drug dependent, those with Munchausen's syndrome, the homeless, and people suffering from psychopathic personality disorders that do not benefit from psychiatric treatment.

It is worth looking at some of these problem areas in detail, as the difficulties that some of these individuals can cause are out of all proportion to the numbers involved.

NFA... The person with nowhere to go

The last two decades have seen a worrying increase in homelessness, particularly among the young. Factors such as the decline of rented accommodation and the policy of discharging large numbers of patients from long-stay mental hospitals without providing sufficient community resources have contributed to this trend. A large proportion of children who have been in the care of local authorities subsequently become homeless indicating a clear failure of the system which government is only now attempting to rectify. There is now a section of the community with no home of their own except a night shelter, hostel, squat, local authority bed and breakfast accommodation or, perhaps, just a cardboard box. For these people, social exclusion is a way of life and A & E is their main source of medical help.

Alcohol abuse is a major problem that affects some people within this group. The prognosis for the 'Skid Row' alcoholic, drinking the day away with fellow 'dossers' on the waste ground and parklands of towns and cities, is very poor indeed.

The 'dossers' form a hard core of A & E regulars. Students often ask 'Surely something can be done for these people?' Society answers by locking them in prison for short sentences due to their drunken behaviour in public, which can often be aggressive. Most of the agencies involved with dossers, however, admit that this is a waste of time, not benefiting the individuals concerned and merely adding to the overcrowding problems in gaols.

There is no easy answer to the problem of drunken vagrancy. Cook (1975), after many years working with alcoholic vagrants in London, wrote: 'One certainly has the feeling that Skid Row has the capacity to absorb any amount of research and social work endeavour, and to remain untouched by it. There is in the Skid Row air as it were a notion of defiance and hopelessness either part of which (or the combination of which) makes reaching out to and helping individuals . . . extremely difficult.' A quarter of a century later Cook's pessimism still seems justified.

The A & E nurse will usually encounter the homeless vagrant when he has fallen over drunk causing injuries to himself such as scalp lacerations, or when a member of the public dials 999 for an ambulance as he has passed out in a public place. 'Drunk again' may be the automatic assumption, however, he could have had an epileptic fit, be in hypoglycaemic coma or be presenting with one of several other medical emergency conditions.

A full assessment should be carried out on reception in A & E, paying particular attention to level of consciousness and airway. Head injury is a common problem, but due to the effects of alcohol extremely difficult to assess. Glasgow Coma Score should be recorded and pupil observations carried out at regular intervals. It is important also to check vital signs, blood sugar levels, and temperature, as hypothermia is a major risk, especially in winter.

If there are no immediate interventions needed, the patient is best laid for his own safety on his side on a mattress on the floor, under observation until he has slept off his alcohol sufficiently to leave.

Aggressive behaviour is unfortunately a possibility due to the alcohol and may occur as the person begins to sober up and become more aware of his surroundings. The police should be called to deal with the person if he does become aggressive and disruptive. A & E departments are not night shelters for vagrant alcoholics; once a person is fit to go, then they must go.

Although this may seem a hard policy on a cold night in February, the nurse should ask what exactly would be achieved by allowing somebody to stay the night in A & E simply because they said they had nowhere else to go. A vagrant alcoholic who has sobered up after a binge in the local park is suffering from far deeper social, psychological and economic problems than a night in A & E can solve. A more constructive long-term approach is to try to forge links with the local voluntary services working in the field, and with Social Services so that advice about helpful points of contact with these agencies may be given.

Psychopathic disorder

'Psychopath' is a term often bandied about in general conversation but usually, like the term schizophrenic, in a totally inappropriate way. However, within the mental health care field there is much debate about its meaning and little agreement. An approximate consensus is offered by Barnes and Frisby (1992) who talk of a person who consistently acts against social norms without showing any recognition of the seriously deviant nature of his/her behaviour, but who is not obviously mentally ill.

Such individuals often live turbulent and troubled lives, satisfying their needs by a whole range of strategies, varying from obtaining their objectives by simply hitting somebody over the head and taking whatever they want, to manipulating an individual (or the system) for their own ends. Their mood can change from one of apparent contrition and regret to extreme aggression and violence in an instant, the constant factor being a desire to get their own way regardless of anybody else and what is right or wrong.

What sort of problems do psychopathic individuals cause in A & E? The more manipulative and passive psychopaths may take drug overdoses and practise DSH. Often they attend A & E in an apparently distressed state claiming that if they are not admitted to a psychiatric ward immediately they will commit suicide. Attention-seeking behaviour is indulged in freely, such as taking their overdose or cutting themselves in front of a waiting room full of people.

The more aggressive psychopath turns up in A & E often with injuries associated with a fight and frequently under the influence of alcohol or else demanding drugs. Their potential for violence is high, especially when they realize that they are not going to get what they want. Disruptive behaviour is common and mental illness is frequently claimed.

In dealing with such a disturbed individual, the first step is to recognize that they are not suffering from a psychotic state which has deprived them of insight. They are fully aware of what they are doing and consequently are fully responsible for the consequences of their actions in A & E. Disruptive behaviour should be dealt with firmly and promptly by asking the person to desist. If they refuse, the danger is that by making too much fuss, the nurse will be merely rewarding the behaviour and thereby leading to its likely repetition. The aim is to deny them the attention that they crave, even if they are swallowing tablets two at a time in front of other patients and relatives. They know exactly what they are doing and must take the consequences (usually little more than a long sleep) and attempts to restrain them physically would only lead to staff getting hurt.

Limits have to be set for such individuals for the protection of other patients in the department whose treatment may be adversely affected by disruptive behaviour. The limits of what is acceptable should be clearly stated at the beginning of the attendance (e.g. no shouting, running around the department or intruding into certain areas) and if the person goes beyond those limits, they should be removed from A & E by the police. Female nurses are just as likely as male nurses to be punched or kicked by aggressive individuals and a policy of zero tolerance to violence should be in place at all times.

Munchausen's syndrome

This syndrome has been described by Bnoch and Trethowan (1979) as individuals 'who obtain admission to hospital with apparently acute illness supported by a plausible but dramatic history which is later found to be full of falsifications. They are subsequently discovered to have attended and deceived staff at many other hospitals and frequently to have discharged themselves against medical advice, often following arguments while under investigation or following a surgical operation.' We have seen earlier that some people may inflict injury upon their children or poison them to gain hospital admission for the child. This is known as 'Munchausen by proxy'.

Such is the highly mobile nature of these individuals that it is almost always to A & E that they present and, unless picked up early, they can consume great amounts of time and energy (and money) having their 'illnesses' treated.

The following five broad categories may be recognized in Munchausen's syndrome on presentation:

1. *The acute abdominal type.* They will manifest acute abdominal symptoms, and some may swallow objects such as razor blades and safety pins in order to obtain the surgery and hospitalization they crave. In well-documented cases individuals have obtained well over 100 admissions and laparotomies numbered in double figures.

2. *The haemorrhagic type.* This is characterized by complaints of bleeding from various orifices: haematuria (coupled with renal colic in order to obtain pethidine), haemoptysis and haematemesis are common. Self-inflicted wounds with needles or razor blades are commonly used to provide the blood to make the samples realistic, e.g. a finger is nicked so that drops of blood can be squeezed into a urine specimen or the back of the tongue may be cut to lend colouring to haemoptysis.

3. *The neurological type.* This type of the syndrome is characterized by very convincing (and some not so convincing) epileptic fits or complaints of migraine. Some individuals may present with a history of trauma, claiming to have suffered a head injury.

4. *The cardiac type.* This type is characterized by a very convincing display of central chest pain that shows considerable knowledge of medical textbooks. Many such patients know that IV diamorphine is administered for chest pain, which may explain their behaviour.

5. *The psychiatric type.* Imitating various forms of mental illness in order to gain admission to psychiatric hospitals is another manifestation of the syndrome.

Some patients maintain a consistent story; others will change their symptoms as they travel. In trying to understand these people, we should not expect a single simple answer. In some cases obtaining drugs is undoubtedly a major feature (e.g. the chest pain type and those feigning renal colic), but there is much more to it than this. They are often attention-seeking, very immature and psychopathic in personality. For others admission to hospital is a way of escaping from the demands of having to cope with the real world outside.

In many Munchausen's patients there appears to be a strong streak of masochism. This fits well into the abdominal type of the syndrome, as they undergo repeated self-induced wounding and may also practise self-mutilation. It has been found that tolerance to unpleasant diagnostic procedures may be high, and their pain thresholds are also high. It is difficult to explain their desire for mutilation, be it by the hand of the surgeon or (sometimes) their own hand, without including a masochistic element in their personality.

The following list of observations should alert the nurse to the possibility that the patient is suffering from Munchausen's syndrome.

1. Any patient presenting alone, who is non-resident in the catchment area of the hospital, who has no apparent injury.

2. A vague reason for being in the area that cannot be readily substantiated, e.g. a long-distance lorry driver says he has left his lorry at a lorry park.

3. If a discreet search of their clothing and effects reveals inconsistencies in their story, such as a different name or address from that given, or evidence of having come from a different part of the country from that which they have stated. There may be evidence of their last port of call such as hospital name tags inside clothes and pyjamas, or evidence of being on the road such as shaving equipment or a change of underwear in a jacket pocket.

4. If the person is known to other A & E departments, locally or in their home area. Check that any address given for their home or GP actually exists.
5. If there are signs of recent IV sites or cut downs. Multiple abdominal scars should rate a very high probability of Munchausen's, if points 1 and 2 are found to be present.
6. If the patient's description of their symptoms is just a little too perfect or textbookish. In practice very few people ever have all the symptoms in the textbook for any given illness.
7. If the patient's manner and behaviour, especially when they think they are not being observed, gives cause for suspicion.
8. If the patient asks for analgesia by the name of a drug.
9. If there is a circular about the person in your department.

What is the course of action when little or no physical signs of illness can be found, and the staff are reasonably sure of the diagnosis of Munchausen's syndrome? The person is neither mentally nor physically ill but suffering from a personality disorder.

There are differing opinions about whether to confront the person in A & E with their Munchausen diagnosis. It is the author's belief that they should be confronted and informed that all hospitals in the area will be circulated at once with their descriptions and details. This should be done over the telephone immediately for your local A & E departments and details of the person added to your own file of Munchausen patients. The effect is to deny the person the attention that they seek by ensuring that they are discovered as soon as possible in other areas, thereby removing the rewards that the individual gets from their abnormal behaviour. In addition, it will also save the hard-pressed NHS considerable time and money. Bnoch and Trethowan come to similar conclusions in their detailed review of the problem, hoping for a decline in the behaviour by denying the rewards that are associated with it.

Such a policy requires cooperation between departments on a national scale to exchange information on these individuals. Computer technology could lead to the development of a central registry with each A & E department having access via a terminal. The scale of the problem, given the itinerant nature of these people, is national; therefore the solution should reflect this characteristic of the problem. Meanwhile departments are recommended to ensure maximum distribution of information concerning Munchausen's patients they come across.

Violence and aggression

For many years A & E staff have not only had to care for the victims of violence but have also become victims themselves. It is only very recently that government and NHS management have begun to take the issue of violence against A & E staff seriously. The publication of a report by the Health Services Advisory Committee (1997) which showed nursing was the most dangerous profession in the UK, with 34% of nurses having been attacked while on duty, acted as wake up call for the Department of Health. A major survey by Jenkins *et al.* (1998) produced data from 233 A & E departments showing that staff were regularly abused and assaulted and that nurses were the most frequent victims. This survey showed documentation of such incidents was poor and perpetrators rarely prosecuted and convicted (only 25% of those arrested by the police in A & E). The problem was greatest in inner city departments. An RCN survey revealed that 47% of a sample of 1000 nurses had been physically attacked during the last year, although this included nurses from areas other than A & E (Kydd, 1998). Violence and aggression are therefore major problems for A & E nursing staff.

The origins of aggression and violence in the human species are the subject of much debate and many theories. Suffice it to say that it is a complex phenomenon whose origins lie in a potent mix of biological, psychological and social factors (Saines, 1999). Even the terms 'aggression' and 'violence' are used to mean different things by different people. Some would use the word violence to mean a physical act such as hitting or throwing an object at someone but others use it to mean any act which places another person at risk, including verbal abuse. Medical texts often urge doctors to 'treat aggressively' but they do not mean hurling abuse and insults at the patient!

Violence occurs in many different settings and with many different types of actors. The following list enumerates just some of them and all may be seen in A & E:

1. Domestic/family violence.
2. Associated with organic disease, e.g. post-head injury or hypoglycaemic state.
3. Associated with psychosis, e.g. schizophrenia.
4. Due to the effects of drugs, e.g. hallucinogenics and alcohol.
5. Professional violence, the mugger.
6. Groups such as football hooligans.
7. Sexual violence, rape.
8. Individual loss of control – violence in response to a situation, heavily influenced by role playing and stereotypes.

The victims of all these types of aggression and violence, and their perpetrators, end up in A & E. An understanding of the psychological processes that are involved in aggressive and violent behaviour will help us to help our patients, and prevent us from being counted among the next victims ourselves.

It is very rare for violence to erupt spontaneously without any warning and reason. There are opportunities, therefore, for intervention before violence occurs which will allow nurses to defuse the situation and lower the temperature.

A major cause of aggression in A & E, is patients' unrealistic expectations, particularly relating to waiting times. This view is supported by the survey carried out by Jenkins *et al.* (1998). They found that unrealistic expectations, lengthy waiting times, alcohol and other recreational drug usage were indeed the main factors associated with violence and aggression.

Good communication with patients will therefore remove a great deal of frustration stemming from unreal expectations and also improve staff–patient relationships. A visual display of approximate waiting times gives valuable information to the patient and good communication can avoid many unpleasant situations by preventing misunderstandings. The welcome expansion of nursing roles has allowed many experienced A & E nurses to see and treat patients with a range of minor injuries without the need for lengthy waits to

see a casualty officer. It is imperative that nurses working in such expanded roles should have a thorough educational preparation for the role. Walsh (2000) has pointed out that the North American use of the term Emergency Nurse Practitioner (ENP) means a nurse with a degree level nurse practitioner education who is able to act as a first point of contact for most patients in A & E. This is different from the common UK usage of the term ENP which means acting as a first point of contact for minor injuries only, without necessarily having undertaken degree level preparation for the role.

Departments should think about the provision of facilities to keep people amused while they are waiting; toys, magazines, piped radio, a TV or a video (well secured to the wall!), a public phone and a drinks machine would all be desirable. Generally nurses should look at the waiting environment provided in A & E and ask if it is really satisfactory – especially if patients have to wait there for 3 or 4 hours with a painful injury.

If, however, you are confronted by an aggressive individual, what then? Self-awareness is crucial as it may be your behaviour that is contributing to the other person's aggression. Consider also how you are responding to that aggression. A lack of self-awareness can make the situation a lot worse by leading to either a defensive or condescending attitude towards the patient or even avoidance of the patient (Morcombe, 1999). You cannot avoid communicating with another person even if you say nothing. Your body posture and facial expression can still speak volumes. Self-awareness is therefore about more than what you say and how you say it.

Ward (1995) reminds us that some nurses do not reflect upon their own communication and interpersonal skills sufficiently to realize that they may, albeit unwittingly, actually antagonize patients. There is a natural tendency to blame patients always for violent and abusive outbursts. This is missing a golden opportunity to improve practice and reduce the future incidence of violence. As Ward puts it: ' …failure to explore the behaviours of all those involved in violent or aggressive events is both short sighted and therapeutically counterproductive' (Ward, 1995, p. 89).

There should always be a debriefing after an incident both to support the staff involved and honestly to try to see if lessons could be learned. It is not a case of victim blaming, but rather of reflecting honestly on how you handled a situation. It may well be that you did all that could be reasonably expected of a nurse in the circumstances, but it may also be that there was something about your behaviour or tone of voice that contributed to the outburst. We talk a lot in nursing about being reflective practitioners, if ever there was a case where this rhetoric should be put into practice it is picking up the pieces after a violent outburst.

There are several things that you can do to prevent an aggressive situation from getting out of hand. First, keep your voice to its normal pitch and volume. When shouted at, it is easy to shout back, but do not. It only raises the temperature immediately. There is nothing wrong with telling yourself repeatedly to control yourself; it is a feedback mechanism that works.

Body positioning is critically important. Stand just a little more than an arm's length (the patient's arm) away. This is far enough to give you the chance to escape any sudden grab or punch, but not so far away as to suggest disinterest in the patient's problem. Standing too close, on the other hand, crowds the person's individual space and is very threatening, so try to keep just beyond arm's length from the patient at all times.

Your posture should be slightly oblique to the patient. Standing square on is very confrontational, especially if you have your arms in the traditional nursing position of folded across the chest.

The correct stance is with one leg slightly behind the other. The back leg should be the dominant one and should be straight with your weight fully on it, while the leading leg should be slightly flexed at the knee. This position poses minimal threat, but coupled with the distance you have placed between yourself and the aggressor, gives you the best chance of avoiding a kick or a blow. Avoid standing with your feet too far apart as this invites a kick to the groin.

In this particular situation, prolonged eye-to-eye contact can be construed as very provocative and should therefore be avoided. Only engage in brief eye-to-eye contact and in between concentrate your attention at a point about level with the second shirt button down. This still conveys interest and gives you the best chance of seeing a punch or grab with your peripheral vision, while not threatening the aggressor with direct eyeball-to-eyeball contact (Figs 18.1–18.3).

Finally, you should be aware of any suspicious bulges in jacket pockets that may be potential weapons such as bottles, and of any potential weapons in the immediate environment of the patient. Do not carry pointed scissors and, whatever sort you do use, keep them well out of view. They have been used on a number of occasions to assault nursing staff. The practice of wearing a stethoscope draped around the back of the neck should be discontinued as it makes it very easy for an assailant to restrain a nurse in a potentially life-threatening manner.

Verbal contact with the patient will often

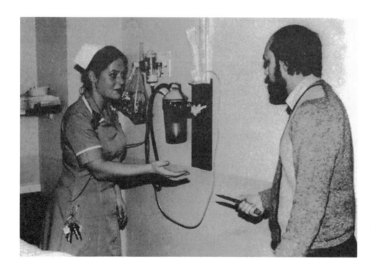

Fig. 18.1 The patient in A & E with a weapon. The wrong approach: the nurse has allowed the patient to get between her and the outside of the cubicle. She is holding out her hand demanding the knife and she is making eye-to-eye contact. This is confronting and threatening to the patient and may cause him to respond violently and he may use the knife to inflict serious harm.

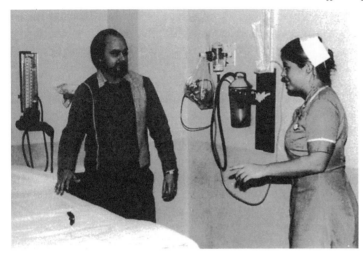

Fig. 18.2 The right approach. The nurse is keeping to the outside of the cubicle and is asking the patient to place the weapon on neutral territory before attempting to remove it. She is keeping at a safe distance (arm's length) and avoiding eye-to-eye contact.

allow the situation to be brought under control. Try to avoid an immediate confrontational attitude – a them and us situation. Explain that you are there to try to help. What can you do? What is the patient's problem? Keep your sentences short and simple as there is less chance of misunderstanding and this allows the patient plenty of time to have their say without having to interrupt you. Kinkle (1993) recommends the nurse to follow a strategy of 'verbal venting', allowing the patient to say their piece without interruption, even if there is a strong urge to defend verbally another member of staff who is coming in for serious criticism during such an outburst.

The person should be interviewed individually if possible, without friends and relatives who are often the cause of more trouble than the patient. When a group of rowdy individuals brings one of their mates to A & E, the best policy is to ask the rest to leave. They will accomplish nothing in the department except be disruptive and endeavour to impress each other with acts of bravado, depending on the pecking order in the group. Such behaviour is well documented in studies of group violence. Allowing such a group to remain in the department will only lead to trouble; therefore they should be asked to leave and if they refuse, the matter referred to the security service or the police.

One of the most effective ways of defusing a situation is simply by passing on information. People are far less likely to get angry if they

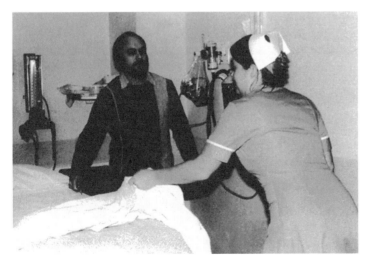

Fig. 18.3 If attacked with a weapon, the nurse should try to smother it with a blanket or anything else available, while retreating rapidly to safety and calling for help.

know what is going on, how long they will have to wait, and why.

However, there are some situations in which, despite all these measures, violence still erupts or, to be more precise, passes from being verbal to physical. In many cases, the patient will smash some physical objects, throw a chair at a wall or window, but then become calmer again having 'let off steam' as it were. Therefore, if a patient indulges in an outburst against property, they are best left to break whatever it is they have in mind. Probably that will be the end of the episode and if you do intervene the result will be a violent struggle in which you will become the object of the person's aggression. Broken windows are easier to repair than a broken arm.

The police should always be contacted in these circumstances as staff may become the next target of the person's aggression. Furthermore, prosecution for serious damage to hospital property should always be part of a zero tolerance policy.

If the person challenges a male member of staff to a fight, going perhaps through the ritual of removing the coat, issuing threats and insults, then violence is less likely to occur, provided the situation is handled correctly. Allow the person to have a 'moral' victory by backing off. The ritual having been fulfilled, physical contact is less likely. While the patient is boasting of his victory and swaggering around the department, the police can be on the way. Remember it is usually the winner of the last battle who wins the war.

At the end of the day, however, a direct assault on a member of staff may occur. A & E staff should be taught breakaway techniques. They can only be learnt properly in a practical workshop but Ward (1995) offers the following useful points:

- If grabbed from behind a sharp stamp on the toes or shins will give you a chance to escape
- If grabbed in a bear-hug from behind force apart the little fingers, this will break the hold
- If grabbed from the front, placing your head on the assailants chest/shoulder will avoid a head butt
- If grabbed in a strangle hold from the front rubbing as hard as you can with the knuckle of your 3rd finger on the sternum will be so painful it will usually break the hold.

Staff should always wear personal alarms for their own safety. Modern devices not only have a panic button to press in case of attack but will automatically alarm if placed in a horizontal position so even if you cannot reach the panic button it will still go off if you are knocked out of an upright position. When intervention is needed (as in such a situation), the basic premises of military strategy still hold good, i.e. concentration of force in time and space coupled with the element of surprise. This means that you should ensure sufficient pairs of hands to do the job of taking down an assailant (ideally at least three people). Plan the move to be simultaneous so as to overwhelm the person, and if possible distract his attention or approach from the rear. This way the risk of injury to staff and patient is minimized. Although the situation in which direct physical intervention is required is unpredictable and, therefore, hard and fast rules cannot be made, the nurse would do well to adhere to these basic principles.

All incidents should be documented and all assailants prosecuted as part of a zero tolerance policy. There should be in-service training for all staff in the skills required to handle aggressive patients and real investment in security equipment (CCTV, alarms etc.) and security staff. This investment will be recouped by the Trust as a result of reduced staff sickness, turn over and damage to property.

References

Barnes C, Frisby R (1992) Personality disorders. In Brooking J, Ritter S, Thomas B (eds) *A Textbook of Psychiatric and Mental Health Nursing*. Edinburgh: Churchill Livingstone.

Bnoch MD, Trethowan WH (1979) *Uncommon Psychiatric Syndromes*. Bristol: John Wright and Sons.

Cook T (1975) *Vagrant Alcoholics*. London: Routledge & Kegan Paul.

Health Services Advisory Committee (1997) Violence and aggression to staff in health services. Norwich: HMSO-HSE books.

Jenkins M, Rocke L, McNicholl B, Hughes D (1998) Violence and verbal abuse against staff in the A&E department; a survey of consultants in the UK and Republic of Ireland. *Journal of Accident and Emergency Medicine*, **15**:262–5.

Kinkle S (1993) Violence in the E. D. *American Journal of Nursing*, July, 2–43, 52–3.

Kydd P (1998) Pinpointing the problem of violence. *Emergency Nurse*, **6**:8, 8–10.

Morcombe J (1999) Interpersonal approaches to managing violence and aggression. *Emergency Nurse*, 7:1, 12–16.

Saines J (1999) Violence and aggression in A&E: recommendations for action. *Accident and Emergency Nursing*, 7:8–12.

Walsh M (2000) *Nursing Frontiers*. Oxford: Butterworth-Heinemann.

Ward M (1995) *Nursing the Psychiatric Emergency*. Oxford: Butterworth-Heinemann.

Chapter 19

SEXUAL PROBLEMS IN A & E

Sexually transmitted disease

Patients sometimes present at A & E, often in a very distressed condition, thinking that they are suffering from some form of sexually transmitted disease. It is essential to know something of the more common types and their presenting symptoms in order that an assessment of the patient's problems may be made.

Table 19.1 shows the numbers of people attending clinic in 1996 compared to 1993 according to the main types of sexually transmitted disease (STD). The reduction in numbers that occurred in the late 1980s–early 1990s has been reversed with a 20% increase between 1993–6. This suggests that the effects of safer sex public education campaigns may be wearing off, which bodes ill for the spread of HIV.

Patients usually come to A & E when the local department of genitourinary medicine is closed, and very often refuse to give details of their complaint to the receptionist, usually because of embarrassment. A sensitive approach to triage is essential in such circumstances and it helps if the nurse is the same sex as the patient.

Table 19.1 New cases of STD, England, 1993–96 (in thousands)

Disease	1993	1996
Syphilis	1.3	1.2
Gonorrhoea	12.0	14.4
Herpes simplex	25.5	27.6
Chlamydia	34.0	44.7
Wart virus	84.7	97.8
Others	196.5	238.6
Total (except HIV/AIDS)	354.0	424.3

Source: Health and Personal Social Services Statistics, England (1998)

In assessing the patient, privacy is important, and the nurse should try to set the patient at ease and then ask them to explain the nature of their problem. Many people are not familiar with the medical words used to describe sexual function and anatomy, therefore the language used may involve slang and some rather crude terms. It is important to obtain a description of the symptoms and how long they have been present for. It is essential to find out how many sexual partners the patient has had over the last 4 weeks. If the patient has been monogamous during that period with their regular long-term partner, the implication is that their partner has not, which can have a very damaging effect on their relationship. You also need to find out what types of sexual practices have taken place as the throat or anal region may be at risk of infection, whether homosexual activity has taken place and whether condoms have been used. As in other illnesses, the psychological and social sides of the problem must not be overlooked. Great care and sensitivity is required in talking, for instance, to a married woman who has suddenly developed a vaginal discharge, two weeks after her lorry driver husband has returned from a trip to Europe.

The two most common complaints that patients present with are a discharge (vaginal or urethral) or ulceration of the genitalia. The significance of these complaints is as follows:

1. *Urethral discharge in males.* This is almost always pathological and can be broadly classified into either gonococcal or non-gonococcal, the most common non-gonococcal causes being *Chlamydia trachomatis, Ureaplasma urealyticum, Trichomonas vaginalis* and *Candida albicans* organisms (Adler, 1998). If uncircumcised males are suffering from Candida infection, they will reveal the site of the infection clearly upon retraction of the foreskin. However, the origin of the discharge in the other

conditions is not so easily located. The incidence of gonorrhoea fell sharply in the late 1980s and early 90s as a result of safer sex campaigns but is beginning to increase again. Approximately 20% of infections are acquired homosexually (Steadman, 1998).

A useful test is to ask the man to pass 60–120 ml of urine into a glass container, and then to finish off passing his urine into another glass container. If there is infection of the anterior urethra, the first specimen will be hazy, containing threads or specks of pus, while the second specimen will be clear. If, however, they are both hazy this indicates that the infection involves other parts of the urinary tract, e.g. cystitis or nephritis. If a patient is being advised to attend the genitourinary medicine clinic with a urethral discharge, advise him not to pass urine for at least 4 hours before attending. The two glass test will almost certainly be carried out and this period of time allows the discharge to collect within the urethra, making interpretation unambiguous (Adler, 1998).

2. *Vaginal discharge.* This can be either pathological or non-pathological. Some degree of discharge from the vagina occurs in all women, the amount varying along a continuum. It is important to ascertain, therefore, what the normal discharge is like and why this condition is different. The woman should be reminded that a normal vaginal discharge may increase and be only noticed premenstrually, at time of ovulation or when using the contraceptive pill or an IUD. A discharge therefore does not automatically imply a disease process.

If the discharge is pathological in origin, the most likely cause is *Candida albicans* (which some authorities do not consider to be an exclusively sexually transmitted disease), while other organisms that might be responsible are *Neisseria gonorrhoeae, Trichomonas vaginalis* and *Chlamydia trachomatis.* Cervical lesions may also produce a vaginal discharge whether they are infective (herpes or warts) or not (neoplasm, polyps).

3. *Genital ulceration.* In practice, there tend to be two types of ulcer found – ulcers that are multiple and painful (usually genital herpes caused by the herpes simplex virus type 1 or 2) and those that occur singly and are painless (usually syphilis). Single painful ulcers are rare and may be due to tuberculosis while multiple painless ulcers are also rare, usually only seen in secondary syphyllis.

In taking a history, the key points mentioned in asking about a discharge should be covered. In addition, you should ask about the number of ulcers and whether they are painful, how their appearance relates in time to sexual intercourse, possible trauma and any other lesions elsewhere on the body. Diagnosis of the infecting organism on clinical findings is very uncertain, therefore careful microbiological examination and culture are required, which is why departments of genitourinary medicine (GUM) insist that A & E departments do not treat these cases, but rather refer them on to the specialist clinic.

In all cases of sexually transmitted disease the usual policy is not to treat the patient but to tell them instead to attend the GUM clinic the following day or the next Monday, and it is probably true to say that no physical harm will come to the patient. However, when nurses are passing this information on or reinforcing what the casualty officer has said, they need to remember that the patient will be very anxious and considerable reassurance is needed that this wait is for the best. Abstinence from sexual activity is to be strongly recommended until attending clinic when it is next open. One of the most important reasons for the patient attending the clinic rather than receiving treatment in A & E is the need for the patient's sexual partners to be traced – a role that A & E units cannot take on. Various forms of sexually transmitted disease produce no symptoms, or symptoms which can be and are ignored. For example, rectal gonorrhoea is often symptomless and, given the often multiple nature of homosexual encounters, it is therefore very important indeed to trace contacts as they may not know that they have been infected. (If symptoms do appear they consist of anal pain and discomfort, painful defecation and a blood-stained or purulent discharge.) Oropharyngeal gonorrhoea likewise is often asymptomatic.

The reader will be aware that there are various forms of sexually transmitted disease besides those described so far (e.g. genital warts caused by the human papillomavirus), but this is not a textbook on genitourinary medicine. What matters is that the nurse can show sympathy and understanding for what is a very distressing condition *for the patient*. If the most likely cause of the problem is sexual transmission, the most appropriate place of treatment is not A & E but the outpatient clinic of the department of genitourinary medicine. Telephone calls to the A & E department in the middle of the night are another manifestation of the anxiety felt by persons who think they may have acquired such a disease. Such calls should be dealt with tactfully and with due understanding, the patient being advised to attend the appropriate clinic and abstain from sexual activity meanwhile.

HIV/AIDS

While most forms of STD can be treated and cured, the exception, AIDS, remains, and the fear of having contracted this disease is understandably likely to produce extreme anxiety. By December 1997 there had been 15 074 reported cases of AIDS in the UK, 89% of whom were men (Adler, 1998). Although homosexual men remain the biggest single group at risk, the percentage of new HIV cases acquired through heterosexual activity has remained around the 30% level throughout the 1990s (Health and Personal Social Statistics for England, 1998).

A patient who phones or presents at A & E in a greatly distressed state, worried that because of some casual sexual adventure he or she may have contracted AIDS, should be treated sympathetically. There is little that can be done except to emphasize the need for sexual abstinence and to encourage an early visit to the STD clinic. It will help if the unit can pass on the phone number of useful agencies such as the Samaritans, or the local Gay Switchboard.

Infection with HIV may produce a transient feeling of being ill similar to glandular fever, 2–6 weeks later. The patient may not notice any malaise at all. However, antibodies to HIV usually develop 2–6 weeks after infection but it may take up to 3 months. Testing is carried out therefore 3 months after possible exposure (Steadman, 1998). This has to be explained to the patient in A & E who, because of their fear and anxiety may be demanding an instant test.

The discussion about HIV should remind the nurse of the fundamental rule that in dealing with all body fluids nurses must take great care and beware sharp objects, needles etc. to avoid the risk of accidentally contracting any blood-borne disease such as hepatitis B or AIDS. The principles of universal precautions should be observed at all times. Although IV drug users and homosexuals engage in high-risk behaviour, the nurse should remember that *anybody* could have AIDS or hepatitis.

Sexual orientation

Homosexuality is not a sexual problem but rather a sexual choice. A significant proportion of the population is homosexual or bisexual and, as a consequence, a significant proportion of A & E patients will be gay/lesbian. In many cases this probably will not be recognized, but in other situations the person may display behaviour that is more in keeping with their sexual orientation. It is perfectly natural for a gay man to comfort his partner after an accident or sudden illness. This is a sexual orientation that the nurse has no right to censure. Unfortunately, there is still homophobia among some nurses who need to examine their own attitudes towards gay and lesbian patients.

Society still broadly disapproves of homosexuality, which places many homosexuals under great pressure. Some are more able to live with these pressures than others, while others again are just unable to come to terms at all with their homosexual tendencies, especially if they are married. The result is a great deal of stress in the lives of many homosexuals which, coupled with the often transient nature of homosexual relationships and, therefore, a lack of stability and support, may lead to a higher incidence of unhappiness and anxiety than in other sections of the population. The nurse must therefore display the same caring approach to any patient, whatever their sexual orientation.

One other situation that may be encountered is the patient who prefers to dress in accordance with the opposite sex. This may vary in extent from occasional cross dressing of a fetish nature (usually involving underwear) for sexual gratification through to a person who wishes to live as a member of the opposite sex because they are convinced that is their correct gender (trans-sexual). There are various stages in between these two extremes and many transvestites choose to dress regularly as women without desiring to change sex. Most are heterosexual although some may be bisexual or gay.

A trans-sexual may be so disturbed and depressed at his situation, particularly if he feels he is receiving little help from the health service in attaining his goal of gender re-assignment, that serious self-harm or suicide may be attempted. A more likely presentation is the person who refuses to undress for no apparent reason, he is of course wearing 'inappropriate' underwear. A transvestite may have the misfortune to suffer an accident or acute episode of illness while out 'dressed' and be very embarrassed at being brought to A & E. The patient requires a non-judgemental, caring approach just like any other. Discreet assistance with resolving the problem such as access to male clothing and confidentiality are required. Extreme anxiety may be present in such a situation and the nurse should ensure that as few people as possible know about the patient's predicament. This will build up the trust and cooperation that is needed to treat the injuries sustained by the patient most effectively. It is also possible to get phone calls late at night from trans-sexuals and trans-vestites who are desperate for help. Ensure you have the number of the local Samaritans available and if possible the local TV helpline. A useful contact address to pass on is The Northern Concorde, PO Box 258, Manchester M60 1LN – this is a large self-help group for transvestites that can put individuals in contact with other similar groups around the country.

Genital trauma

The sexual acts that people perform in the privacy of their own homes are their own business. However, some practices can occasionally have unfortunate consequences which lead the person, with great reluctance and embarrassment, to the local A & E department.

A common problem is that of a foreign body that has either been retained in the rectum, vagina or urethra, or damage done to any of these organs by such a foreign body. The patient may admit to what is causing the problem (e.g. a carrot or a sex-aid such as a vibrator) or to what was responsible for the injuries sustained which makes treatment much easier. However, such is the embarrassment felt that the patient may not feel able to admit the truth. It is essential to bear this in mind when somewhat reluctant individuals walk into A & E complaining they have not been able to open their bowels for several days or that they are bleeding rectally, or simply complaining of abdominal pain. In such cases, rupture of the bowel is possible with disastrous consequences. Laparotomy to remove the offending object may be necessary; vibrators have been known to reach the transverse colon. Severe rectal damage may also be caused by over-vigorous insertion of the whole fist up to the forearm into the rectum.

A wide variety of foreign bodies may be removed from the vagina, with or without the woman's admission of their presence. Details of the steps necessary for a thorough internal and external examination are given by Kyle and Crumbie (1999) who stress the importance of a good light source, privacy, the correct equipment and a structured approach to what is a very embarrassing procedure for the woman.

Urethral trauma can occur from the passing of objects such as straws or the flexible inside part of a biro. Fresh bleeding from the urethra should raise this possibility even though the patient may not admit to such a practice.

Trauma to the external genitals may be the result of consensual sadomasochistic practices, or may be accidental. The injuries should be treated at their face value unless there is a possibility that they were inflicted against the person's will, in which case discreet questioning when alone with the patient should be undertaken. A not uncommon presentation is a person in handcuffs which usually have been bought from a sex shop. They are cheap imports of very poor quality and consequently unreliable, having a habit of becoming jammed or the key breaks in the lock. They are usually of such low quality metal that they can be sawn through very quickly with an ordinary hacksaw blade. Remember to protect the skin with a wooden spatula inside the cuff as the blade may go through very suddenly inflicting further trauma. Always check to ensure good circulation returns and there is no neurological damage as the cuffs may have been tightly on for several hours.

A common injury is the zip injury to the penis which can be exquisitely painful. Generous analgesia with Entonox will greatly facilitate freeing the penis from the zip. If swelling is present, ice packs should be applied. Injection with local anaesthetic (lignocaine) and gentle manipulation may allow release but, in young boys, it may require a general anaesthetic. Wyatt and Scobie (1994) have reported on a series of 30 boys with this problem seen in A & E. Only a small proportion required a general anaesthetic, no circumcisions were required to free the zip and all recovered without any subsequent complications. This work supports the approach advocated here.

Uncircumcised males who have a tight foreskin run the risk during their first sexual encounters of the foreskin becoming so retracted that it will not resume its normal anatomical position, acting as a tight constriction around the end of the penis leading to swelling and oedema (paraphimosis). This is a very alarming condition and, as with all such sexual problems, the nurse should display great tact and reassurance in dealing with the patient. Ice packs to reduce the swelling together with the use of lubricating gel will in most cases allow the foreskin to be manipulated back to its normal position.

Relatively minor lacerations to the penis can bleed profusely, and the patient may well limp into A & E after several hours of bleeding. Even after suturing, bleeding may occur. Ice packs and firm manual pressure are recommended, although it may take some time finally to stop the bleeding from what is a very vascular organ.

Bruising and swelling of the scrotum are often seen after accidents and are best treated with ice and a scrotal support. The nurse should be alerted, however, by the young man who says that he has severe pain but has no apparent injury. This is the classical presentation of torsion testis which, if not promptly relieved by surgery, can lead to a gangrenous testicle due to the impairment of the blood supply.

References

Adler M (1998) *ABC of Sexually Transmitted Infections*. London: BMJ Books.

Health and Personal Social Services Statistics for England (1998) London: The Stationery Office.

Kyle L, Crumbie A (1999) The female reproductive system. In Walsh M, Crumbie A, Reveley S (eds) *Nurse Practitioners; Clinical Skills and Professional Issues*. Oxford: Butterworth-Heinemann.

Steadman T (1998) *Sexually Transmitted Infections*. London: Stanley Thornes.

Wyatt I, Scobie W (1994) The management of penile zip entrapment in children. *Injury*, 25:59–60.

Evidence based practice

Chapter 20

EVIDENCE BASED PRACTICE IN A & E

You will be frequently regaled with impressive looking research findings by various 'reps' which show how good their equipment is. Alternatively, they will just assert that their equipment is superior to their rivals, drawing upon anecdotal evidence in support of their claims. In order to see through the high pressure sales talk and spend your limited budget wisely, you need objective evidence. On attending a conference you may find different A & E units treat the same problem in very different ways to your unit. This raises questions of which approach is better, not to mention whether it is acceptable to have such a wide variation in practice? Hutchinson and Baker (1999) are of the opinion that the wide variation in practice is such as to include significant adverse effects upon many patients. To grapple with issues such as these you need to be able to understand what is meant by evidence based practice. Most A & E nurses will have heard phrases such as 'evidence based practice', 'clinical effectiveness' and 'clinical governance'. It would be a mistake to dismiss these phrases as just so much jargon that will not make any difference to the real world of busy A & E practice. We are, therefore, concluding this edition with an overview of the key principles involved, demonstrating why the drive for evidence based practice is important for all of us. It will also help you spend your equipment budget with the maximum benefit for all.

What is evidence?

The concept of evidence based practice originated in medicine but its principles are equally applicable to nursing. The most famous definition is that of Sackett *et al.* (1996) who defined evidence based medicine as 'The conscientious, explicit and judicious use of current best evidence in making decisions about the care of individual patients'. There are three key sources of evidence according to Sackett *et al.*, of which research is only one. Equally important are the patient's preferences and the clinical experience of the practitioner.

The A & E nurse, therefore, should be basing practice on a combination of published research, the views and wishes of the patients and the collective wisdom of staff in the department. All that is published is not however gold. The nurse needs to acquire critical appraisal skills in order to distinguish between good research evidence and the not so good. Patient wishes have largely been ignored in the past and it therefore requires a considerable culture shift in health care to take patients seriously. Finally, experience is not a justification for traditional practice or simply following the wishes of the senior sister because she happens to be the senior sister. Learning from experience only takes place through the process of critical reflection upon that experience. The virtues of being a reflective practitioner have been greatly extolled in the nursing literature, it is therefore time to convert rhetoric into practice. These observations suggest that if evidence based practice is to be constructed upon the three pillars of Sackett *et al.*, a great deal of work is needed by A & E nurses.

A key goal of research is to demonstrate cause and effect. For example, that a particular treatment of a wound produces a better effect in terms of wound healing. Research produces other forms of evidence, such as describing the frequency with which something happens or how staff/patients feel about a particular issue. Cause and effect however have traditionally been the main aim of medical research. As we develop the broader concept of evidence based practice (EBP) for all health professionals, that linkage between cause and effect remains very important. It lies at the heart of the concept of clinical effectiveness which may be summarized as a measure of the extent to which interventions do what they are supposed to do (McClarey and Duff, 1997).

Randomized controlled trials and the hierarchy of evidence

Given the focus on establishing cause and effect, it is not surprising to find a hierarchy of evidence is often referred to and top of that hierarchy is the randomized controlled trial or RCT. This is the classical scientific experiment in which an intervention is carried out on one group of patients but not on an equivalent second or control group. If patients are allocated at random to these two groups and all other factors are controlled so as to be equal, then any differences in outcome can, with a high degree of confidence, be assigned to the effects of the experimental intervention. That is the logic of the RCT. Life is never that simple as there may be subtle differences between the groups that the researcher is unaware of. Even the best RCT cannot be said therefore to ever offer 100% proof of any hypothesis. A hypothesis is merely the statement being researched such as dressing A will produce a quicker healing of a wound than dressing B. In practice, research proceeds by disproving hypotheses rather than seeking to prove them.

The RCT is sometimes referred to as the gold standard of evidence when it comes to establishing cause and effect as it allows us to have the maximum confidence that A causes B (but never 100% proof). The RCT is therefore the least biased approach to comparing the effectiveness of treatments and, consequently, if evidence from well carried out RCTs is available, this should form the basis of recommendations for treatment (Hutchinson and Baker, 1999). The RCT is stronger than an experiment where, although there was a control group, there was not random allocation of patients to either the experimental or control group. If you introduce a new burns dressing regimen in your department and compare the results to the A & E department down the road, this is not a true RCT as any patient does not have an equal chance of being in either the experimental or control group. The group they are in is determined by where they live, they do not have a 50:50 chance of being in either group which would be the case if true randomization were present. Observed differences could be due to factors related to the two different geographical areas rather than the type of burns dressing used. If a control group is absent, the evidence derived from such a study is even weaker. You may, for example, decide to stop using sterile saline to irrigate wounds and instead use drinking water from the tap. As a means of deciding how effective your intervention has been you audit notes to find out how many patients with wounds returned with infections over the last year and compare that with the numbers who return from now on, after you have changed to tap water instead of sterile saline. The problem is this could reflect changes in staff and technique, variations in patterns of wounding, or several other factors which you could only eliminate with the aid of randomization and a control group.

The next stage down in the hierarchy is the descriptive study. A survey might reveal that a particular area of your town produces higher rates of attendances as a result of self-poisoning than the rest of your catchment. This is an interesting finding but it is difficult to attribute causality to that observation based purely on such a descriptive study. The weakest form of evidence of all, in terms of causality, is expert judgement. In terms of cause and effect, an 'experts' opinion ranks behind objective research based data, whether that expert is the A & E consultant or senior nurse.

This hierarchy of evidence is much quoted in the medical literature and clinical effectiveness has the concept of cause and effect at its heart. However, as we have said, it only applies to questions of causality. Qualitative research can capture information way beyond the reach of an RCT, such as what it feels like to the patient, what they are worried about or frightened of. This descriptive, qualitative approach allows us to build up evidence from the patient's point of view. Critical reflection allows the nurse to learn from experience and helps validate our own clinical judgement as a source of evidence. The RCT is therefore only the gold standard where evidence linking cause and effect is concerned.

Evidence based care rests upon the

assumptions that clinicians:

- Are involved in delivering care directly to patients that has a real impact upon patient outcomes.
- Assume full responsibility for their practice.
- Draw upon and contribute to a body of knowledge, elucidating best evidence and optimum effectiveness.

Consideration of these points led Kitson (1997) to pose the following key questions which are important for any A & E nurse committed to EBP:

- Can you show that your nursing care makes a difference to patient outcomes? This has perhaps been taken for granted but the challenge of EBP and clinical effectiveness is *to show* that you make a difference. Arguments for improved staffing or more investment in staff training carry much more weight if you can show that the nursing staff in question actually do make a positive difference to patient outcomes.
- Are you in control of your nursing practice? Nursing has embraced the concept of accountability during the 1990s. This means being able to account for your actions, to justify what you did and to be fully responsible for your care. This requires a high level of knowledge and the authority to act in accordance with your knowledge and judgement. EBP therefore requires the nurse to have sufficient authority to be fully responsible for their practice (Walsh, 2000).
- Does nursing have a scientific basis for its practice? Justifying your actions in terms of following orders, doing what we always traditionally do, what you were taught 20 years ago as a student or even what your intuition told you to do, does not add up to EBP. There has to be a scientific *basis* for practice, although putting that basis into action often involves artistry of the highest order. That is where the science and art of nursing meet. Artistry allows you to put science based care into practice.

What makes for good evidence?

Good evidence has several characteristics that distinguish it from weak or poor evidence. The best evidence demonstrates the effectiveness

(where that is appropriate) of whatever intervention is proposed. This allows a cost benefit analysis to be carried out showing how much it will cost to bring in the new procedure and what the benefits are likely to be. The bottom line is usually how much you would expect to save in an average year, which should be more than it costs! A common statistic that occurs in the literature is the number needed to treat (NNT), which is an estimate of the number of patients who need to be treated with the new intervention to prevent one adverse event. The lower the NNT the more effective the intervention. For example, if you are going to invest in the cost of pressure relieving mattresses for your A & E trolleys, how many patients do you have to use them on to prevent one patient developing a pressure sore? If the evidence gives you that kind of information, that is high quality evidence.

Evidence has to be appropriate to your local situation. Solutions that work in a New York ER may not work in Abergavenny or Aberdeen. When reading research findings check whether the sample is similar in key characteristics to your A & E population; consider age, gender, social class, employment status, ethnic and cultural background. When listening to an expert at a conference, ask yourself whether s/he is talking about the same sort of patients and conditions that you have to deal with?

A key question to ask concerns how current the evidence is. There is commonly a delay of at least a year between submission of a research paper and its publication, often longer. A good journal publishes submission dates with its papers in order to let you judge the delay. *The Journal of Advanced Nursing*, for example, publishes submission dates which tell you that the paper was usually submitted over a year before publication. The time between data gathering and submission of the finished paper may be up to a year, consequently research findings 'hot off the press' may already be two years out of date! There is little that you can do about this lag other than be aware it exists and remember that when citing publications from 2 years ago you may actually be referring to data gathered 4 years ago.

In searching for evidence, always use primary sources wherever possible, rather than citations in other papers or books. There are two reasons for this. If a reference is cited from a secondary source, it will be even more out of date than we discussed in the preceding paragraph. This book for example will be published in 2000. The work on it took place in 1999, therefore the most current primary sources we used in updating it were those published in 1998/9, which mostly refer to work undertaken in 1997/8. An even more serious problem, however, concerns the risk of work being quoted out of context and its meanings changed in the process. The more times a primary source becomes used and cited in this way the more likely the game of 'Chinese Whispers' will come into play. A classic example of this concerns Maslow's Hierarchy of Needs which can be found in many pre-registration nursing texts as a rationale for planning nursing care. The original source material dates from the early 1950s and is based upon experiments carried out with young, middle-class, white, American college students who predated Elvis Presley. Maslow's work has been subject to multiple citations of citations of citations and so on with little thought to its original source material. The sample bears no resemblance to the reality of patient populations from mixed ethnic and social class backgrounds found in the UK today, consequently the work lacks validity and currency. The problem is not with Maslow's research, it is with those nurse authors who have repeatedly cited the work in an unthinking and uncritical way from secondary sources!

As we move towards an increasingly complex and patient focused care environment, multi-professional evidence and patient perspectives acquire greater value. Research evidence which draws upon the perspectives of A & E nursing and medical staff has greater validity than only one or the other. The same comment applies to pre-hospital care where the joint findings of paramedic and medical staff, for example, are of more value than the views of one group or the other. The patient's view is one of the three main sources of evidence upon which we should base health care. Good research evidence, therefore, should make explicit patient involvement and their feelings about the care offered. It also goes without saying that the credibility of those who profess to present the evidence has to be examined, whether they be the authors of published papers or standing on conference platforms.

Research has to be both valid and reliable. These two terms are used a great deal in discussions of research methodology. While the average practitioner may not wish to go into great depth about these terms in reading papers there are some simple checks that you should make:

- Reliability means accuracy and consistency of measurement. Has the author demonstrated that whatever tool they have used to measure their variables, such as a questionnaire, is accurate and consistent?
- Validity means that something is measuring what it says it is measuring. Again, has the author demonstrated this? Content validity simply means that a topic area has been fully covered, so a questionnaire that purported to find out about patient's knowledge of out of hours medical services and which failed to ask anything about NHS Direct could hardly be said to have content validity.
- Is the sample big enough and typical enough to be representative of the population the researcher is making generalizations about? The findings contained in a study of 30 patients in a single A & E department cannot be generalized to the whole UK, neither could a study of sports injuries carried out between May and September be generalized to the whole year. Neither would be valid as they are not ultimately measuring what they say they are measuring.

Evidence should never be accepted at face value. It should always be subjected to critical appraisal, checking out the issues raised above. Critical appraisal of evidence requires a structured approach by the reader who should have a clear goal in mind. This systematic approach must be allied with open mindedness. Pause for thought before you begin and reflect upon your own preferences and bias, write them down, be aware of them while reading the evidence. The evidence must be read and considered with an objective rather than a subjective approach. Look for the key points mentioned in the preceding section concerning, for example, currency, reliability, validity, sample size and representativeness. Your final judgement about the evidence should be based upon the reported facts not guesswork or opinion. The evidence may be contrary to what you believe but that does not allow you to reject it simply because you do not like it.

A particularly useful source of evidence is the systematic review which pulls together all the recently published work on a particular topic. The reviewer has done a lot of the hard work for you, rejecting papers that are, for example, out of date, do not constitute primary sources or are lacking in rigour due to problems with sample sizes, reliability or validity. A systematic review may also access evidence that has not been published such as a PhD thesis in a library or results that were not published for whatever reason. The best known and most accessible series of systematic reviews is produced by the York NHS Centre for Review and Dissemination. These are published as effective health care bulletins at regular intervals, each focused on one topic and are distributed free to all NHS Trusts. Your Trust and local library (Postgrad Medical or University) will have the full set. Make it your business to keep up to date with them. The Cochrane Collaboration is a cooperative based in Oxford which keeps a series of systematic reviews updated, although these tend to be of more relevance to doctors than the York reviews. A systematic review should not be confused with a meta-analysis. This latter term refers to statistical techniques which can be used to combine the results from several similar studies to make one big study. The BMJ publishing group has just started publishing a 6-monthly compendium of the best effective evidence for health care under the title 'Clinical Effectiveness'. There is much in this publication that is of relevance to A & E practice (BMJ, 1999).

Making EBP work

To make EBP work in your department involves a lot more than simply finding the evidence and saying 'Right we start on Monday!'. You have to approach the problem as a critical thinker and stay with this mind set as you work your way through the following stages:

- Identify the problem
- Find the evidence
- Transform the evidence into a solution that works for your department
- Transform the solution into action
- Evaluate the change.

Critical thinking means that you can organize yourself, structure knowledge, and work to a plan with a clearly defined goal and timetable. Simply 'Doing something about waiting times' does not meet these criteria. Reducing mean waiting times for patients with minor injuries by 20% over the next 12 months represents a clearly defined goal and timetable which, in turn, allows you to structure your search for evidence. This goal tells you that you need evidence on mean waiting times now in your department. You need to search the literature for measures which have succeeded in reducing waiting times for patients with minor injuries in departments similar to yours, together with evidence of what the patients thought about these measures. You also need to design a system for evaluating any changes you may make.

Problem identification sounds easy. However, you have to be sure that you are all seeing the same problem in the same way. You may be aware that patients with minor injuries and conditions are waiting for long periods and some are complaining aggressively in a threatening way. Some staff may see the problem as not enough doctors, others may blame the patients for attending when they should have gone to their GP or called NHS Direct (so-called 'inappropriate attenders'). Senior medics may blame the junior doctors inexperience and lack of training, as this makes them very slow at dealing with patients. The problem may appear as a lack of nursing staff to others. The problem may also be seen as verbal aggression towards staff, while lengthy waiting times may not be seen as a problem, merely what patients should expect if they all come crowding down here with trivial complaints. Different perspectives see the problem in different ways and the *causes* of the problem become mixed up with the *actual* problem itself. The need therefore is for a clear statement of the problem which all parties are agreed to. The problem should also be worded in such a way as to be soluble (see previous paragraph).

The process of locating the evidence begins in the library with searches of databases such as CINAHL and MEDLINE, systematic reviews such as Effective Health Care Bulletins and use of the Internet. Do remember, however, that while journal articles are refereed, the Internet is unpoliced, therefore, even the most outrageous pseudoscientific rubbish can appear on the net. Patient opinions and experiences are an important source of evidence, which should be gathered where relevant, and the views of all the staff involved should also be sought. Not only is the staff perspective valuable evidence, it also ensures they are involved in the change process from the beginning which makes it more likely that you will achieve a successful outcome.

The hard work really begins once you have found the evidence, as evidence is not a solution. You have to translate the evidence into a practical solution that stands a good chance of working in *your* A & E department and then putting the paper solution into effect on the ground. Change management is a huge topic (Walsh, 2000) which we cannot cover here. Suffice it to say that simply issuing an edict to the effect that starting next Monday we will do something differently often does not achieve anything like 100% compliance. Protocols and guidelines are one way of translating evidence into changes in clinical practice. If they are generated locally, based upon best evidence, this should help increase a sense of ownership and relevance to local problems, which will, in turn, improve the chances of obtaining staff cooperation.

A key statement about guidelines is that they are 'tools not rules' (Hutchinson and Baker, 1999). In other words they are there to guide thinking and decision making, but not to replace these skills. They should not therefore be slavishly followed 100% of the time for all patients. If in the nurse's view there are good reasons to depart from the guidelines then this is permissible. Accountable practice requires the nurse to be able to justify his/her own actions, therefore, you may depart from guidelines in a given clinical situation providing you can justify your decision. That is what being an accountable practitioner is all about.

Perhaps the most crucial step of all is to evaluate the change you have made to practice. There are two elements to evaluation – process and outcome. Process refers to whether or not staff actually are carrying out the change in practice as required and outcome refers to the results obtained. If the change in practice produces no measurable change in outcomes,

this may be because the change in practice actually has not occurred, hence the importance of an evaluating process. A simple audit criterion could therefore be that the new procedure is carried out in accordance with the protocol/guidelines. Only then can you consider effects on outcome as being due to the change in practice. However, you need to be sure there are not other factors which have changed and which could effect outcome measures (intervening variables to use research jargon). Your drop in minor injury attendances might be due to your newly introduced nurse practitioner scheme, but it might also be due to the new NHS drop in centre opened at the local supermarket or a recently closed A & E department 10 miles away re-opening as a nurse-led MIU.

Ultimately, the evaluation of your changes should demonstrate the clinical effectiveness of practice. This requires evaluation, which includes indicators of effectiveness such as reduced waiting times, reduced re-attendance rates, fewer X-rays ordered, more rapid transfer times to wards, shorter delays in administration of anticoagulation therapy, fewer patient complaints, less staff turnover etc. Key questions which are asked about clinical effectiveness are whether:

- The cost can be justified in terms of the health gain expected?
- The same gains could have been achieved at less expense by other means?
- Other health gains could have been achieved for the same cost?

The clinical effectiveness of introducing nurse practitioners into your department could be assessed using these key questions. That means you have to assess the health gains expected, which includes less obvious factors such as reduced staff turnover as staff enjoy more job satisfaction and there is less aggression and threatening behaviour from patients facing lengthy waits. The second question involves a cost comparison between doctors and nurse practitioners (assuming extra doctors actually want to come and work in your department). Such a comparison has to be done carefully to ensure it is fair. If there are very restrictive protocols in place limiting severely the type of patients that NPs can treat, then their cost effectiveness will be greatly reduced. A good honours degree level education is essential to allow NPs to treat a wide enough range of patients to be cost effective. The exact nature of the treatment should also be considered. If the NP goes on to administer the treatment him/herself, then s/he will see fewer patients per hour than a doctor, however, there will be less demand on other nursing staff than with a conventional medical service, so there will be savings elsewhere. The final question has to be addressed openly as it is possible that our own professional agendas get in the way here. The medics may be keen to construct an argument for another consultant post, while the nursing staff may be arguing for NP posts as part of their own professional agenda. The key question here is what is best for the patient rather than the professional group involved?

Clinical governance is concerned with allowing clinical staff to take charge of the quality agenda. It is therefore potentially very empowering. It is also concerned with holding clinical staff accountable for the effectiveness and quality of the care they deliver, which some may find threatening. Either way it cannot be ignored. Clinical effectiveness is therefore a key tool in meeting the clinical governance agenda and relies heavily upon evidence based practice. These are all likely to be dominant themes in A & E over the lifetime of this edition. Nurses should therefore engage with this agenda. The introduction provided in this chapter is merely intended to get you started, there is a great deal to be done in this field which could be potentially very beneficial for nursing and our patients. The challenge is to *show* nursing makes a difference in A & E, rather than merely take it as read.

References

BMJ (1999) *Clinical Effectiveness*, **1**, June 1999. London: BMJ Publications.

Hutchinson A, Baker R (1999) *Guidelines in Clinical Practice*. Oxford: Radcliffe Medical Press.

Kitson A (1997) Evidence Based Nursing. *Paper delivered at Evidence Based Practice Conference*, BMJ/RCN, London, November 1997.

McClarey M, Duff L (1997) Clinical effectiveness and evidence based practice. *Nursing Standard*, **11**:51, 31–5.

Sackett D, Rosenberg W, Muir Gray J, Haynes R, Richardson W (1996) Evidence based medicine: what it is and what it isn't. *BMJ*, **312**:71–2.

Walsh M (2000) *Nursing Frontiers*. Oxford: Butterworth-Heinemann.

INDEX